PSYCHOTOMIMETIC DRUGS

**Workshop Series of Pharmacology Section
National Institute of Mental Health
No. 4**

PSYCHOTOMIMETIC DRUGS

Proceedings of a Workshop Organized by the Pharmacology Section, Psychopharmacology Research Branch, National Institute of Mental Health Held at the University of California, Irvine, on January 25–26, 1969.

Edited by

Daniel H. Efron, M.D., Ph.D.

Chief, Pharmacology Section, Psychopharmacology Research Branch, National Institute of Mental Health, and Clinical Professor of Psychopharmacology, Department of Psychiatry, University of Maryland School of Medicine

RAVEN PRESS • New York

The opinions expressed and any conclusions drawn are those of the participants of the meeting upon which this book is based, and are not to be understood as necessarily having the endorsement of, or representing the viewpoints of, the Public Health Service of the U.S. Department of Health, Education and Welfare.

© 1970 by Raven Press Books, Ltd. All rights reserved. This book is protected by copyright. No part of it may be duplicated or reproduced in any manner without written permission from the publisher. Made in the United States of America.

Standard Book Number 911216-07-3
Library of Congress catalog card number 73-89388

Preface

The revolution in the area of psychotropic drugs has as a by-product the enormous development of so-called *psychotomimetic compounds*. One has to admit that some psychotomimetic substances were used a long time ago, *e.g.,* Asclepiades (128–56 B.C.), a Bithynian physician, claimed that *"papaver alienationem facit"*—that poppy juice ingestion causes mental derangement.[1] But the new era of psychotropic drugs brought with it the isolation of active substances from natural sources, their syntheses and the creation of many and much more active compounds. I shall mention only some of those which have been known for a long time: peyote (*Lophophora Williamsii,* a Mexican dumpling cactus), from which mescaline was isolated; teonanacatl, a compound used by the Aztecs and obtained from a mushroom, *Panaeolus campanulatus;* soma, whose identity is unknown but which, according to a new theory advocated by R. G. Wasson,[2] is a mushroom, fly agaric (*Amanita muscaria*); iboga (*Tabernanthe iboga*) roots; coca (*Erythroxylon coca*) leaves; quat (from *Catha edulis,* an Ethiopian plant); seeds of *Piptadenia peregrina,* and many more.

The use of these psychotomimetic substances in ancient times was either for religious, ceremonial or recreational purposes. They were used in a very restricted way and, one may say, in an *orderly* fashion. Their use was limited in frequency, in dosage and in the age of users. The new era brought with it the use of psychotomimetic drugs on a much larger scale with no restrictions on the frequency, the dosage or in the user's age. In other words, many people started to abuse the compounds and to use them in a disorderly manner as well as to use drugs of unknown pharmacology and activity. The newer times also brought with them the so-called "experimenting" with drugs by people who do not possess enough knowledge in this area and, what is even worse, enough maturity to judge these "experiments." Hard scientific data are lacking in many cases.

Even the terms used to describe these drugs are not well established and do not always cover the same spectrum of activity. The term most frequently

---

[1] Caelius Aurelianus: *On Acute Diseases and on Chronic Diseases.* University of Chicago Press, Chicago, 1950.
[2] R. G. Wasson: *Soma—Divine Mushroom of Immortality.* Harcourt, Brace & World, New York, 1968.

used (and used also in this publication) is *psychotomimetic drug* or *psychotomimetic compound*. This name means that a drug causes a state that mimics naturally occurring psychosis, although this contention is not really true. Another term is *hallucinogenic drug*, which indicates that the drug causes hallucinations—but we know that this is not always the case. Some scientists use the term *psychotogenic*. It is also rather arbitrary as to which compounds are put in this category.

The problem of psychotomimetic compounds is a "hot" one because of its social, political and even economic implications. But these were not the aspects that we wanted to stress during this workshop, and these considerations did not influence the selection of the participants. We deeply believe that only the accumulation of more scientific data, the distribution of existing data and the establishment of new directions for research can enable us to have a profound understanding of the mechanism of action of these compounds. This, in turn, will enable us to solve the other problems. We were trying to organize a multidisciplinary meeting with the participation of neurologists, pharmacologists, physiologists, psychiatrists, psychologists, *etc.*, who will help bring new points of view and show new possibilities for research in this difficult area.

To make possible a structure around which free, uninhibited and unlimited discussions could develop, we had to limit both the number of participants and the number of presentations. This workshop was held in conjunction with the meeting of the Preclinical Psychopharmacology Research Review Committee of the National Institute of Mental Health whose members also participated in it. During the meeting new data and new approaches were presented and discussed. I feel that the results will contribute to a better understanding of the field.

The workshop was divided into four sessions. Each paper was followed by a discussion, the last paper of each session by a combined discussion of the given paper and general discussion of the session. At the end of the meeting we held a general discussion of all proceedings, and a summary of the workshop was given. The editor feels that the discussions contributed greatly toward the stated goals of the workshop. They brought out new ideas, new data (*e.g.*, on marihuana), possibilities of new methodology (*e.g.*, predicting hallucinations), *etc*. Therefore, the discussion is included verbatim with only some editorial changes. In one case, where the given paper could not be printed for reasons beyond the control of the editor, the discussion, because of the extensive amount of information in it, is included nonetheless. The editor begs the indulgence of the reader if some parts of this discussion refer to statements not printed in this book, but this was the only way that it could be presented.

Because of the multidisciplinary nature of this workshop, problems of terminology and the extent of discussion, no restrictions were imposed on the participants with regard to nomenclature used, order of material or uniformity of presentation and reference listing. The diversity of form and style of the various presentations and statements were not altered for publication.

I would like to extend our deep appreciation to the University of California at Irvine and especially to its Vice Chancellor for Academic Affairs, Dr. Roger W. Russell, for his gracious hospitality and help in organizing this meeting. I would also like to thank his staff, and especially Mrs. Nancy Collett, for their assistance. Many special thanks are due Dr. Albert A. Manian of the Pharmacology Section, Psychopharmacology Research Branch, N.I.M.H. for his invaluable help in preparing this manuscript.

I would like to express my appreciation to the publisher, Raven Press, and its Director, Alan M. Edelson, for their help and effort in publishing this book in the shortest possible time and in giving it the most desirable aesthetic appearance.

Finally, I would like to express my deepest thanks to all speakers, discussants and participants in the workshop. The success of the meeting as well as the stimulation of new developments in the area of psychotomimetics should be attributed to their knowledge and contributions. It is entirely their success!

Daniel H. Efron

Bethesda, Maryland
September 15, 1969

Contents

SESSION I: CHEMISTRY
Alfred Burger, Ph.D. and Bo Holmstedt, M.D., Co-Chairmen

Chemistry and Structure-Activity Relationships of the Psychotomimetics   21
Alexander T. Shulgin, Ph.D.

Discussion 38

Steric Models of Drugs Predicting Psychedelic Activity 43
Solomon H. Snyder, M.D. and Elliott Richelson, M.D.

Discussion 59

Stereochemical and Membrane Studies with the Psychotomimetic Glycolate Esters 67
Leo G. Abood, Ph.D.

Discussion and Chairmen's Closing Remarks 74

SESSION II: PHARMACOLOGY
Daniel H. Efron, M.D., Ph.D. and Peter Waser, M.D., Ph.D., Co-Chairmen

Biochemical and Metabolic Considerations Concerning the Mechanism of Action of Amphetamine and Related Compounds 83
Fridolin Sulser, M.D. and Elaine Sanders-Bush, Ph.D.

Discussion 94

Pharmacological Studies of 5-Methoxy-N,N-dimethyltryptamine, LSD and Other Hallucinogens 105
Peter K. Gessner, Ph.D.

Discussion 118

Mechanism of the Facilitating Effects of Amphetamine on Behavior . . 123
Larry Stein, Ph.D. and C. David Wise, Ph.D.

Discussion 145

The Combination of Gas Chromatography and Mass Spectrometry in the Identification of Drugs and Hallucinogens 151
Bo Holmstedt, M.D.

Discussion 153

Turnover of Monoamines in Brain Under the Influence of Muscimol and Ibotenic Acid, Two Psychoactive Principles of *Amanita Muscaria* . . 155
Peter G. Waser, M.D., Ph.D. and Petra Bersin, M.D.

Discussion 162

SESSION III: PHYSIOLOGY, NEUROPATHOLOGY, and NEUROCHEMISTRY
Morris A. Lipton, M.D., Ph.D. and Wallace D. Winters, M.D., Ph.D., Co-Chairmen

LSD and Mescaline: Comparison of Effects on Single Units in the Midbrain Raphé 165
George K. Aghajanian, M.D., Michael H. Sheard, M.D. and Warren E. Foote, Ph.D.

Discussion 170

Visual Information Processes: *Discussion* 178

The Separation of Retinal and Central Processes in Vision 183
Bela Julesz, Ph.D.

Discussion 188

Drug Induced States of CNS Excitation: A Theory of Hallucinosis . . 193
Wallace D. Winters, M.D., Ph.D. and Marshall B. Wallach, Ph.D.

Discussion 214

SESSION IV: CLINICAL CONSIDERATIONS
    a. Model Psychosis
    b. Therapeutic Use and Therapeutic Potential
Daniel X. Freedman, M.D. and Louis J. West, M.D., Co-Chairmen

The Relevance of Chemically-Induced Psychoses to Schizophrenia . . 231
Morris A. Lipton, M.D., Ph.D.

CONTENTS

Discussion 240

DOET (2,5-Dimethoxy-4-Ethylamphetamine) and DOM (STP) (2,5-dimethoxy-4-methylamphetamine), New Psychotropic Agents: Their Effects in Man 247
Solomon H. Snyder, M.D., Herbert Weingartner, Ph.D. and Louis A. Faillace, M.D.

Discussion 263

Children's Reactions to Psychotomimetic Drugs 265
Lauretta Bender, M.D.

Discussion 271

DMT (N,N-Dimethyltryptamine) and Homologues; Clinical and Pharmacological Considerations 275
Stephen Szara, M.D.

Discussion 284

Psychosis Induced by the Administration of *d*-Amphetamine to Human Volunteers 287
John D. Griffith, M.D., John H. Cavanaugh, M.D., Ph.D. and John A. Oates, M.D.

Discussion 294

Effects of Marihuana Smoking on Sensory Thresholds in Man . . . 299
Donald F. Caldwell, Ph.D., Steven A. Myers, M.D. and Edward F. Domino, M.D.

Discussion 308

GENERAL DISCUSSION, SUMMARY AND CLOSING REMARKS

General Discussion 325

Summary of the Workshop 345
Morris A. Lipton, M.D., Ph.D.

Closing Remarks 349

Author Index 353

Subject Index 357

Participants and Guests

LEO G. ABOOD, Ph.D.
Center for Brain Research and Department of Biochemistry
University of Rochester
Rochester, New York 14627

GEORGE K. AGHAJANIAN, M.D.
Department of Psychiatry
Yale University School of Medicine
New Haven, Connecticut 06519

LAURETTA BENDER, M.D.
Consultant in Child Psychiatry
New York State Department of
   Mental Hygiene
Creedmoor State Hospital
Queens Village, New York 11724

JOHN BIEL, Ph.D.
Department of General Pharmacology
Abbott Laboratories
North Chicago, Illinois 60064

ALFRED BURGER, Ph.D.
Department of Chemistry
University of Virginia
Charlottesville, Virginia 22901

J. CYMERMAN CRAIG, Ph.D.
Department of Pharmaceutical
   Chemistry
University of California Medical
   Center
San Francisco, California 94122

PARTICIPANTS AND GUESTS

JOHN DALY, Ph.D.
Laboratory of Chemistry
National Institute of Arthritis and
  Metabolic Diseases
National Institutes of Health
Bethesda, Maryland 20014

WILLIAM DEMENT, M.D.
Department of Psychiatry
Stanford Medical School
Palo Alto, California 94305

SIDNEY P. DIAMOND, M.D.
Department of Neurology
Mt. Sinai School of Medicine
New York, New York 10029

EDWARD DOMINO, M.D.
Department of Pharmacology
University of Michigan School of
  Medicine
Ann Arbor, Michigan, and
Lafayette Clinic, Detroit, Michigan
  48207

DANIEL H. EFRON, M.D., Ph.D.
Pharmacology Section
Psychopharmacology Research
  Branch
National Institute of Mental Health
Chevy Chase, Maryland 20015

DANIEL X. FREEDMAN, M.D.
Department of Psychiatry
University of Chicago School of
  Medicine
Chicago, Illinois 60637

PETER K. GESSNER, Ph.D.
Department of Pharmacology
State University of New York
  at Buffalo School of Medicine
Buffalo, New York 14214

PARTICIPANTS AND GUESTS

JOHN D. GRIFFITH, M.D.
Department of Psychiatry
Vanderbilt University School of
  Medicine
Nashville, Tennessee 37203

ANTHONY J. HANCE, Ph.D.
Department of Pharmacology
University of California School of
  Medicine
Davis, California 95616

LEON HARMON, Ph.D.
Bell Telephone Laboratories, Inc.
Murray Hill, New Jersey 07974

BO HOLMSTEDT, M.D.
Department of Toxicology
Karolinska Institutet
Stockholm 60, Sweden

MILTON H. JOFFE, Ph.D.
Abuse and Liabilities Branch
Division of Drug Sciences
U.S. Department of Justice
1405 Eye Street
Washington, D.C. 20537

BELA JULESZ, Ph.D.
Bell Telephone Laboratories, Inc.
Murray Hill, New Jersey 07974

IRWIN J. KOPIN, M.D.
Laboratory of Clinical Science
National Institute of Mental Health
Bethesda, Maryland 20014

CONAN KORNETSKY, Ph.D.
Division of Psychiatry
Boston University School of Medicine
80 East Concord Street
Boston, Massachusetts 02118

PARTICIPANTS AND GUESTS

VICTOR G. LATIES, Ph.D.
Department of Radiation Biology
   and Biophysics
University of Rochester
Rochester, New York 14620

GERARD LEHRER, M.D.
Division of Neurochemistry
Department of Neurology
Mt. Sinai School of Medicine
New York, New York 10029

JEROME LEVINE, M.D.
Psychopharmacology Research
   Branch
National Institute of Mental Health
Chevy Chase, Maryland 20015

MORRIS A. LIPTON, M.D., Ph.D.
Department of Psychiatry
School of Medicine
University of North Carolina
Chapel Hill, North Carolina 27515

ARNOLD LUDWIG, M.D.
Mendotta State Hospital
Madison, Wisconsin 53704

ARNOLD V. MANDELL, M.D.
Department of Psychiatry
University of California School of
   Medicine
Irvine, California 92664

ALBERT A. MANIAN, Ph.D.
Pharmacology Section
Psychopharmacology Research
   Branch
National Institute of Mental Health
Chevy Chase, Maryland 20015

HUMPHRY F. OSMOND, M.D.
Bureau of Research in Neurology
   and Psychiatry
Princeton, New Jersey 08540

PARTICIPANTS AND GUESTS

ROGER W. RUSSELL, Ph.D.
University of California
Irvine, California 92664

ALEXANDER T. SHULGIN, Ph.D.
Consultant
1483 Shulgin Road
Lafayette, California 94548

VAN SIM, M.D.
Medical Research Laboratories
Edgewood Arsenal, Maryland 21010

IRVING SIMOS, Ph.D.
National Institute of Mental Health
Chevy Chase, Maryland 20015

SOLOMON H. SNYDER, M.D.
Departments of Pharmacology and
    Psychiatry
The Johns Hopkins University School
    of Medicine
Baltimore, Maryland 21205

LARRY STEIN, Ph.D.
Wyeth Laboratories
Philadelphia, Pennsylvania 19101

FRIDOLIN SULSER, M.D.
Psychopharmacology Research
    Center
Department of Pharmacology
Vanderbilt University School of
    Medicine
Nashville, Tennessee 37203

STEPHEN SZARA, Ph.D.
Section on Pharmacology
Division of Special Mental Health
    Research
National Institute of Mental Health
St. Elizabeth's Hospital
Washington, D.C. 20032

PARTICIPANTS AND GUESTS

HANS-LUKAS TEUBER, Ph.D.
Department of Psychology
Massachusetts Institute of Technology
Cambridge, Massachusetts 02139

SANFORD UNGER, Ph.D.
Maryland Psychiatric Research Center
Baltimore, Maryland 21228

EARL USDIN, Ph.D.
Pharmacology Section
Psychopharmacology Research
  Branch
National Institute of Mental Health
Chevy Chase, Maryland 20015

PETER G. WASER, M.D.
Department of Pharmacology
University of Zürich
Zürich, Switzerland

LOUIS J. WEST, M.D.
Department of Psychiatry, Neurology
  and Behavioral Sciences
University of Oklahoma Medical
  Center
Oklahoma City, Oklahoma 73104

WALLACE D. WINTERS,
  M.D., Ph.D.
Department of Pharmacology
University of California School of
  Medicine
Los Angeles, California 90024

VIRGINIA L. ZARATZIAN, Ph.D.
Pharmacology Section
Psychopharmacology Research
  Branch
National Institute of Mental Health
Chevy Chase, Maryland 20015

SESSION I

CHEMISTRY

Alfred Burger, Ph.D. and Bo Holmstedt, M.D., Co-Chairmen

CHEMISTRY AND STRUCTURE-ACTIVITY RELATIONSHIPS OF THE PSYCHOTOMIMETICS

Alexander T. Shulgin, Ph.D.

Consultant
1483 Shulgin Road
Lafayette, California 94548

This meeting is a discussion of the psychotomimetics, and since no one has yet defined the word, and I am the first to speak, I will define it. The first voice heard is the one that is argued against later.

The definition of the word is worthy of a few minutes. This entire group of materials can be arranged in a variety of ways. They could be, for example, considered from the point of view of their site of action. Thus, if you will classify a chemical as active at a cellular level or at a molecular level, you can argue that this is its primary site of action, and all such materials can be classified depending upon their action at this specific site. Secondarily, they have an action upon man, which is incidental to its classification. A material may be primarily cytolytic, and only incidentally cure some bacterial infection in man.

Quite separately, you can take all of the compounds assembled in the *U.S. Pharmacopoeia* and arrange them on the basis of their action on the human organism. The primary classification would describe the action on the intact individual, and only secondarily would it suggest how this action came to be. For example, a material may be a contraceptive and it is classified as such in the drug manuals. It is incidental whether it is a contraceptive because it inhibits ovulation or because it disturbs the cervical mucosa.

I would like to suggest a third way of organizing these materials. The psychotropic materials, as a special entity in the drug classification, can only be defined by their effect upon the interrelationships between people. This definition involves relationships such as mood, which, after all, have no

22 CHEMISTRY AND STRUCTURE-ACTIVITY RELATIONSHIPS

absolute value. One can only evaluate a change in mood relating one person to another in his society, or even to himself at some separate time. One has a tenuous assignment of sanity, for sanity is a statistical thing. You have to have three people to decide which one is insane. It is a minority concept. The specific terms, sanity, insanity, psychosis and psychotomimetic, must be defined at a social or human level of interaction. This classification describes the general term "psychotropic," which is literally from the Greek $\psi v \chi \eta$, the mind or the soul, and the turning or changing of it.

One is confronted with an apparent paradox regarding sanity in the definition of psychotomimetics. When one changes from a real environment to a different environment, and this second environment seems as real as the first but is different from the first, then there seems to be no absolute way of determining which of the two real worlds is the "real" real world.

The psychotropic chemicals were subdivided into five groups some thirty or forty years ago by Lewin (1927). These form a useful way of cataloging psychotropic chemicals. They are presented in a circular form which allows a convenient classification of chemicals, for many of these drugs have more than one action.

The first of his classifications was an area known as "Excitantia," literally, chemicals that cause excitement and stimulation. Included here are such synthetic materials as amphetamine, methedrine and Ritalin. Here also are such natural materials as caffeine and khat.

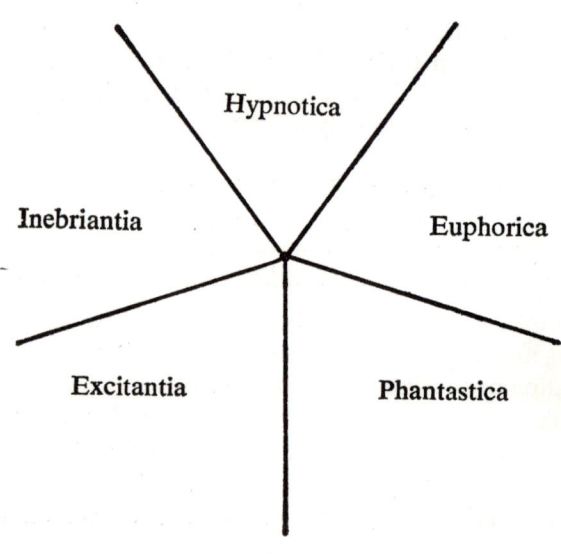

The adjacent and very closely allied classification is entitled "Inebriantia." Here one finds inebriants which cause intoxication in the social sense, rather than in the pharmacological sense. There is a host of organic compounds known to all: ethanol, chloroform, ether, the various materials that have an initial phase of excitement and that cause mental distortion and mental depression, leading quite smoothly into the area of "Hypnotica," the third classification.

This region is best characterized by the barbiturates. In this area one finds the first challenge to the meaning of the real world. There is a replacement of reality with amnesia or confusion. Here, in addition to the sedatives and anesthetics, there are drugs such as atropine, scopolamine, benactyzine, phencyclidine, and other delusional and mentally deranging psychotropic chemicals that will be discussed later in this meeting.

Adjacent to "Hypnotica" is the area entitled "Euphorica," best illustrated by the opiates, in which there is a replacement of the unremembered and unrecalled "not" world with a synthetic substitute that circumvents all problems. This satisfies the user without any constructive benefits.

The last of Lewin's classifications, the one which fascinated him most, is the "Phantastica." This is the area which we will discuss during the next two days. Here, one replaces a real world with an alternate real world which is equally real and yet different. We must return to this philosophic argument: How can one determine which of these two is the "real" real world? There are people in South America, for example, who use the native drug ayahuasca, and who live as much of their lives as possible in a drug-modified world. They consider that state the real world, and it is only when the body becomes purged of these chemicals that they inhabit what we accept as our real world. They consider our world an idyllic heaven, but they soon return to their drugged state which is their real world, whereas ours is the escape world. Which of these two exclusive states is real?

The class of "Phantastica," thus defined, is presented as a working definition of the term "psychotomimetic." The word psychotomimetic is from "psychoto," implying the origin of psychosis, and "mimetic," meaning the imitation of it. This is, admittedly, a controversial definition because in many ways these compounds do not imitate psychosis, but produce some recognizable symptoms. They have been called the hallucinogens as another synonym, but this is questionable, as hallucinations are rare things. They have been called psychedelics, but this name reflects some anticipation of virtue. Whatever they are, these are the classes of compounds which cause a change of reality but still allow recall.

I would like to discuss briefly the several principal families of compounds that fall into this "Phantastica" classification. (See Usdin and Efron, 1967, for leading references.) Several of these families will be talked about at length by others, therefore I will not go into detail on those. These various families can be organized quite nicely from the chemically complex to the chemically simple, from the polycyclic to the monocyclic, from the very potent to the relatively non-potent compounds. Interestingly, in the same arrangement, the compounds are ranked from those which are without apparent relationship to known metabolic pathways, progressively to the compounds that can be more and more easily rationalized as being involved in known metabolic schemes. It is with the simplest of these families, with the compounds related to mescaline, that I will discuss recently evolved structure-activity relationships.

The first of these families contain the compounds related to the ergot alkaloids. LSD (Fig. 1a) is among the most potent of all of the compounds

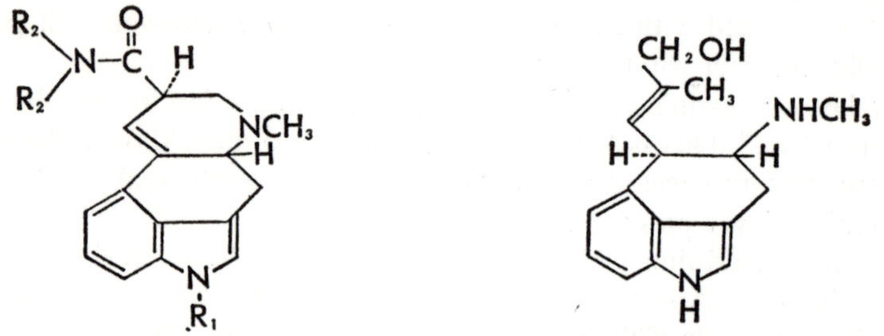

(a) LSD: $R_1 = H$
$R_2 = C_2H_5$

(b) Chanoclavine

FIG. 1.

known in this area, and among the most widely publicized of the materials. The compound is an indole. Through much of this discussion there will be a continual reference to indoles or to the tryptamine nucleus, which is, with very few exceptions, present. I shall not elaborate much on the structure-activity relationships of these. Most changes in the structure of LSD lead to a loss of potency; very few changes appreciably increase it. Methylation or acetylation of the indole nitrogen at R_1 and replacement of the diethyl group with the pyrrolidine ring, $R_2 = -(CH_2)_4-$, are modifications that, to a large extent, do not change the activity of the compound. LSD appears to be of nearly optimum structure as it stands, as no single structural variation grossly increases its activity. Conversion of either of the asymmetric positions to the corresponding isomers, bromination of the nucleus of the indole, removal of one of the ethyl groups, or the replacement of the two ethyl groups with methyls, all reduce the potency of the compound.

This compound does not occur as a natural material, although there are closely related natural psychotomimetic substances. Ololiuqui is a name for the seeds of various *Convolvulaceae,* such as *Rivea corymbosa* and *Ipomoea spp.,* the morning glory. For example, there are analogs of lysergamide itself, and compounds wherein the carboxyl group in ring D is reduced to the carbinol. Chanoclavine (Fig. 1b) represents materials present in the natural product, in which the D ring is actually open. The morning glory contains a large variety of these indole alkaloids, very few of which have had any individual clinical evaluation. Most experiments have employed the entire mixture, which to a large extent produces an LSD-like response.

Ibogaine (Fig. 2; $R_1 = OCH_3$, $R_2 = H$) is another example in the family of psychotomimetics, with complex structures and no resemblance to known metabolic materials. It is not a highly potent compound. It is, however, a material that has been widely used in Africa and has had sufficient improper

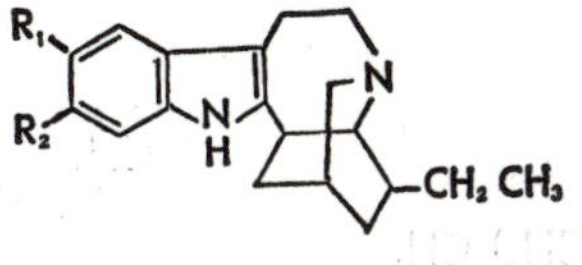

FIG. 2.

use recently in this country that it has now been added to the federal government's list of dangerous drugs. It has a reputation in the native usage of causing alertness, immobility, and attention that can be maintained for hours or even days. This allows the user to stalk game with minimum motion and without a need for food. I believe the compound may allow the native to think that he has been motionless for a long period, because this property has not been objectively observed in controlled studies. The analog with the methoxy group in the indolic-6 position, similar to the harmala alkaloids rather than to serotonin, is known as tabernanthine (Fig. 2; $R_1 = H$, $R_2 = OCH_3$). It is a local anesthetic, but it has shown no central effects.

The next class of compounds to be discussed is a bit simpler in structure. It is the group from the plant *Cannabis sativa,* and its active components are known as the cannabinoids. They are characterized by either a three-ring system or a system that can be easily converted into a three-ring system. The totally aromatic compound is cannabinol (Fig. 3a), and it displays the carbon skeleton common to the group. All the materials found in the native plant have an amyl group in the 5-position of the resorcinol.

It is worth a moment here to discuss the numbering systems employed

26 CHEMISTRY AND STRUCTURE-ACTIVITY RELATIONSHIPS

with these compounds. One hears continuously of the chemistry of delta this-or-that tetrahydrocannabinol, and it sounds as if there are dozens of possible isomers known. In reality, there are only a few, but they can be numbered in several different manners. The ring system itself is quite often numbered according to *Chemical Abstracts*. This is shown with cannabinol (Fig. 3a). The aromatic hydroxyl group establishes the number 1 position, numbers 5 and 6 are in the heterocyclic ring; and numbers 7, 8, 9 and 10 complete the third ring which is in this case aromatic, but which in the active compound is tetrahydrogenated. A severe disadvantage to this numbering system becomes apparent when one notes that many of the compounds that are present have the center ring open. This results in a diol system with some form of unsaturation in the isopropyl group, as seen in cannabidiol (Fig. 3b). As a consequence, the above numbering system is totally invalid. Two additional numbering methods exist, one based on a benzopyran skeleton and one on a diphenyl nucleus, but they both have the same limitation, *i.e.*, applicability to only one of the two types of systems found in the cannabinoids.

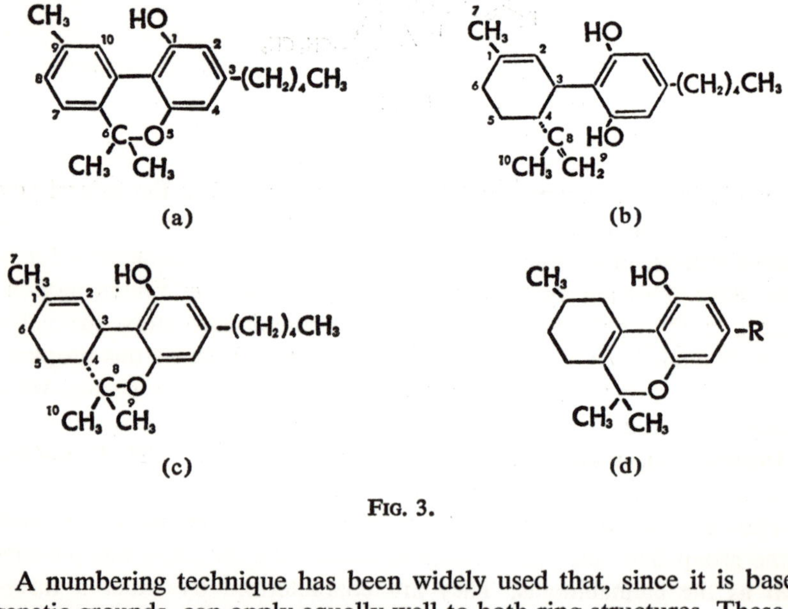

FIG. 3.

A numbering technique has been widely used that, since it is based on biogenetic grounds, can apply equally well to both ring structures. These compounds can be considered as resulting from an amalgamation of a terpene and a resorcinol. A terpene, the left-hand ring in Fig. 3, is numbered from the carbon carrying the methyl group as number 1, progressing with sequential carbons about the ring. The methyl group becomes number 7 and the isopropyl group picks up the remaining three numbers. On that basis the ring on the left-hand side of Δ^1-tetrahydrocannabinol, component of cannabis, is numbered 1 under the methyl group as shown in Fig. 3c. The virtue of this procedure is that it applies to all compounds, whether the oxygen ring is closed or open.

As to structure-activity relationships in this family, the most complete study that has been reported concerns variations of the unnatural Δ^3-tetrahydrocannabinol. This work by Adams and a number of graduate students appeared twenty-one years ago (1948). Parallel studies, complementary to Adams's, were reported by Todd in England at about the same time. Of all the structural points in the molecule that were investigated, the one that led to the greatest variation in activity was the amyl group on the 5-position of the resorcinol moiety. I will not go deeply into the complete SAR studies of this work because of time limitations, and I want to talk at some length about the simplest family, the mescaline analogs. However, I will mention that variations in the identity of "R" in Δ^3-tetrahydrocannabinol (Fig. 3d) have led to a range of biological potency that spans over three orders of magnitude. A maximum in activity was reported for a branched chain 9-carbon system. These materials proved to be many times more potent than the natural compounds, both in animal tests and in man.

This is, however, a whole chapter in its own right. I will just add that in the last two or three years, six independent syntheses have appeared, from Israel, Germany, Switzerland and this country, that describe preparations of compounds with the double bond located in the natural position. This suggests a possible series of studies that could couple the recently developed synthetic skills in double-bond orientation with the knowledge that "R" is a very sensitive point in the molecule. This whole family of compounds, with the unconjugated double bond and the variation in "R," is totally unexplored and could very well justify new research interests in the area of the cannabinoid compounds.

The area of *Cannabis* chemistry has recently been reviewed by Mechoulam (1967).

I will be brief in the discussion of the next family of compounds as they will be discussed at length later on this morning. These are materials related to *Datura*. The carbon skeleton of the natural alkaloids is shown in the parent compound, atropine (Fig. 4a). The chemical relationship here to acetylcholine (Fig. 4b), a neural transmitter to which it is an antagonist, is the first suggestion of similarity to metabolic systems. Hyoscyamine is the *l*-isomer of atropine, and is the form which is present in the plant. The epoxide of this is

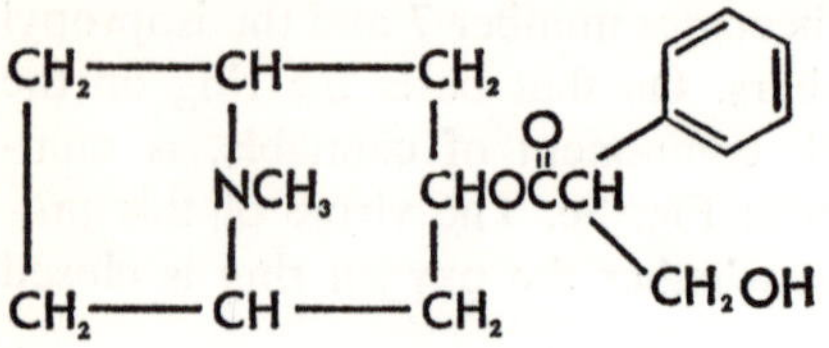

28   CHEMISTRY AND STRUCTURE-ACTIVITY RELATIONSHIPS

(a) Atropine

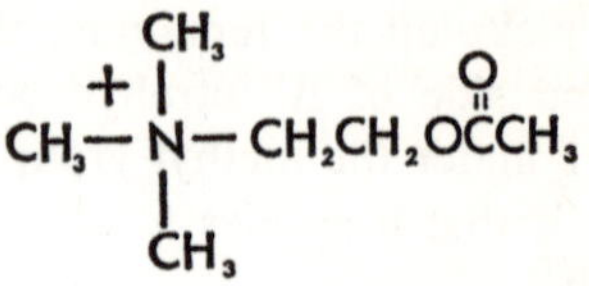

(b) Acetylcholine

FIG. 4.

hyoscine, or *l*-scopolamine. This group represents the biologically active belladonna alkaloids. It has prompted many synthetic studies, evolving materials such as ditran and benactyzine. These will be talked about later, but I would again caution that although these have commonly been called psychotomimetics, they lead to more of a delusional state with amnesia rather than to an intoxication with recall that is the mark of the other psychotomimetics being discussed here.

Another family is a group of alkaloids found in species of both *Banisteriopsis* and *Peganum*. The carbon skeleton of this family is shown in harmaline (Fig. 5a; $R_1 = H$, $R_2 = OCH_3$). This is an indole, and here again, one could see a resemblance to serotonin (Fig. 5b) which is a hydroxy

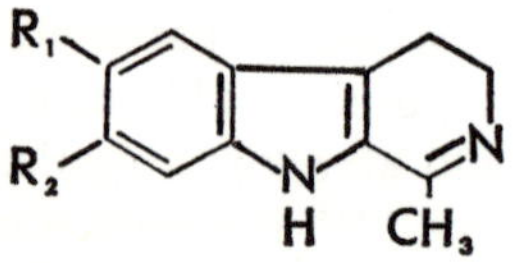

(a)

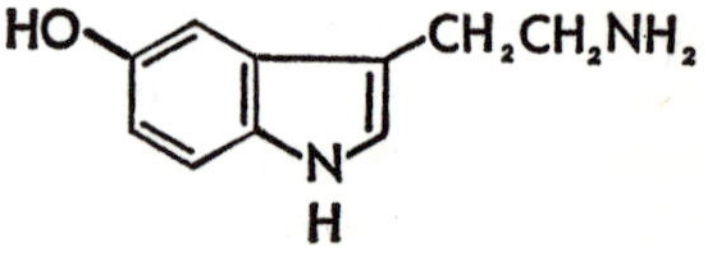

(b) Serotonin

FIG. 5.

substituted tryptamine. The methoxy group in this case is in the position it was in tabernanthine from *Tabernanthe iboga,* as mentioned earlier. This compound occurs in the native drug ayahuasca along with the totally aromatic derivative harmine, and its tetrahydro derivative, tetrahydroharmine. This group of compounds constitutes the principal active constituency of these natural plants, but later on today there will be a talk by Dr. Holmstedt discussing some of the other materials that have been found in the plant. There are interesting analogs in which the methoxy group is found in the indolic 5-position.

Materials with the indole-5-methoxy substitution but with the intact harman tricyclic ring system are not known in nature. The direct analogy to harmaline would be 6-methoxyharmalan (Fig. 5a; $R_1 = OCH_3$, $R_2 = H$), the totally aromatic system is 6-methoxy harman, and its tetrahydro derivative would be 6-methoxytetrahydroharman. McIsaac has advanced a hypothesis that such chemicals could be generated in the pineal gland, say from melatonin by dehydration or from the corresponding methoxy ether of serotonin by the addition of acetaldehyde. As far as I know, these have not been confirmed as components of the intact brain, although spectrophotometric evidence suggests their presence. Yet these materials, the hydrogenation products of 6-methoxy-harman, are two or three times more potent as psychotomimetics than the natural analogs with the methoxy group in the indolic-6 position. Since the chemical mechanisms for their generation *in situ* are certainly present, it is intriguing to speculate that such materials might arise in the abnormal synthesis or metabolism of melatonin.

The next family of psychotomimetics is represented by the indolealkylamines, and they are chemically very close to normal metabolism and normal metabolites. The simplest compound is N,N-dimethyltryptamine (Fig. 6;

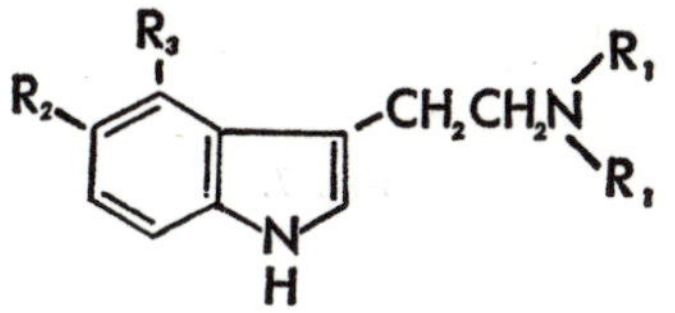

FIG. 6.

$R_1 = CH_3$, $R_2 = R_3 = H$; DMT). This material has been found in a number of snuffs through many areas of South America and the Caribbean. The 5-methoxy-N,N-dimethyltryptamine ($R_1 = CH_3$, $R_2 = OCH_3$, $R_3 = H$) is also a snuff component, and a recently discovered compound of the *Banisteriopsis* group mentioned earlier. Neither of these two materials is active in man orally, only parenterally. The diethyl and dipropyl homologs of DMT have been evaluated in man and the potencies and their interrelationships will be discussed later by Dr. Szara.

The 4-hydroxy compound is the compound psilocin, and it and its phosphate ester, psilocybin (Fig. 6; $R_1 = CH_3$, $R_2 = H$, $R_3 = OH$; $R_1 = CH_3$, $R_2 = H$, $R_3 = OPO(OH)_2$, respectively) are the active components of the teonanacatl mushroom of Mexico. Psilocybin is stoichiometrically equivalent to psilocin. Mention should be made here of the 5-hydroxy compound, bufotenine (Fig. 6; $R_1 = CH_3$, $R_2 = OH$, $R_3 = H$). It is N,N-dimethyl serotonin, and has been found in both animals and plants. It has been claimed to be a psychotomimetic, and has been added to the federal government's list of dangerous drugs, but I feel that this claim could not withstand serious challenge. The material is definitely biologically active; it has been shown to be present in human metabolic schemes, and there is a very close chemical relationship to serotonin, from which it could certainly arise by well known processes.

In the remaining time I would like to discuss the last of these families of psychotomimetics, the simplest of all. These stem from peyotl, the cactus *Anhalonium lewinii* (*Lophophora williamsii*), found in the southwest part of the United States and the northern part of Mexico. The principal compound present in it, and the presumed active principle, is the compound, mescaline, 3,4,5-trimethoxyphenylethylamine (Fig. 7a). Here there is a very close relationship to the neurotransmitter, norepinephrine (Fig. 7b), which is itself a

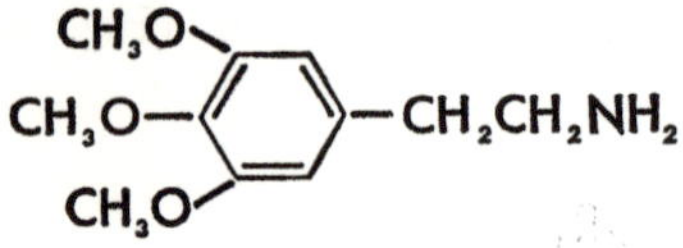

(a) Mescaline 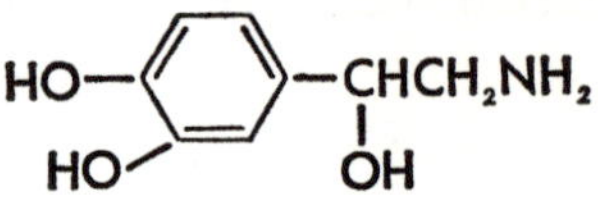   (b) Norepinephrine

FIG. 7.

trihydroxylated phenethylamine. The three oxygens are methylated in the case of mescaline, whereas the third hydroxy group of norepinephrine is a benzylic hydroxy group. Mescaline, although one of the least active of all the psychotomimetics, is actually one of the best studied. It has served as a basis for the evaluation of several groups of derivatives. These have been designed to challenge different quadrants of the molecule, and to establish what role they play in generating the psychotomimetic syndrome.

Hopefully, from this there may come some understanding of their relationships with neural metabolic pathways. After all, the whole rationalization behind studies of this type is that perhaps one could observe a disruption, presumably in the norepinephrine path, which would lead to the accumulation within the organism of some compound not normally there, some compound that might generate the symptoms of a spontaneous endogenous psychosis.

The data to be discussed in the remainder of this presentation are all assembled in the accompanying Table I. Vertically, the various compounds are presented in accord with today's discussion, and the lettered abbreviations will

TABLE I

	Compound	Ring position	M.U.	Chain length	Quinone to OCH₃	Quinone to ortho-H	Ortho	Meta	(OCH₃)₂ → —OCH₂O—
"natural"	Mescaline	3,4,5	"1"						
	TMA	3,4,5	2.2	3 →² 4 (<2)					
	MMDA	3,4,5	2.8	3 → 2 (1)					
	MMDA-2	2,4-5	12						
	MMDA-3a	2,3-4	10						
	MDA	3-4	3						
	DMMDA	2,3,4,5	12						
	DMMDA-2	2,3,4-5	5						
	Tetra-MA	2,3,4,5	6						
	DMA	3,4	<1	3 → 2 (<0.2)					
	TMA-2	2,4,5	17	3 → 2 (1)					
	4-MA	4	5	3 → 2 (<1)					
"unnatural"	TMA-3	2,3,4	<2						
	TMA-4	2,3,5	4		*				
	TMA-5	2,3,6	13		*				
	TMA-6	2,4,6	10						
	2,4-DMA	2,4	5		**				
	2,5-DMA	2,5	8		**				
	EMM *OEt*	2,4,5	<7						
	MEM *OEt*	2,4,5	15						
	MME *Et*	2,4,5	<7						
	DOM *Et*	2,4,5	80	3 → 2 (<15)					
	DOET *Et*	2,4,5	—	→ 4 (<15)					

* Signifies compounds with a 1, 2, 4 orientation of oxygen.
** Signifies the compounds that are *para*, 2, 4, or 2, 4, 6 oriented.

be defined during their description. Sequential columns elaborate their comparisons with regard to structural parameters.

One of the first changes that was made in the structure of mescaline was the incorporation of the side chain found in amphetamine, the α-methyl homolog of phenylethylamine. This compound, α-methyl mescaline or 3,4,5-trimethoxyamphetamine, brings together the structures of a sympathomimetic amine and a psychotomimetic one. It is the second entry in the table, with the convenient code TMA. The use of "A" with this and most of the compounds to be discussed during the remainder of this paper is inaccurate. Amphetamine, like aspirin, is the name of a single compound, and cannot have functional groups attached to it. These substituted derivatives properly should be called variously substituted phenylisopropylamines, as this is the proper chemical name for amphetamine. Therefore, "A" here and through the code letters of the table should be thought of as standing for phenylisopropylamine. With that we will probably continue calling them amphetamines, for it is a convenient nomenclature.

TMA, and all of the compounds that follow it in the first column of the table, have α-methyl groups, with certain exceptions that I will mention. Mescaline alone is a phenethylamine. The second column of the table lists the substitution positions of the oxygens on the phenylisopropylamine (amphetamine) moiety. All groups are methoxyls unless italicized; a single number in italics indicates the position of the grouping listed immediately after the compound; two numbers in italics indicate that a methylenedioxy ring is in that position. The third column is a measure of the relative potencies of each in man, compared against mescaline as a reference with unit potency. The mean effective level of mescaline is taken to be 3.75 mg/kg of the free base. All of these mescaline unit (M.U.) values must be held with a fair amount of reservation. Although most were established through rather extensive clinical trials, one must recognize that there is a wide variation between individuals and with a given individual from day to day. I would say that ±25% would indicate the degree of uncertainty in these M.U. values.

TMA (Fig. 8a; 3,4,5-trimethoxy) shows about a two-fold increase in potency over mescaline. If a three-carbon chain is more effective than a two-

Fig. 8.

carbon chain, then an obvious extension is to the four-carbon chain. The α-substituent was extended in a study of homologs, but the next immediate compound, α-ethyl mescaline, already showed a decrease in psychotomimetic activity. On the basis of this initial study it appears that three is an optimum carbon-chain length. This will be borne out as we get further into this compilation. The function of the α-methyl group may only be to make the amine group less amenable to deamination by enzymatic attack.

There is a compound in nature that has the same atomic skeleton as TMA, but no nitrogen; this is the essential oil, elemicin (Fig. 8b; 3,4,5-trimethoxy). It is interesting that it is a component of nutmeg, and nutmeg has a reputation for producing peculiar mental effects. A logical step was to inquire into nutmeg and to analyze its aromatic ether fraction. This approach with nutmeg and several related natural products has resulted in the first dozen or so amphetamines in the table. They have been called the "natural" amphetamines since their ring substitution patterns are those of natural oils from which, to a large extent, they have been chemically derived.

The most prevalent essential oil in the aromatic fraction of nutmeg is the methylenedioxy counterpart of elemicin, myristicin (Fig. 8b; 3-methoxy-4,5-methylenedioxy). This served as a template for the synthesis of the next compound in this series, 3-methoxy-4,5-methylenedioxy amphetamine. This material, MMDA ("M" for methoxy, "MD" for methylenedioxy), has an increase of about 50% in potency, providing a compound that is about three times as active as mescaline itself. There is quite a change in the qualitative nature of the intoxication. A continuation of this study of the "natural" amphetamines led to the study of materials with the number, the orientation and the identity of substituents of various essential oils.

The first of the structural rearrangements involved the relocation of the methoxy group. The 2,4,5-orientation is found in oil of *Calamus,* and the 2,3,4-orientation is found in oil of *Crowei*. The two corresponding amphetamines are MMDA-2 and MMDA-3a (Fig. 8a; 2-methoxy-4,5-methylenedioxy and 2-methoxy-3,4-methylenedioxy, respectively). Their potencies were increased five-fold, about ten times the potency of mescaline.

Another modification, other than rearranging the methoxy group, is the removal or addition of methoxy groups. Demethoxylation leads to a compound derived directly from safrol, known as methylenedioxyamphetamine (MDA). On the other hand, the addition of a methoxyl group to MMDA leads to bases that are structurally related to apiole and dillapiole.

These compounds (DMMDA and DMMDA-2; 2,5-dimethoxy-3,4-methylenedioxy; and 2,3-dimethoxy-4,5-methylenedioxy, respectively, were prepared, and they have the potencies shown. They are an order of magnitude more potent than mescaline. The third tetraoxygenated amphetamine based on natural oils is 2,3,4,5-tetramethoxyphenylisopropylamine (Tetra-MA). The essential oil counterpart is found in oil of parsley and oil of *Calamus;* the derived amine has a potency of 6 M.U. Dimethoxyamphetamine, DMA (Fig. 8a; 3,4-dimethoxy-) is a direct analog of methyleugenol. This base appeared to be without biological activity, the only one of the natural orientations that is not active. The compound, TMA-2, with a 2,4,5 orientation, is derived from the essential oil asarone, and is the most potent of all materials that have been found within this "natural" system.

The next logical step was to complete those series that were mentioned above. For example, in the trimethoxyamphetamines, the 3,4,5-isomers were related to elemicin, and the 2,4,5 was based on the compound asarone. This left four more isomers possible, the 2,3,4, the 2,3,5 and 2,3,6, and the 2,4,6 counterparts. The first of these, TMA-3, has been found to be inactive, but the other three are quite active. None of them, however, exceeds the 2,4,5-trimethoxy orientation in potency. Two of the "unnatural" dimethoxyamphetamines have been prepared, the 2,4- and 2,5-dimethoxyphenylisopropylamine (2,4-DMA; 2,5-DMA). They have a potency of about five times that of mescaline.

With most of these compounds, the style and the qualitative nature of the intoxication has been found to vary quite radically from one to another, and, therefore, the device of jamming them all into the common mold of mescaline potency has serious limitations. However, I have mentioned earlier the flexibility expected with these numerical values. The trimethoxy compound with a 2,4,5-orientation appeared to be the most potent of this group, and all possible ethyl homologs of this compound, TMA-2, were prepared. Three monethoxy compounds were evaluated in clinical trials. Only the compound with the ethoxy group in the para-position retained biological activity. The appearance of ethoxy groups in either of the other two positions led to a decrease in biological activity.

All this brings into emphasis the substituent that is located in the 4-position. This position could well be sensitive in man to some extent, for it is known in certain animal species to be a principal location for detoxification of amphetamine by hydroxylation. Perhaps these materials display different biological activity due to the substituent in the 4-position. We know that hydrogen in this location provides an active compound, 2,5-dimethoxyamphetamine. A methoxyl group at this position leads to the most active compound mentioned, and this potency is not lost with the ethoxy homolog. It seemed obvious that the blocking of this position with a group that would be biologically unavailable to metabolism, such as a methyl group which cannot be either easily removed or oxidized to a hydroxy group, could grossly change its biological nature. It could be argued that such a compound might be more potent because now it cannot be cleared through detoxification. On the other hand, one could argue that the compound could not only be without potency, but also that it might serve as a competitive antagonist to the known potent materials, and so actually serve as a prophylactic agent against them.

The first of these two possibilities proved to be the case. This compound is DOM, and it proved to be about eighty times as potent as mescaline in activity and to be extremely long-lived in activity as well. An obvious departure from this compound was the extension in length of this 4-alkyl chain, leading to the specific compound 4-ethyl-2,5-dimethoxyamphetamine, known as DOET. It was originally called DOE ("E" for ethyl, as "M" was for methyl), but this code name turned out, unfortunately, to be a synonym for methamphetamine, and the "T" was rapidly added to keep confusion and undesirable association from occurring in the literature. This ethyl compound does not have a potency listed in the table. Dr. Snyder will deal at length about it specifically. It has a dual action. At low levels it serves as an energizer, and it is being clinically evaluated from that point of view in his laboratories. It is only at higher levels that there are psychotomimetic effects. Thus, it is more potent in the sense of biological activity, and less potent in terms of mescaline units.

This brings to an end the listing of compounds and their relative activities. In the space I have left I would like to take this body of data and see what can be done from the consideration of structural parameters. In this way, insight could be gained concerning metabolic products that might not normally be present in the organism but whose presence might produce these mental changes artificially.

Chain length has already been mentioned. The column in the table entitled "chain length" lists those effects. These and subsequent data are presented in a recent analysis (Shulgin *et al.*, 1969; see also references contained therein). In TMA, a chain length of three is twice as active as mescaline. Extending the chain to four leads to a decrease in the activity below that found with the chain length of three. This length appears to be optimum. The two-carbon analog of 3,4-dimethoxyamphetamine is the compound DMPEA, dimethoxyphenylethylamine. This is the substance related to the pink spot of schizophrenic urine. It has been shown to be inactive even at levels five times that of mescaline, *i.e.*, it has an activity of <0.2 M.U. Since DMA is less than 1 M.U. no information can be gleaned. When TMA-2 undergoes a change in chain length from three to two, the biological activity of the compound drops down to that of mescaline itself, a full order of magnitude of change. A similar change occurs with 4-methoxy amphetamine. Progressing from a chain length of three to two, the compound decreases from a drug much more potent than mescaline to one distinctly less potent. The one remaining example is with

DOM itself. Both the two and the four chain compound have been synthesized, both have been evaluated, and both are less active than the three carbon chain. All this evidence tends to affirm that a three carbon chain is indeed an optimum chain length.

Suggestions have been advanced that these materials may show biological activity by virtue of the fact that they may either imitate or form indoles during the course of their metabolism. In the formation of an indole, the nitrogen must have access to the aromatic ring. This can be achieved by attack on the ortho-methoxyl group in a ring with substitution allowing quinone formation or on the ortho-hydrogen of an oxidized ring in a direct nucleophilic attack. This proclivity to form a quinone at a methoxy group would be maximum if the oxygen orientations were such as to allow quinone formation, either ortho or para. A 1,2,4-arrangement of the three oxygens would provide a maximum opportunity for reaction, whereas there would be a minimum possibility if the oxygens were arranged meta to one another, in a 1,3,5-pattern. There are five compounds that have a 1,2,4 orientation of oxygen, and these are indicated by a * in the table. The compounds that are para, 2,4, or 2,4,6-oriented are indicated by **. Presumably the former would be most able to form a quinone intermediate by methoxy displacement, and the latter least able to form it. Yet these two groups of compounds encompass the same range of biologic activities. On this basis, one can conclude that quinone formation through an ortho methoxy group is not a likely explanation.

At the ortho-hydrogen, however, a totally different argument presents itself, for an attack at this position would involve an intermediate of quinone form, one amenable to nucleophilic attack. The addition of methoxy groups to the parent molecule would make this style of reaction more probable. These compounds have been compared on the basis of the addition of a methoxy group to a reference material. These references and the consequences of methoxylation are summarized in the next column of the table. The only structural requirement is that there should be an oxygen located para to the displaced hydrogen. The table looks like an unsuccessful football play by Knute Rockne as it is presented. Nonetheless, it is apparent that there is a large number of plusses, implying that the activity has generally gone up with the addition of a methoxy group. Thus, there is some encouragement given to the argument that this type of an intermediate might be involved, reflecting the differences in basicity resulting from the addition of a methoxy group. This analysis is compromised by the fact that methoxy groups are being added at different positions to achieve this overall inductive effect.

It is interesting to go through the same data considering the specific position at which a methoxy group is added. The comparison of compounds without an ortho-methoxy group in relationship to counterpart compounds with one is shown in the next column of the table. A large number of plusses is apparent, only one unchanged, and no minusses. In almost every instance, a given compound in comparison with an analogous material that is substituted with an ortho-methoxy group shows the latter to be more active. Quite the opposite is observed with the addition of a group in the meta position. In general, the addition of a meta-methoxy group to a parent compound decreases its activity.

The parallel presentation for para-substitution is not presented, as it is not fair. Almost all of these compounds are para-substituted. There are only a very few instances in which you can compare materials with and without a para group. The one remaining analysis that is given in the table is a comparison between dimethoxy compounds and their methylenedioxy counterparts. In most cases, the methylenedioxy analog was a compound that is slightly more potent.

What can one conclude from all of this? The ultimate purpose of this study is to look at what compounds might be present in the human, not through normal metabolism, but generated through some idiosyncratic or pathologic state. This material might result from some norepinephrine pathway deviation, and might be a biologically active agent. Although it appears that a chain length of three carbons is optimum, this may merely reflect the defense of the amino group to deamination. As three-carbon chains are virtually unknown in animal metabolism, it is probable that the two-carbon chain of the norepinephrine metabolism is a more likely structure for such an agent. An increase in the number of methoxy groups leads to an increase in the potency of a compound, but this must be more carefully analyzed. The addition of ortho groups increases activity, the addition of meta-methoxy groups decreases it, and although the para substituent is not essential, it certainly is of much importance.

Accepting that this abnormal agent is going to be related to the norepinephrine scheme, it is possible that some dimethoxy material, perhaps dimethoxyhydroxyphenethylamine, could be involved. Since 6-hydroxylation can occur *in vivo,* perhaps some 6-hydroxy or 6-methoxy analog of norepinephrine metabolites might be expected. This is a 2,4,5-orientation that has proved to be the most potent of the orientations studied. These materials, dimethoxyphenethanolamine or the 6-hydroxy analogs of the various metabolic intermediates, represent a series of compounds that could be implicated in abnormal metabolism.

How can one challenge these proposals? Paradoxically, the most direct way of challenging this entire group will fail, for if you have a material that is suspected of being an endogenous psychotogen, you cannot assay it in normal human subjects because the normal subject is, indeed, normal for the very reason that he has the machinery for disposing of such a compound. Therefore, one must distort such a compound in some way that will make it a valid challenge. One way would be through the introduction of a methyl group α to the amine function. This would lead to a series of variously substituted ephedrines, presumably less susceptible to MAO attack. Possibly the replacement of the methoxy group in the para position with a methyl group would interfere with metabolic disposition.

A chemical explanation of mental illness is only one of several that are possible, but the fact remains that there are some aspects of mental illness that can be duplicated chemically. A hypothesis of an endogenous psychotogen certainly deserves this type of further investigation, and the compounds which are implicit in these combinations of ring substitutions, of chain length variations and in degrees of oxygenation could very well provide the tools that can challenge this hypothesis.

REFERENCES

Adams, R., MacKenzie, S. Jr. and Loewe, S.: Tetrahydrocannabinol Homologs with Doubly Branched Alkyl Groups in the 3-Position. XVIII. *J. Am. Chem. Soc., 70:* 664 (1948).

Lewin, L.: *Phantastica; Narcotic and Stimulating Drugs, Their Use and Abuse.* London, Routledge & Kegan Paul (1931) (Translated from the second German Edition, p. 30–31 (1927).)

McIsaac, W. M.: A Biochemical Concept of Mental Disease. *Postgrad. Med. 30:* 111 (1961).

Mechoulam, R. and Gaoni, Y.: Recent Advances in the Chemistry of Hashish. *Fortsch. Chem. Org. Natur. 25:* 175 (1967).

Shulgin, A. T., Sargent, T. and Naranjo, C.: Structure-Activity Relationships of One-Ring Psychotomimetics. *Nature, 221:* 537 (1969).

Usdin, E. and Efron, D. H.: *Psychotropic Drugs and Related Compounds.* U.S. Dept. of Health, Education and Welfare. Public Health Service Publication No. 1589. January 1967.

DISCUSSION

DR. BURGER: Thank you, Dr. Shulgin, for an excellent, comprehensive and thought-provoking presentation.

DR. DOMINO: I'd like to ask about the phencyclidines. In your discussion, Dr. Shulgin, you mentioned Sernyl or phencyclidine in relationship to atropine-like compounds, but pharmacologically, of course, they are quite different. Phencyclidine is really a sympathomimetic and in large doses is used as an anesthetic. A lot of people would even argue that it is not a psychotomimetic, but at least the psychiatrists I'm associated with feel that phencyclidine is, indeed, the best drug model of the primary symptoms of schizophrenia of any psychotomimetic we have.

Since this is a phenylmethylamine derivative, I wonder if you could comment a little bit further about phencyclidine and where you would place it in your scheme.

DR. SHULGIN: Generally I had placed it much closer to the atropine group, not so much on chemical structure or pharmacological structure, as in the use and misuse of it. There's been quite a flurry of what has been called synthetic THC in and around the West Coast, and probably in the East Coast markets, too. I have assayed several samples of this material, and with one exception they have been phencyclidine. Apparently this has enough of a psychopharmacologic similarity to the tetrahydrocannabinol type of psychotomimetic that it can be sold and disguised verbally as being that, and this is believed. On the other hand, as you mentioned, the excessive usage of it leads to an anesthetic state, and in this way it is very much like the use of twilight sleep in the atropine group. So, in general, I have tended to put it along with the other synthetics related to the *Datura* group, but this is quite arbitrary. Primarily one observes behavioral changes rather than pharmacological ones.

DR. MANDELL: Dr. Shulgin turned me on about an idea that never occurred to me until hearing his talk. His work suggests that we may be able to get rid of the indole concept in LSD and other indole containing hallucinogens. If what Dr. Shulgin is saying about mescaline is true, then we might conceive of the benzene ring in an indole getting electron donor effects from the pyrrole ring.

If what he said was true about the 3-carbon ring structure being the essential link to an active amine nitrogen, in the structure of LSD we can get to the 6-nitrogen in two ways. This structural concept may join together the mescaline and the indole bag by throwing them together with just three very simple and economical structural requirements: (1) the possibility of a high molecular energy level in a single aromatic system; (2) a three carbon chain and (3) a nitrogen. This kind of concept is clear for the phenylethylamine hallucinogens; perhaps it is true for LSD as well. Perhaps the very high potency of LSD is due to the rigidity of holding the 6-nitrogen in place while still maintaining the 3-carbon chain. The 6-nitrogen may be activated by non-bonded resonance with its methyl group.

It never occurred to me until you started playing around with the mescaline story. But, as you know, the pyrrole ring donates electrons, perhaps very much like the methoxy group in mescaline would. This line of thought could marry then in one model, the mescaline theorizing with the indole theorizing. That's off the top of my head. What do you want to do with it?

DR. SHULGIN: It's certainly appealing to think that you have two sites of basicity in the molecule, one a diffuse π-system with its molecular-orbital definition, and perhaps a somewhat more localized base in the form of a lone nitrogen pair. If you do have these two sites, they may define the successful attachment to some reaction site somewhere. If there is an optimum separation as well as an optimum localization, then a rigid configuration, if it were the right one, would produce a more effective approach to this site.

DR. MANDELL: And the sigma bonds would hold that tight?

DR. SHULGIN: You might make a birdcage structure that would be very specific by adding a third methylene branch in some way.

DR. CRAIG: Perhaps I should tell Dr. Mandell how much I agree with him, because we have already made substantial progress on the syntheses of both of these.

Now if, in addition to leaving out the pyrrole, you change the 6-membered ring to the indene structure, a 5-membered ring, then the substance becomes a phenylethylamine in both directions, as well as being rigid. We have almost completed the syntheses on both of these LSD compounds. I don't know if they will be any good, but it seemed something that ought to be done.

DR. LEHRER: I wonder if you could comment on the question of transport of these substances into the brain. It's known that indoles and catechols are more easily transported into the brain as the corresponding amino acids; and I wonder whether some of the mescaline series of drugs might not get into the brain more easily as the amino acids, and then become decarboxylated?

DR. SHULGIN: The only one I know that's been studied that way is the actual analog of mescaline itself, trimethoxyphenylalanine. It was synthesized in England and reported in the J.C.S., where it was stated that, "Pharmacology will follow." And about two years later, not having found it, I wrote, and was told, oh, yes, there was absolutely nothing of interest. Other than that, I know of no amino acid studies in this area that would challenge that. It would be a fairly simple series to make, I would think.

DR. BIEL: I don't know if they get decarboxylated.

The question I had was in regard to bufotenine. You ascribed rather low activity to it.

DR. SHULGIN: As far as being a psychotomimetic. There is no question but that it's biologically active, however.

DR. BIEL: Himwich recently published the correlation between the appearance of bufotenine in the urine of schizophrenics and a gradual improvement as urinary bufotenine levels went down or disappeared altogether. Does this alter the picture at all?

DR. SHULGIN: No. There's no question that bufotenine is a metabolite. It's been found not as an artifact but as a genuine component of urine.

I would mention that in the human trial with it (I think it was given intravenously), a whole series of symptoms was observed, but I would hardly call any of them psychotomimetic in nature. That's my only reason for downgrading it. It's not the potency but the nature of the action. It's a highly potent compound.

DR. DOMINO: People turn blue. There are marked cardiovascular effects.

DR. GESSNER: We do have some preliminary data which make us believe that the reason bufotenine is not found to be active is because it simply does not get into the brain. If you put an O-acetyl group on it, it gets into the brain, and then it's hydrolyzed back to bufotenine. It's quite active.

DR. SHULGIN: You haven't done it in humans yet?

DR. GESSNER: No.

STERIC MODELS OF DRUGS PREDICTING PSYCHEDELIC ACTIVITY

Solomon H. Snyder, M.D. and Elliott Richelson, M.D.

*Departments of Pharmacology and Psychiatry
The Johns Hopkins University School of Medicine,
Baltimore, Maryland 21205*

INTRODUCTION

Correlation of the structure of drugs with their pharmacological activities is important both for predicting the activity of new compounds and for affording insight into mechanisms of action. Among psychedelic drugs of the LSD, mescaline and psilocybin classes, there are striking differences in potencies of compounds with slight variations in structure. Even more interesting, some compounds of dissimilar structures produce similar effects in man. Thus mescaline produces subjective effects which are essentially the same as those of LSD, although chemically it differs markedly from LSD and more closely resembles other drugs, for instance, amphetamine, whose effects are dissimilar.

Unfortunately, studies of structure-activity relationships of psychedelic drugs are more difficult than for many other drugs, since there are no simple chemical or *in vitro* systems for evaluation of pharmacological activity. *In vivo* studies of psychedelic drug action may not always reflect their true potency at receptor sites. Instead, apparent potency may be determined by the ability of the compound to resist metabolic degradation or by its enhanced capacity to pass the blood-brain barrier. For example, adding an alpha methyl substituent to mescaline produces a compound, TMA (3,4,5-trimethoxyamphetamine), which is about twice as potent as mescaline. Its enhanced potency is presumably due to a decreased susceptibility to deamination provided by the alpha methyl group. Even after penetration into the brain, drug activity may be determined by regional, cellular or subcellular variations in its localization. For instance, we found that there are differences in the regional localization of LSD in the monkey brain, with highest concentration in visual reflex areas and hypothalamus, regions which could be the sites of the compound's psychotropic action (Snyder and Reivich, 1965).

In spite of these limitations, there appear to be enough instances of differences in psychedelic drug activity which do not appear to be simply attributable to differences in metabolic degradation or access to the brain, that it might be possible to deduce the structural elements which are most crucial for psychedelic activity.

The first well known structure-activity hypothesis about the actions of LSD was the anti-serotonin concept (Gaddum, 1953; Woolley and Shaw, 1954) which suggested that LSD acts by blocking serotonin receptors in the brain, so that active analogs could be predicted by their antagonism to serotonin in simple smooth muscle preparations. However, some compounds did not fit into this scheme. For instance, 2-bromo-LSD is more potent as a serotonin antagonist than is LSD, yet it is quite weak or inactive as a psychedelic agent (Cerletti and Rothlin, 1955). Cerletti (1959) found a correlation between the psychotropic actions of LSD derivatives and central sympathetic stimulation. Quite recently, Aghajanian et al. (1968 and personal communication) have shown that potent psychedelic agents all slow the firing of serotonin neurons in the brain at very low doses, while related drugs which are not psychedelic lack this action.

Earlier, we described a correlation between the psychedelic action of drugs and their electronic configuration so that, within steric classes of compounds, potency was related closely to the energy of the highest occupied molecular orbital (HOMO), an index of the electron donating capacity of the π or resonating electrons of the molecule (Snyder and Merril, 1965; Snyder and Merril, 1967). In LSD, the π electrons at C-9-10 can resonate with the electrons of the indole ring to produce a more energetic HOMO than in a simple tryptamine derivative. This model (Snyder and Merril, 1965) would predict that reduction of the C-9-10 double bond should reduce psychedelic activity, as is in fact the case with dihydro-LSD and lumi-LSD. Since the HOMO energy of indoles such as LSD is localized at C-2, one would predict that substituents at C-2 should reduce activity, as is known to occur with 2-bromo-LSD and 2-oxy-LSD. Although this model predicted the activity of psychedelic drugs within a given steric class, it could not compare compounds of different structural classes. Thus, chlorpromazine has an extremely energetic HOMO but is not psychedelic.

Recently, in making molecular models (Dreiding-Stereo models (Swissco)) of psychedelic compounds of tryptamine, phenylethylamine and phenylisopropylamine classes, we observed that they can all approximate a conformation simulating in part rings A, B and C of LSD (Fig. 1). In the more potent derivatives, certain structural features might permit the stabiliza-

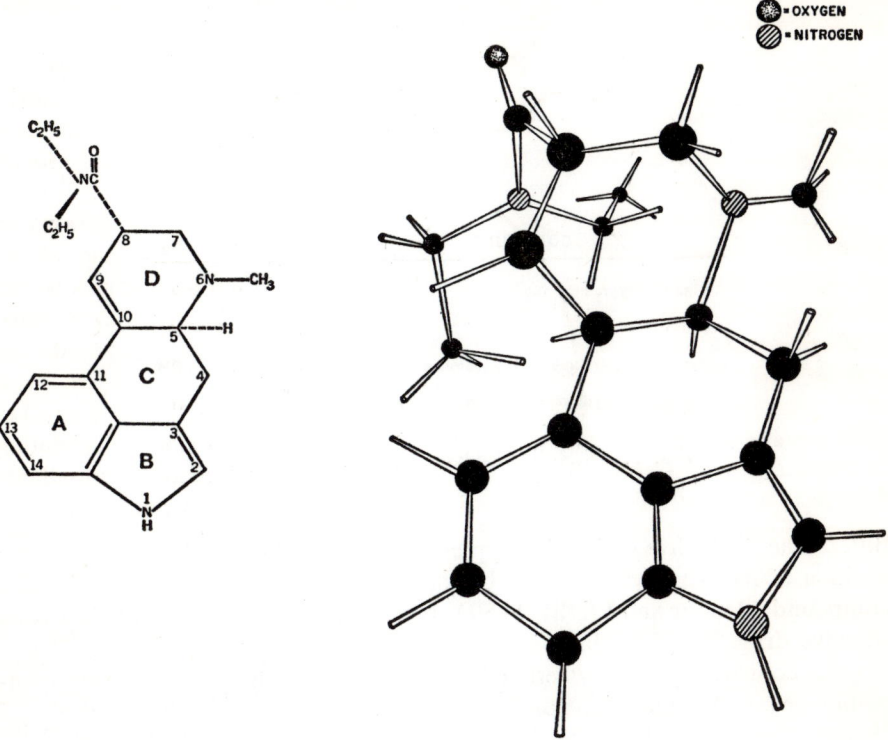

Fig. 1. *d*-Lysergic acid diethylamide (LSD).

tion of the hypothetical "active" conformation, enabling the prediction of the psychotropic activities of a large number of psychedelic drugs.

In the following formulation, potency of psychedelic drugs will refer primarily to the minimally detectable dose in humans or ED50 in animals and expressed as mescaline units (M.U.), defined as the effective dose of mescaline divided by the effective dose of the compound evaluated.

TRYPTAMINE DERIVATIVES

Among the N,N-dimethylated derivatives there are some marked differences in activity with small variations in structure. Psilocin (4-hydroxy-dimethyltryptamine) (Fig. 2) is the most potent agent, about 31 M.U.

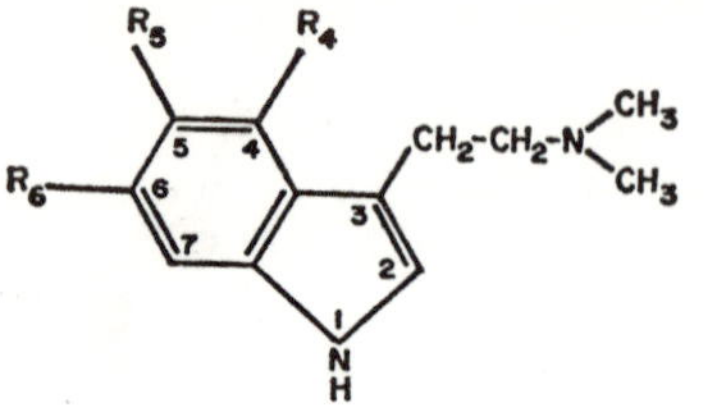

FIG. 2. N,N-dimethylated tryptamine derivatives.

COMPOUND	R_4	R_5	R_6
Dimethyltryptamine	H	H	H
Bufotenine	H	OH	H
6-Hydroxy-N,N-Dimethyltryptamine	H	H	OH
Psilocin (4-Hydroxy-N,N-Dimethyltryptamine)	OH	H	H

Bufotenine (5-hydroxy-dimethyltryptamine) differs from psilocin only in the position of its hydroxyl grouping, but appears to be inactive as a psychedelic compound (Turner and Merlis, 1959). N,N-dimethyltryptamine (DMT) is an effective drug, but only about ⅛ as potent as psilocin (Szara, 1957). There is some controversy as to whether its actions are due to the unchanged compound or to a metabolite, possibly a 6-hydroxylated derivative (Szara and Hearst, 1962; Rosenberg, et al., 1963). When 6-hydroxydimethyltryptamine was administered to humans it did not produce psychotropic effects (Rosenberg et al., 1963). It is probable that of the hydroxylated tryptamines, 6-hydroxydimethyltryptamine would most readily be metabolically conjugated and rapidly excreted, explaining its lack of psychotropic activity.

All of the tryptamine derivatives possess the indole moiety of LSD (rings A and B). The side chain of these compounds can fold back on the indole ring to approximate the C ring of LSD. However, since the side chain is freely rotating it may assume a great number of other conformations. The C ring conformation would be attained more frequently if there were some means of its stabilization. In the molecular model of psilocin (Fig. 3), the amine moiety of the side chain approaches the hydroxyl group of the benzene ring and physically permits hydrogen bonding between the two groups. Such hydrogen bonding with the hydrogen of the 4-hydroxyl and the tertiary amine nitrogen would stabilize an 8 membered ring which, in three dimenions, would resemble ring C of LSD. The distance separating groups forming the bonds would be 1.7 Å, which is in the range of values seen for strong hydrogen bonds. Such intramolecular hydrogen bonding could not take place for bufotenine or DMT. Thus, the structure of psilocin, the most potent psychedelic tryptamine, favors

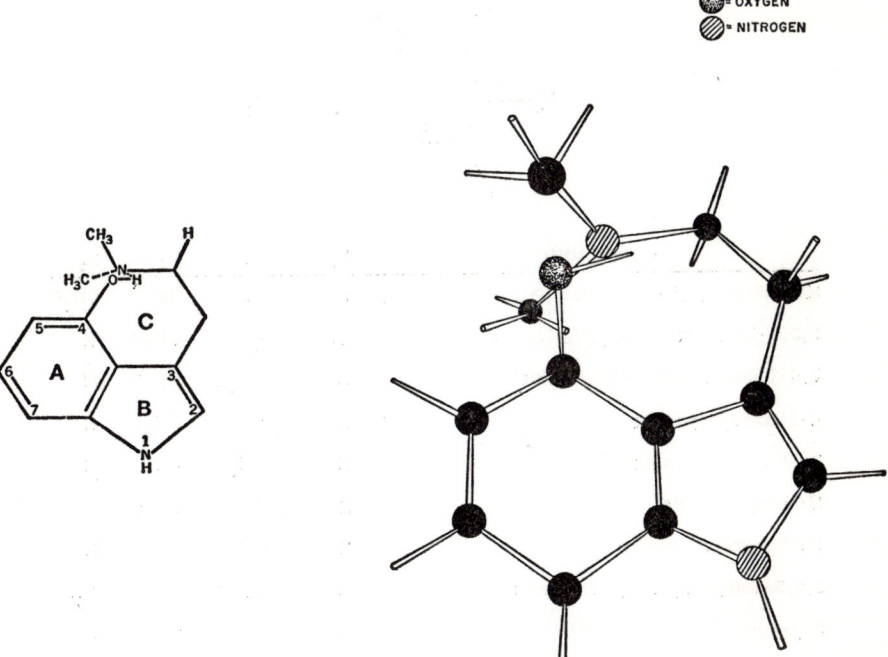

FIG. 3. 4-Hydroxy-N,N-dimethyltryptamine (psilocin).

the LSD conformation more than the less potent tryptamines. Stabilization of psilocin's C ring in this way requires that the amine grouping be nonprotonated, which would be the case if the hypothetical receptor site were lipid-like. If, at the receptor, psilocin's amine group were protonated, as may occur at physiologic pH in aqueous solution, this type of hydrogen bonding would not be feasible. In this case, the protonated amine could interact with the oxygen of the 4-hydroxyl grouping, stabilizing the C ring. In addition to fostering a resemblance to ring C of LSD, the conformation described here for psilocin would also make it more lipid soluble. Interestingly, P. Gessner (personal communication) has found that psilocin is more lipid soluble than bufotenine.

PHENYLETHYLAMINES

The only phenylethylamine structure known to be psychedelic is mescaline (3,4,5-trimethoxyphenylethylamine) (Figs. 4 and 5). Numerous investigators have suggested that the side chain of phenylethylamine molecules might

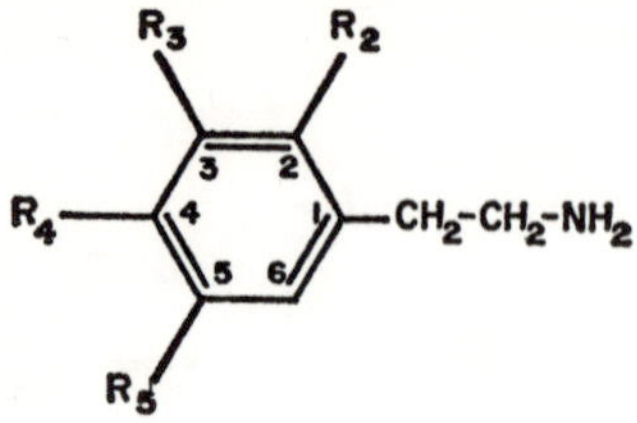

COMPOUND	R₂	R₃	R₄	R₅
Mescaline (3,4,5-Trimethoxyphenylethylamine)	H	CH₃O	CH₃O	CH₃O
2,3,4-Trimethoxyphenylethylamine	CH₃O	CH₃O	CH₃O	H
3,4-Dimethoxyphenylethylamine	H	CH₃O	CH₃O	H
4-Methoxydopamine	H	OH	CH₃O	H
3-Methoxydopamine	H	CH₃O	OH	H
Methoxytyramine	H	H	CH₃O	H
Methoxymetatyramine	H	CH₃O	H	H
3,4,5-Trihydoxyphenylethylamine	H	OH	OH	OH
Dopamine	H	OH	OH	H
Tyramine	H	H	OH	H
Metatyramine	H	OH	H	H
Phenylethylamine	H	H	H	H

FIG. 4. Phenylethylamine derivatives.

fold down toward the ring, resembling the indole nucleus (rings A and B of LSD). Such a conformation might conceivably be stabilized by hydrogen bonding between the hydrogen of the amine side chain and π electrons of the benzene ring at C-2 or C-6. Inasmuch as the extent of this type of interaction would depend on the negative π charge at positions 2 and 6, it is interesting that of all 6 isomeric trimethoxyphenylethylamines, the negative π charge at C-2 and C-6 is greatest in mescaline (Merril and Snyder, in preparation), indicating that ring B could be formed more readily in mescaline than in the other isomers. The only other trimethoxyphenylethylamine which has been examined for activity in man, to our knowledge, is 2,3,4-trimethoxyphenylethylamine, which would not as readily form ring B. This is inactive in man (Slotta and Muller, 1936). In order for the amine side chain to interact with

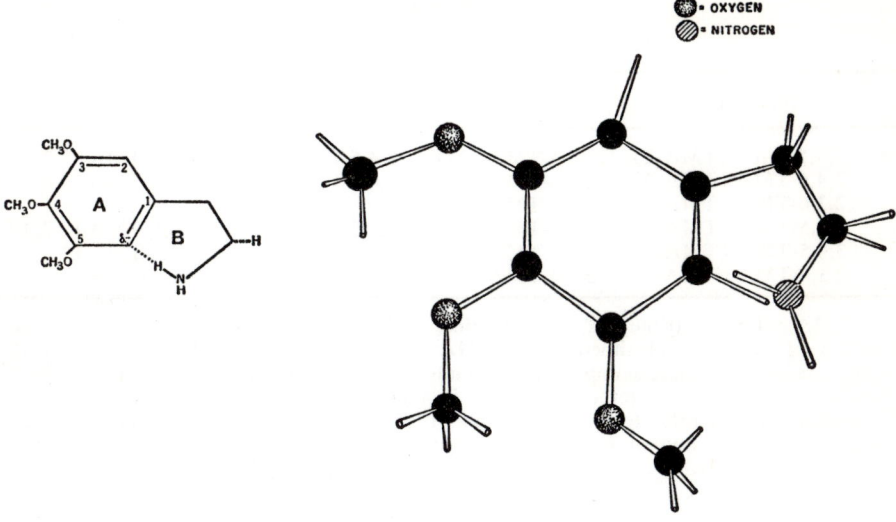

Fig. 5. 3,4,5-Trimethoxyphenylethylamine (mescaline).

π electrons of the ring, it would have to assume a position above the plane of the ring, and accordingly would not be coplanar with the benzene ring as in a true indole structure. It is unclear whether or not such a configuration could interact with indolic receptor sites.

AMPHETAMINES

A large number of trimethoxyamphetamines and methoxymethylenedioxyamphetamines have been synthesized and evaluated in man (Shulgin, 1964; Shulgin et al., 1969). There are marked differences in potencies among the six isomers of trimethoxyamphetamine (Table 1 and Fig. 6). Thus 3,4,5-trimethoxyamphetamine (TMA), the amphetamine analog of mescaline, is about twice as active as mescaline, while 2,4,5-trimethoxyamphetamine (TMA-2) is about 18 times as active, and 2,3,4-trimethoxyamphetamine (TMA-3) is inactive. Since both active and inactive TMA derivatives are metabolized at similar rates and penetrate the blood brain barrier to a similar extent (Mitoma, personal communication), the marked discrepancies in potency cannot be explained by differences in these parameters.

Just as with the phenylethylamines, the side chain of the amphetamine derivatives could approach the benzene ring to approximate ring B of LSD

TABLE I
Structure-activity of trimethoxy-amphetamines

Efficacy	Steric model	Man	Monkey	Rat
Potent	2,4,5-TMA (TMA-2)	2,4,5-TMA (17)	2,4,5-TMA (5.4)	2,4,5-TMA (7.2_u) (4.0_s)
	2,4,6-TMA (TMA-6)	2,3,6-TMA (13)	2,4,6-TMA (3.2)	3,4,5-TMA (4.0_u) (1.5_s)
	2,3,6-TMA (TMA-5)	2,4,6-TMA (10)		
Weak	2,3,5-TMA (TMA-4)	2,3,5-TMA (4)	3,4,5-TMA (1.8)	2,4,6-TMA (1.7_u) (1.0_s)
	3,4,5-TMA (TMA)	3,4,5-TMA (2.2)	2,3,5-TMA (1.1)	2,3,4-TMA (1.6_u) (0_s)
	2,3,4-TMA (TMA-3)	2,3,4-TMA (<2)	2,3,4-TMA (0.7)	

TMA refers to trimethoxyamphetamine, and the preceding numbers refer to the location of methoxy substituents. The TMA designations in parentheses are the code names assigned to these compounds by Shulgin (1964, and personal communication). Numbers in parentheses refer to potency in mescaline units as explained in the text. Subscripts u and s refer to data of Uyeno (1968) and Smythies et al. (1967), respectively. Monkey and human data were obtained by Uyeno et al. (1968) and Shulgin et al. (1969), respectively.

(Figs. 7 and 8). In addition, in isomers with methoxy substituents at C-2 or C-6, an interaction could take place between the hydrogen of the amine side chain and the oxygen of the methoxy group at C-2 or C-6 to form a 7 membered ring that, sterically, closely resembles ring C of LSD (Figs. 7 and 9). Thus, it would be possible for certain of the trimethoxyamphetamines to form both rings B and C of LSD even though no one molecule could assume more than a two ring conformation at any one time.

As with the phenylethylamines, if the amine side chain were to interact with the electron cloud of the benzene ring, the negative π charge at positions 2 and 6 would be important parameters. This negative π charge would be greatest in compounds with 3,4,5-trimethoxy substituents. However, this type of interaction would probably be fairly weak and has not been utilized for prediction of psychotropic activity in the present model.

In the formation of ring C by trimethoxyamphetamines with the hydrogen of the amine (or its proton, if the molecule be protonated) and the methoxy groups at C-2 or C-6, an interaction considerably stronger than described above for the B ring might be expected. The capacity of methoxyamphetamines to form the C ring appears to predict psychotropic potency. In approximating the C ring conformation, the methoxy group at C-2 must fulfill a relatively rigid spacial arrangement. Molecular models show that if there is a methoxy group at C-3 ortho to the methoxy group at C-2, the free rotation of the methoxy at C-3 sterically would hinder the ability of the C-2 methoxy to assume its required arrangement. This steric hindrance would interfere with

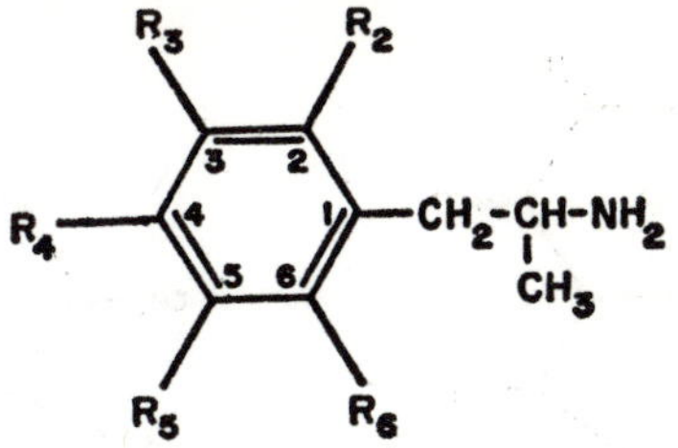

COMPOUND	R_2	R_3	R_4	R_5	R_6
TMA	H	CH_3O	CH_3O	CH_3O	H
TMA-2	CH_3O	H	CH_3O	CH_3O	H
TMA-3	CH_3O	CH_3O	CH_3O	H	H
TMA-4	CH_3O	CH_3O	H	CH_3O	H
TMA-5	CH_3O	CH_3O	H	H	CH_3O
TMA-6	CH_3O	H	CH_3O	H	CH_3O
DOM	CH_3O	H	CH_3	CH_3O	H
DOET	CH_3O	H	CH_3CH_2	CH_3O	H
DMMDA	CH_3O	O-CH$_2$-O		CH_3O	H
DMMDA-2	CH_3O	CH_3O	O-CH$_2$-O		H
MMDA	H	O-CH$_2$-O		CH_3O	H
MMDA-2	H	O-CH$_2$-O		H	CH_3O
MMDA-3a	CH_3O	O-CH$_2$-O		H	H
MDA	H	O-CH$_2$-O		H	H
DMA	CH_3O	H	H	CH_3O	H

FIG. 6. Amphetamine derivatives.

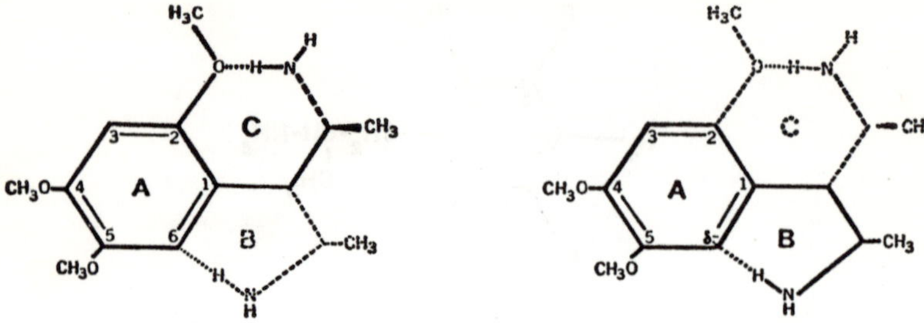

FIG. 7. 2,4,5-Trimethoxyamphetamine (TMA-2).

the formation of ring C in compounds possessing methoxy groups at both C-2 and C-3, *i.e.*, TMA-4 and TMA-3. Compounds with methoxy groups at C-2 or C-6 whose ability to approximate the side chain amine is not hampered by methoxy substituents at C-3 or C-5 respectively should be quite potent. These predictions (Table I) correspond closely to the potency of these com-

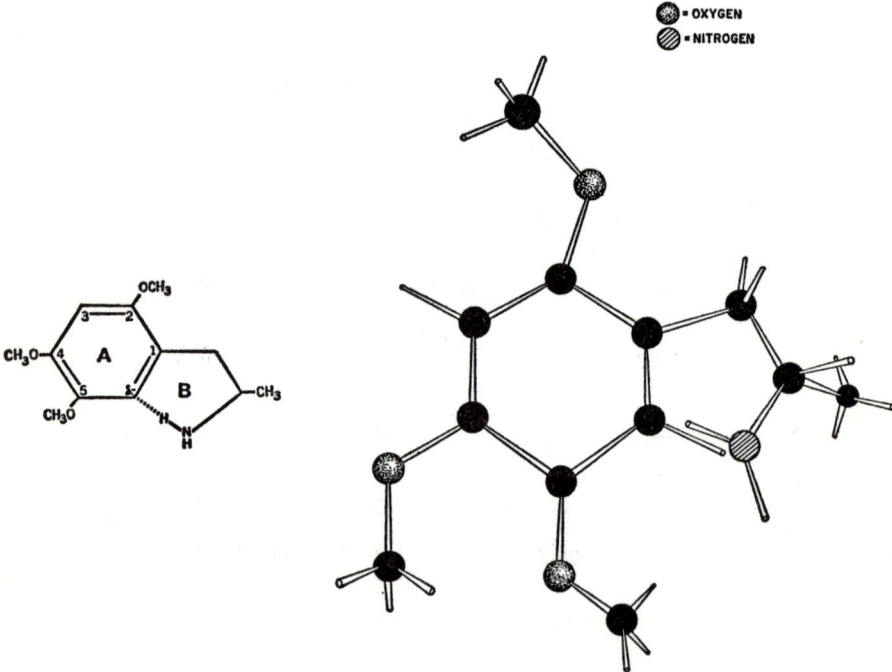

FIG. 8. 2,4,5-Trimethoxyamphetamine (TMA-2).

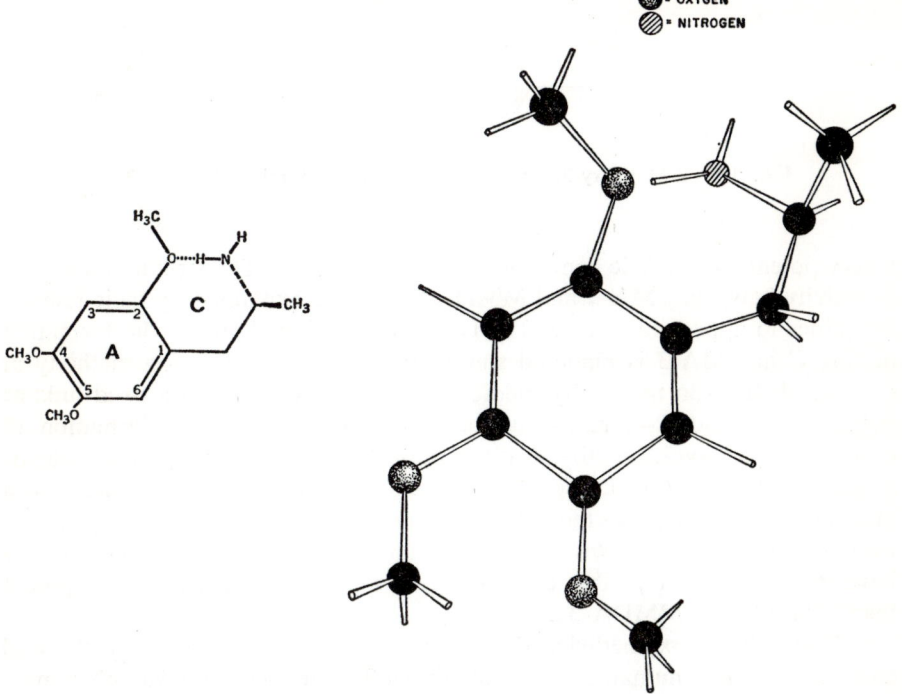

FIG. 9.   2,4,5-Trimethoxyamphetamine (TMA-2).

pounds evaluated in man and in squirrel monkeys. Interestingly, the relative potency of the trimethoxyamphetamines in rats differs somewhat from their rank-order in man and monkey.

METHOXYMETHYLENEDIOXYAMPHETAMINES

These compounds are analogs of the trimethoxyamphetamines in which methylenedioxy groups replace two adjacent methoxys (Fig. 6). 3-Methoxy-4,5-methylenedioxyamphetamine (MMDA), the analog of TMA, has a potency of 3 M.U., similar to TMA. 2-Methoxy-4,5-methylenedioxyamphetamine (MMDA-2), the analog of TMA-2, has a potency of 12 to 20 M.U. (Shulgin, 1964; Shulgin et al., 1969), similar to TMA-2. 2-Methoxy-3,4-methylenedioxyamphetamine (MMDA-3a) (Figs. 6 and 10), is the analog of TMA-3. Although TMA-3 is inactive as a psychedelic agent, MMDA-3a is

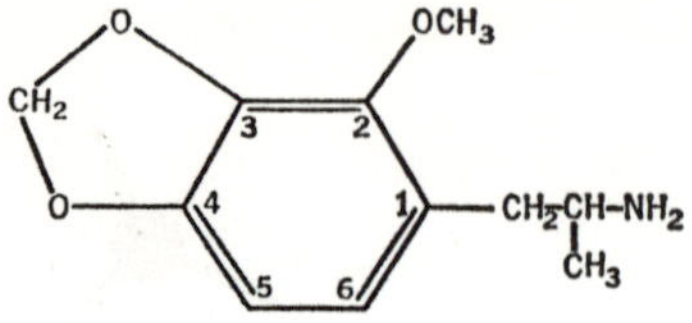

FIG. 10. 2-Methoxy-3, 4-methylenedioxyamphetamine (MMDA-3a)

a very potent psychedelic compound (12 to 20 M.U.). The striking difference in activity between TMA-3 and MMDA-3a can be explained by their relative capacities to approximate ring C of LSD. As mentioned above, the formation of ring C in TMA-3 is hindered sterically by the freely rotating methoxy at C-3. In MMDA-3a the methylenedioxy substituent constitutes a fixed linkage between C-3 and C-4, removing the steric hindrance to the formation of ring C. 4-Methoxy-2,3-methylenedioxyamphetamine would be predicted to be a weak psychedelic agent, because its methoxy group at ring C-2 is fixed in a methylenedioxy bridge to the substituent at ring C-3 and, accordingly, is not available for interaction with the side chain. Recently, Shulgin *et al.* (1969) have demonstrated that this compound, in man, is considerably less potent than MMDA-2 or MMDA-3a.

Two dimethoxymethylenedioxyamphetamines have been synthesized and tested in humans. 2,5-Dimethoxy-3,4-methylenedioxyamphetamine (DMMDA) (Fig. 11) is equivalent to MMDA-3a with an additional methoxy

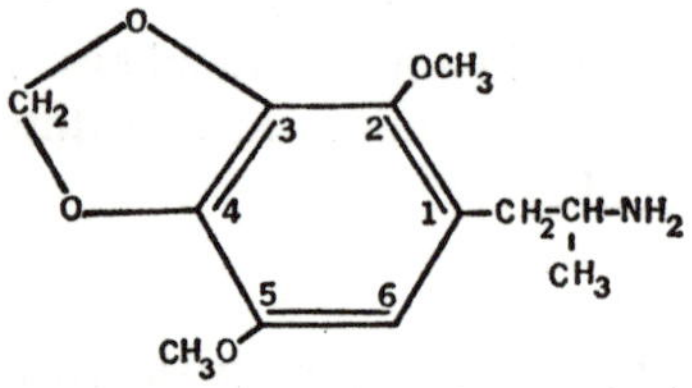

FIG. 11. 2,5-Dimethoxy-3,4-methylenedioxyamphetamine (DMMDA).

grouping at C-5. As with MMDA-3a, both rings B and C can be readily formed. DMMDA is an active psychedelic agent, with a potency of 12 M.U. 2,3-Dimethoxy-4,5-methylenedioxyamphetamine (DMMDA-2) (Fig. 12) differs from DMMDA only in the position of the methylenedioxy bridge. However, it is less than half as potent (5 M.U.) as DMMDA (Shulgin *et al.*, 1969). The decreased potency is readily explicable in terms of the relative

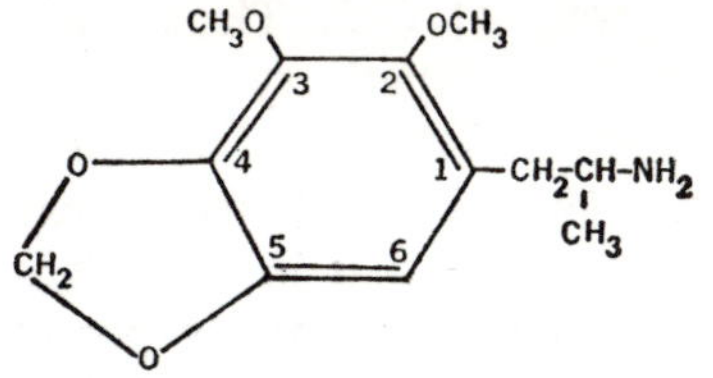

FIG. 12. 2,3-Dimethoxy-4,5-methylenedioxyamphetamine (DMMDA-2).

capacity of the methoxy at C-2 to form ring C with the side chain amine. In DMMDA-2, just as in TMA-3, there is a freely rotating methoxy group at C-3 that sterically would hinder interactions between the methoxy at C-2 and the side chain.

The three methoxymethylenedioxyamphetamines which our model predicts to be active are indeed potent in man (Table II), while the two which our model predicts to be relatively weak are considerably less potent.

TABLE II

Structure-activity of methoxymethylenedioxyamphetamines

Efficacy	Steric model	Man
Potent	2,4-5-MMDA (MMDA-2)	2,4-5-MMDA (12)
	2,3-4,5-DMMDA (DMMDA)	2,3-4,5-DMMDA (12)
	2,3-4-MMDA (MMDA-3a)	2,3-4-MMDA (10)
Weak	2,3,4-5-DMMDA (DMMDA-2)	2,3,4-5-DMMDA (5)
	2-3,4-MMDA (MMDA-3)	2-3,4-MMDA (3)

MMDA and DMMDA refer to methoxymethylenedioxyamphetamine and dimethoxymethylenedioxyamphetamine, respectively. Hyphens between numbers preceding compounds indicate methylenedioxy bridges. Lettered designations in parentheses refer to code names assigned by Shulgin (1964) and Shulgin *et al.* (1967). Numbers in parentheses are psychotropic potency in mescaline units, as reported by Shulgin *et al.* (1969).

DIMETHOXYAMPHETAMINES

When this model was first proposed (Snyder and Richelson, 1968), only one of the dimethoxyamphetamines had, to our knowledge, been evaluated in man for psychotropic potency. As with the other amphetamine analogs, our model would predict that the potent isomers would be those containing a methoxy grouping at C-2 whose interaction with the side chain would not be hindered by a methoxy group at C-3. Thus, we would predict that 2,5-dimethoxyamphetamine and 2,4-dimethoxyamphetamine should be relatively potent, while 3,5-dimethoxyamphetamine, 3,4-dimethoxyamphetamine and 2,3-dimethoxyamphetamine should be relatively weak (Table III). Recently, Shulgin et al. (1969) have shown that in man, 2,5-dimethoxyamphetamine and 2,4-dimethoxyamphetamine are relatively potent (8 M.U. and 5 M.U. respectively), while 3,4-dimethoxyamphetamine is inactive.

TABLE III

Structure-activity of dimethoxyamphetamines

Efficacy	Steric model	Man
Potent	2,5-DMA	2,5-DMA (8)
	2,4-DMA	2,4-DMA (5)
Weak	3,5-DMA	3,4-DMA (<1)
	3,4-DMA	
	2,3-DMA	

DMA refers to dimethoxyamphetamine. Numbers in parentheses are psychotropic potency in mescaline units reported by Shulgin et al. (1969).

There is at least one methoxyamphetamine whose activity is not explained by the above model. Thus, 4-methoxyamphetamine, which could not readily form ring C, is moderately active in man (Shulgin et al., 1969) and quite potent in rats (Smythies et al., 1968).

Recently, 2,5-dimethoxy-4-methylamphetamine (DOM) (Fig. 6 and 13) has been used widely by the "hippie" population and was designated by them as STP. This compound is analogous to TMA-2 (2,4,5-trimethoxy-

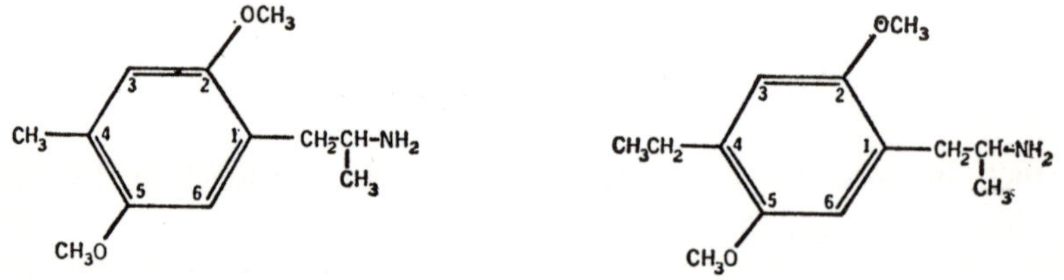

FIG. 13. 2,5-Dimethoxy-4-methylamphetamine (DOM) and 2,5-dimethoxy-4-ethylamphetamine (DOET).

amphetamine) in which the methoxy grouping at C-4 has been replaced by a methyl substituent. This compound was first synthesized by A. Shulgin (personal communication) with the rationale of preventing possible metabolic degradation by demethylation of the methoxy group at C-4 with subsequent excretion of the hydroxylated derivatives as water soluble conjugates. We have administered DOM to normal control volunteers and estimated its potency as about 50 to 100 M.U., approximately 5 times as active as TMA-2 (Snyder et al., 1967; Snyder et al., 1968). The possibility that the increased potency of this compound is related to a slower metabolic degradation than in the trimethoxyamphetamines is supported by its relatively prolonged action (F. Meyers, personal communication). Schweitzer and Friedhoff (1967) and Sargent et al. (1968) have shown that 3,4-dimethoxyphenylethylamine is degraded by demethylation at C-4. The methyl group at C-4 in DOM would prevent this metabolic route, and may account for its increased potency. DOET (2,5-dimethoxy-4-ethylamphetamine) appears to be slightly more potent in man than DOM (Snyder et al., 1968; Snyder et al., in preparation).

In a previous study, we performed molecular orbital calculations for a number of psychedelic compounds, and described a correlation between their potency and the energy of their highest occupied molecular orbital. This index is a relative measure of the ability of the π electrons in the highest molecular orbital of compounds to be transferred to acceptor molecules. This correlation was valid only for compounds which first fulfilled whatever steric considerations were required for psychedelic activity. If both molecular orbital energetics and the steric considerations described here are predicters of psychedelic activity, we would expect the molecular orbital calculations to be predictive only after the compound has satisfied the requirements of the steric model. For instance, 4-methoxy-psilocin possesses a more energetic highest occupied orbital than psilocin (Snyder and Merril, 1965), and, if steric considerations are insignificant, it should be a more potent psychedelic agent than psilocin. However, introduction of a methyl group at the number 4 position (assuming that the nitrogen of the amine side chain is not protonated), according to the steric model, would yield a psychedelic agent less active than psilocin. We are unaware of any studies in humans of 4-methoxypsilocin, but in behavioral tests in rats and monkeys, 4-methoxypsilocin is somewhat less potent than psilocin (Uyeno, personal communication).

Similarly, lysergic acid derivatives all possess optimal steric features for psychedelic activity according to the present model. Some of their variations in potency, such as the ineffectiveness of 2-bromo-LSD, lumi-LSD and dihydro-LSD, are predicted by the electronic model (Snyder and Merril, 1965; Snyder and Merril, 1967). The alterations in potency associated with stereo-isomerism of LSD or changes in its diethylamide chain are not predicted by either the steric or electronic models.

Acknowledgment: This research was supported in part by N.I.H. grant 1-RO1-NBO-7275 and by FDA Contract 68.8. Solomon H. Snyder is a recipient of N.I.M.H. Research Career Development Award K-3-MH-33128.

REFERENCES

Aghajanian, G. K., Foote, W. E. and Sheard, M. H.: Lysergic acid diethylamide: sensitive neuronal units in the midbrain raphé. *Science 161:* 706–708 (1968).
Cerletti, A. and Rothlin, E.: Role of 5-hydroxytryptamine in mental diseases and its antagonism to lysergic acid derivatives. *Nature 176:* 785–786 (1955).
Cerletti, A.: Discussion. In: *Neuropharmacology,* edited by P. B. Bradley, P. Deniker, and C. Raduco-Thomas, p. 117. Elsevier, Amsterdam (1959).
Gaddum, J. H.: Antagonism between lysergic acid diethylamide and 5-hydroxytryptamine. *J. Physiol. 121:* 15P (1953).
Rosenberg, D. E., Isbell, H. and Miner, E. J.: Comparison of a placebo, N-dimethyltryptamine, and 6-hydroxy-N-dimethyltryptamine in man. *Psychopharmacol. 4:* 39–42 (1963).
Sargent, T. W., Israelstam, D. M., Shulgin, A. T., Landow, S. A. and Finley, N. N.: A note concerning the fate of the 4-methoxy group in 3,4-dimethoxyphenethylamine (DMPEA). *Biochem. Biophys. Res. Comm. 29:* 126–130 (1967).
Schweitzer, J. W. and Friedhoff, A. J.: The metabolism of ^{14}C-3,4-dimethoxyphenylethylamine. *Biochem. Pharmacol. 15:* 2097–2103 (1966).
Shulgin, A. T.: Psychotomimetic amphetamines: methoxy 3,4-dialkoxy-amphetamines. *Experientia 20:* 1–4 (1964).
Shulgin, A. T. and Sargent, T.: Psychotropic phenylisopropylamines derived from Apiole and Dillapiole. *Nature 215:* 1494–1495 (1967).
Shulgin, A. T., Sargent, T. and Naranjo, C.: Structure-activity relationships of one-ring psychotomimetics. *Nature 221:* 537–540 (1969).
Slotta, K. H. and Muller, J.: Über den Abbau des Mescalins in mescalina inlicher Stoffe in Organismus. *Zeitschr. Physiol. Chem. 238:* 14–22 (1936).
Smythies, J. R., Johnston, V. S., Bradley, R. J., Benington, F., Morin, R. D. and Clark, L. C.: Some new behaviour-disrupting amphetamines and their significance. *Nature 216:* 128–129 (1967).
Snyder, S. H. and Merril, C. R.: A relationship between the hallucinogenic activity of drugs and their electronic configuration. *Proc. Natl. Acad. Sci. U.S.A. 54:* 258–266 (1965).
Snyder, S. H. and Reivich, M.: Regional localization of lysergic acid diethylamide in monkey brain. *Nature 209:* 1093–1095 (1966).
Snyder, S. H. and Merril, C. R.: A quantum-chemical correlate of hallucinogenesis. In: *Amine Metabolism in Schizophrenia,* edited by H. Himwich, S. S. Kety and J. R. Smythies, pp. 229–245. Pergamon Press, New York (1966).
Snyder, S. H., Faillace, L. and Hollister, L.: 2,5-Dimethoxy-4-methyl-amphetamine (STP): a new hallucinogenic drug. *Science 158:* 669–670 (1967).
Snyder, S. H., Faillace, L. A. and Weingartner, H.: DOM (STP), a new hallucinogenic drug, and DOET: effects of low doses in man. *Amer. J. Psychiat. 125:* 357–364 (1968).
Snyder, S. H. and Richelson, E.: Psychedelic drugs: steric factors that predict psychotropic activity. *Proc. Natl. Acad. Sci. 60:* 206–213 (1968).

Szara, S.: The comparison of the psychotic effect of tryptamine derivatives with the effects of mescaline and LSD-25 in self experiments. In: *Psychotropic Drugs,* edited by S. Garattini and V. Ghetti, p. 460. Elsevier, Amsterdam (1957).

Szara, S. and Hearst, E.: The 6-hydroxylation of tryptamine derivatives, a way of producing psychoactive metabolites. *Ann. N.Y. Acad. Sci. 96:* 134–141 (1962).

Turner, W. J. and Merles, S.: Effects of some indolealkylamines on man. *Arch. Neurol. Psychiat. 81:* 121–129 (1959).

Uyeno, E. T.: Hallucinogenic compounds and swimming response. *J. Pharmacol. Exp. Therap. 159:* 216–221 (1968).

Uyeno, E. T., Otis, L. S. and Mitoma, C.: Behavioral evaluation of hallucinogenic trimethoxyamphetamines in squirrel monkeys (*Saimiri Sciureus*). *Comm. Behav. Biol. A1:* 83–90 (1968).

Woolley, D. W. and Shaw, E.: A biochemical and pharmacological suggestion about certain mental disorders. *Proc. Natl. Acad. Sci. U.S.A. 40:* 228–231 (1954).

DISCUSSION

DR. BURGER: Thank you, Dr. Snyder. I want to start this brief discussion by expressing a little concern about your representation of the hydrogen-bonded indole nitrogen which made it a 5-membered ring in your case, but which actually turns out to be the analog of the tetrahydroisoquinoline.

DR. SNYDER: It would be six membered. You're right.

DR. BURGER: There is, of course a vast difference between tetrahydroisoquinolines and indoles. I wonder whether you want to comment on that.

DR. SNYDER: Right. Because you're adding another hydrogen in all of these rings. These rings are one atom larger than they appear to be just from the simple pictures drawn here, and these would not fit exactly.

You're referring to arranging it to look like an indole.

DR. BURGER: No. You put the hydrogen in the position of the carbinol, and Grollman at Albert Einstein has already shown that you can put hydrogen in the position of such a ring with oxygen in between it and stimulate, for instance, tetrahydroisoquinoline very beautifully. So, I'm in doubt as to whether your representation about that ring is correct.

DR. SNYDER: I'm not sure which ring you're talking about.

DR. MANDELL: I think Dr. Burger is referring to your B ring representation rather than to your C ring.

DR. BURGER: Yes, but, you see, the hypothesis was that three rings of LSD had been simulated, *i.e.,* the A, B, and C rings, and you see, by the time you throw the B ring completely out, you don't have any similarity.

DR. SNYDER: Right. You're quite correct that the simulated indole ring formed by the methoxyamphetamines is not a 5-membered ring. There's an extra atom in the ring.

DR. BURGER: There's another member there.

DR. SNYDER: Exactly. What I was presenting was a model which would explain certain structure-activity relationships. Actually, the indole moiety is not an important part of the model. It has no predictive value in this model but is put in because of the widely held hypothesis that phenylethylamines may simulate indoles sterically and at receptor sites.

DR. BURGER: That's all right, provided you don't refer to three rings being similar in those compounds, *i.e.,* if you just say that the A and the C ring are similar, but omit mention of the B ring altogether.

DR. SNYDER: In spite of certain dissimilarities, it still is conceivable that phenylethylamines could simulate indoles at receptor sites in the brain. We don't know what goes on at the mysterious and mystical receptor site.

DR. MANDELL: Dr. Snyder's emphasis on the C ring gets up out of the many structure-function hypotheses involving an artificially constructed indole nucleus from physico-chemical interactions of various phenylethylamines. An indole is essentially a large aromatic system with π clouds above and below a sigma bonded planar structure; a sandwich in which electron clouds are the pieces of bread. The characteristic maneuver for planar chemists is to bend a substituted phenylethylamine around using hydrogen bonds to make what in two dimensions looks like an indole nucleus. In three dimensions, however, the side chain would bend up out of the plane of the benzene nucleus and would not look like an indole at all.

By eliminating the indole model we're all thinking about and focusing on the C ring as Dr. Snyder did, with an oxygen atom sticking out unhindered, he has made a far more rational story about steric models of hallucinogens, using LSD as a model, than what we have always talked about in terms of A and B relationships, resulting in our taking phenylethylamines and bending them around. I think he's made a very important contribution in that sense.

DR. SNYDER: You were saying that if you were going to form that indole-like structure, the nitrogen atom would be out of the plane of the ring?

DR. MANDELL: Yes, and it's not going to be an indole at all; it's not going to be a sandwich. It's going to be a sandwich, with some portion swinging around. In eliminating the B ring from consideration, it returns us to Shulgin's structure-function model.

DR. BURGER: You're quite right. It's nice to compare the A and C rings; then I think we should not say anything about the B ring.

DR. MANDELL: I don't think he said anything about the B ring. He tried to ignore it, except in the case of psilocybin which brought nitrogen and oxygen too close together. The amount of energy would be prohibitive to overcome the van der Waals forces.

DR. BURGER: Let's set it straight again that the A and C ring are being compared; nothing's being said about the B ring.

DR. DOMINO: I'd like to return to a discussion of phencyclidine. Dr. Snyder, are you familiar with it? It's basically a phenylmethylamine derivative. Consider the A and C rings. If you replace that oxygen with a carbon, you end up with the phenylmethylamine series which is the phencyclidine series of psychotomimetics.

DR. SHULGIN: What is the compound you're talking about?

DR. DOMINO: Sernyl. It's a phenylmethylamine derivative. I'm going to twist phencyclidine into the A-C ring model of Dr. Snyder as follows:

2-Methoxyamphetamine   Phencyclidine

DR. BIEL: There is only one methylene group between the phenyl and the nitrogen.

DR. SHULGIN: There's just a single carbon atom.

DR. BIEL: Your piperidine ring is directly bonded to the cyclohexane ring.

DR. DOMINO: What I'm saying is that phencyclidine is a phenylmethylamine derivative.

DR. KORNETSKY: I'd like now to get a little bit off chemistry for a moment. Dr. Snyder made a statement concerning cross-tolerance between most of these psychotomimetic drugs. I was wondering if you were referring mainly to the amphetamine-like drugs or to all psychotomimetics? I do not believe this has been well documented. In fact, in many of these drugs, tolerance is somewhat weird. I wonder if you could comment on this?

DR. SNYDER: I was referring to Harris Isbell's studies in which I believe he showed the cross-tolerance of LSD, mescaline, and psilocybin.

DR. KORNETSKY: Cross-tolerance to the amphetamines?

DR. SNYDER: No, although Dr. Leo Hollister showed cross-tolerance between mescaline and DOM (STP). It is extremely interesting that there is cross-tolerance between LSD and mescaline but no cross-tolerance to d-amphetamine. Yet there is cross-tolerance to the methoxylated amphetamines.

DR. SZARA: On the other hand, it was shown by Isbell that there's no cross-tolerance between dimethyltryptamine and LSD.

DR. SNYDER: That finding may be explained by the relatively shorter action of dimethyltryptamine.

DR. GESSNER: I'd like to make two points. The first one is in respect to cross-tolerance. Perhaps one can put too much emphasis on this. For one second, let's switch away from the agents under discussion and think of hypnotics. These show very nice development of cross-tolerance plus physical dependence, and, indeed, it might be a very fetching hypothesis to say that they all exert their hypnotic effects by a common mechanism because they have cross-tolerance to each other.

On the other hand, one recent theory is that all they do is to cause a temporary chemical interruption of nervous transmission, a temporary chemical denervation. We know that denervated tissue becomes more sensitive. We know that there's an increase in receptor sensitivity in denervated tissue. Possibly all we're seeing is that, in the presence of the hypnotic, the target tissue becomes more sensitive to the action of whatever is the transmitter, and as the hypnotic is withdrawn this extra sensitivity is what gives rise to a withdrawal effect.

When we see cross-tolerance among psychotomimetic drugs, we might justifiably say that they act on the same system, but not necessarily that they have to act on the same receptor.

My other comment was with respect to psilocin. This is a compound which puzzled me for a long time. I couldn't quite understand why it was active. I found that the lipid solubility of this compound is some 20 or 30 times greater than bufotenine, and all we're doing here is changing the hydroxy group position from 5 to 4! Perhaps some such explanation as you gave might explain this increased lipid solubility of the compound, which otherwise doesn't make too much sense.

One extra word of warning regarding psilocin: the compound decomposes very rapidly. Solutions of it go blue in a matter of a relatively short time, and in those instances where we explored this, these solutions are just as active.

O'Brien at Cornell, working with psilocybin, has also shown this development, *i.e.,* some sort of blue pigments. And he has shown that this occurs much more readily in the presence of tissue. So, perhaps there is formation of some sort of condensation which is still active.

DR. SNYDER: When you say "active," you mean in rats?

DR. GESSNER: Yes.

DR. SNYDER: I wonder if you would comment about the lipid solubility.

DR. DALY: I think that a good explanation for the lipid solubility is that there is hydrogen bonding between the phenolic group and the amine group. I wonder whether you have tested any 2-hydroxyamphetamines with methoxy groups in other positions? According to your model they should be very active psychotomimetics. If they didn't cross the blood-brain barrier, you could use the technique Dr. Gessner used with bufotenine, that is, making the O-acetyl derivative. In the case of norepinephrine, we found that the O-triacetyl derivative passes into the brain, and then the ubiquitous esterases hydrolyze it to norepinephrine.

If I could make one more comment: We always look at similarities when formulating a theory, but it seems very striking that in the tryptamines you require the tertiary amine for psychotomimetic activity, whereas in the amphetamines, to my knowledge, the primary amine is always required. I wonder if either Dr. Snyder or Dr. Shulgin would like to comment on that?

DR. SHULGIN: One specific comment: In the phenylethylamine family, the N, N-dimethyl homolog of mescaline is not active in man.

DR. DALY: Yes, I know. Have any others been studied?

DR. SHULGIN: No.

DR. SNYDER: With N-dimethylated amphetamines there are no hydrogens on the amine nitrogen to interact with the oxygen of the 2-methoxy, although the amine could be proteinated and still interact.

DR. DALY: Then it would seem that the monomethyl derivative should be studied to see if it is active; but it seems that the primary amine is necessary for activity in the amphetamine series.

DR. SNYDER: One other thing. The decreased psychotropic activity of alphaethyl derivatives may be explained by the steric hindrance for interaction of the amine and the 2-methoxy group.

DR. DALY: What of the alpha, alpha-dimethyl compounds?

DR. SHULGIN: None of these have yet been synthesized, as I said earlier. I might mention one thing concerning the tryptamines. N-Monomethyltryptamine is distinctly less active than N, N-dimethyltryptamine.

DR. DALY: The same is true in the 5-methoxy series.

DR. SHULGIN: The monomethyl derivative is less active than the dimethyl counterpart?

DR. DALY: Yes. Much, much less.

DR. BURGER: Then you have a similar situation with Hofman's alkaloids in that the N-methyl compound was considerably less active than N, N-dimethylene derivative.

DR. MANDELL: You mean at the 6-position?

DR. BURGER: This was in the amides of the LSD series.

DR. BURGER: It is Dr. Domino's idea that phencyclidine is a phenylethylamine derivative with a quaternized arm on the carbon, and perhaps Dr. Domino wants to comment on that?

DR. DOMINO: We previously heard that in the case of amphetamine or mescaline compounds the A and C rings were critical. In the course of this discussion it occurred to me that if we replaced the oxygen atom with a carbon we'll end up with phencyclidine derivatives. I tried to make that point previously. Those of you who are chemists can explore this further. As I've drawn the structure of phencyclidine, we have an A ring, and part of a C ring. The only point I wanted to make is that basically the distance between the phenyl ring and the nitrogen in the case of the mescaline series is somewhat larger because of hydrogen bonding than in the case of the phencyclidines where the distance between the phenyl ring and the nitrogen is one carbon. So it doesn't quite fit, but at least it's something to think about.

DR. BURGER: You should take into account, probably, the fact that the phenethylamine-type distance has been distorted due to the distortion of this carbon.

DR. DOMINO: Would that increase the distance or reduce it?

DR. BURGER: It would reduce it.

DR. DOMINO: So, it wouldn't fit the theory as well.

DR. SULSER: May I come back to Dr. Biel's reply to Dr. Lehrer's question? I couldn't quite understand why you said that alpha-methylated amino acids would have difficulty in getting decarboxylated in brain. If I intend to increase the brain level of, *e.g.,* metaraminol, which does not easily cross the blood-brain barrier, I administer alpha-methyl-*meta*-tyrosine. This alpha-methylated amino acid enters the brain very easily and is decarboxylated to alpha-methyl-tyramine, then beta-hydroxylated to form metaraminol, which can displace norepinephrine stoichiometrically.

DR. BIEL: Many of the phenyl-substituted amino acids do not get decarboxylated. It's not the question of the alpha-methyl group on the side chain, but the substitution on the phenyl ring. For instance, alpha-methyl-tyrosine itself is not easily decarboxylated, in contrast to the alpha-methyl-*meta*-tyrosine.

DR. SULSER: It is decarboxylated.

DR. BIEL: Eventually, but not as readily as alpha-methyl-*meta*-tyrosine. So, there already you have one difference.

DR. LEHRER: Are those both the *l* forms? Because certainly the *d*-amino acids can't be decarboxylated.

DR. BIEL: It all depends on what you have on the phenyl ring.

DR. EFRON: When you say *twice as potent,* or *40 times as potent*—what test are you relating it to?

DR. SNYDER: For most of the methoxylated amphetamines I'm referring to data in man of Dr. Shulgin and of Dr. Claudio Naranjo. A large number of the methoxylated amphetamines have been assayed in behavioral tests in squirrel monkeys. These are tests of visual discrimination of circles of different sizes using the Wisconsin General Test apparatus.

But for the human potency data and its reliability, Dr. Shulgin can answer better than I.

DR. SHULGIN: As I mentioned earlier, the potency value given is the mean between a threshold level that is subjectively assignable and an extreme level, objectively determined, a level beyond which there apparently is no further disruption of sensory integrity. The mean of those two values represents the effective level. An individual may vary by 25 percent one way or the other on different days. This is why it takes a score of subjects to get a number that has any reliability at all.

DR. EFRON: Subjective sensory discrimination in man?

DR. SHULGIN: In man, yes.

DR. FREEDMAN: Can I make an obvious methodological point about scaling these things in animals? It really depends on what measures you are going to take, because a drug like LSD will show no effect on certain tests. At a dosage closer to a hundred times less than that dosage it may show an effect, let's say, on tests involving negative reinforcement. So, what the scaler has to do is to rely on the human potency to find out whether or not his scales and his tests and his dose ranges are the reliable predictors or correlates of the effects in man. And I don't know—has Uyeno published the squirrel monkey data, for example?

DR. SNYDER: Yes. (Uyeno, E. T. (1968): Hallucinogenic compounds and swimming response. *J. Pharm. Exp. Therap. 159:* 216, 1968; Uyeno, E. T., Otis, L. S. and Mitoma, L. Behavioral evaluation of hallucinogenic trimethoxyamphetamines in squirrel monkeys. *Comm. Behav. Biol. A1:* 83 (1968)).

DR. LEHRER: I wonder about the visual discrimination of circles of different sizes being used as a criterion. Recently at our institution, Schilder and the Pasils have shown that if you train monkeys to discriminate between a circle and a triangle, and then present them under certain conditions with very small triangles arranged in a circle, or very small circles arranged in a triangle, then if the monkey is trained to go to a circle, he will go to the triangle made up of circles, and if he is trained to the triangle, he'll go to the circle made up of little triangles. Therefore, under certain conditions, there may be a distortion or focus of attention on less obvious parts of the environment; particularly where these drug effects in man are concerned, certain of these phenomena might well appear. I wonder whether we have to consider this type of phenomenon in evaluating the drug's effect?

DR. SHULGIN: One thing may be added here. If you are consistent in the use of the same monkey, at least you know that his ability to achieve this is not a dose-dependent response, and you have eliminated one variable. And to this end, very much of our work has been with a limited group of subjects who are quite experienced. We very definitely prefer to employ experienced subjects. So, at least the monkey is, so to say, kept constant.

DR. BIEL: Getting back to the subject of phenylethylamines, by all rights of structure-activity relationships the 4-methoxy-dimethyltryptamine should really be the most potent member of this series, and I'm wondering whether anyone in this group has made it or knows anything about its potency? Perhaps Dr. Holmstedt could comment?

DR. HOLMSTEDT: It was made after we discovered the 5-methoxy-dimethyltryptamine in plant material used for hallucinogenic purposes. The Sandoz people synthesized this compound, and there has even been some data about it published in review articles, mostly on their effects on spinal reflexes. There's been no study in man or behavioral studies in monkeys, to my knowledge.

DR. GESSNER: Sandoz published the synthesis of it some years back but never gave any pharmacological data. We were curious, and so we synthesized it and tested it. In conditioned avoidance responses in rats, it's relatively active. There are, however, some 5-methoxy derivatives which are more active than this. I will come back to this in my own presentation later in this meeting.

DR. KORNETSKY: I would like to make a comment. This morning there was a somewhat cavalier attitude displayed toward the activity end of the structure-activity problem. I think some of the discussion we have just been having demonstrates the need for a little more attention to it. It is very important that the work on the activity side be as thoughtful and careful as the thoughtful and careful chemical work on structure side. Behavior is not a unitary function, and one has to define it as carefully as one defines those scribblings I see on the blackboard.

DR. BURGER: Our next lecturer is Dr. Abood of the University of Rochester, who will speak to us on stereochemistry and membrane mechanisms of some hallucinogens in the series of glycolate esters in which he has done pioneer work together with Dr. Biel.

STEREOCHEMICAL AND MEMBRANE STUDIES WITH THE PSYCHOTOMIMETIC GLYCOLATE ESTERS

Leo G. Abood, Ph.D.

Center for Brain Research and Department of Biochemistry,
University of Rochester, Rochester, New York 14627

INTRODUCTION

For many years, Abood and Biel (Abood *et al.*, 1959; Abood and Biel, 1962), and later on many others (Adamski and Cannon, 1965; Freiter *et al.*, 1968; Buehler *et al.*, 1965), became involved in the synthesis and the pharmacological properties of the glycolic acid esters. In an effort to understand the relationship between psychotomimetic properties and chemical structures, many hundreds of derivatives have been made. The compounds are generally esters of a heterocyclic imino alcohol and a glycolic acid, and possess strong anticholinergic properties.

A representative compound is N-methyl-4-piperidyl benzilate, which has the structure displayed in Fig. 1. Both the acidic and basic moiety have been extensively investigated from the standpoint of certain quantifiable behavioral and pharmacological tests in animals, tests which have been shown to correlate well with psychotomimetic potency in human subjects (Abood and Biel, 1962). The various tests are summated into what is termed a "behavioral disturbance index" (BDI) (Gabel and Abood, 1965; Abood, 1968). One of the tests is a measure of the hyperactivity peculiar to the centrally active anticholinergics. Another is a measure of the ability of the drugs to disrupt the performance of mice in a swim maze. The third one is the so-called "peep" test, which takes advantage of the peculiar head-bobbing, head-swaying activity that the drugs produce in rats and which is apparently related to exploratory activity characteristic of rodent behavior.

These data have been quantitated, and they correlate extremely well with the efficacy of these compounds to produce in human subjects confusion,

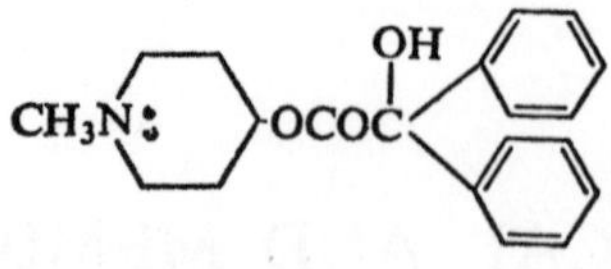

FIG. 1. N-methyl-4-piperidyl benzilate.

delirium, hallucinations and many of the other parameters that are associated with psychosis-like behavior (Abood and Biel, 1962). The greater the BDI, the more potent the compound.

STEREOCHEMICAL RELATIONSHIPS TO DRUG POTENCY

The discussion here does not focus on the acidic part but on the basic portion of the molecule. It is concerned with certain stereochemical aspects of the heterocyclic imino group insofar as they influence the ability of the nitrogen group to interact with an electrophilic center on a presumptive receptor (synaptic) site.

The hypothesis has been advanced that psychotomimetic potency is related to the availability of the non-bonded electron pair on the heterocyclic nitrogen (Gabel and Abood, 1965; Abood, 1968). If anything prevents the non-bonded electron pair from attaching to this electrophilic center, either because of unfavorable conformational forms of the ring structure or because of substituents in the ring, the compound is less effective biologically. Among the most potent compounds are the quinuclidine esters, where the configuration of the N-ring is fixed and the non-bonded electron pair most readily available (Fig. 2).

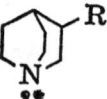

FIG. 2. Quinuclidine esters.

The two most stable conformers of 1-methylpiperidine are the two "chair" forms in which the methyl group can be either equatorial (Fig. 3) or axial (Fig. 4). Although the non-bonded electron pair on nitrogen usually has a steric requirement similar to a hydrogen atom, its steric requirement

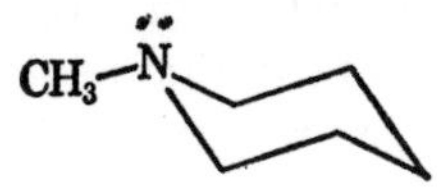

FIG. 3. 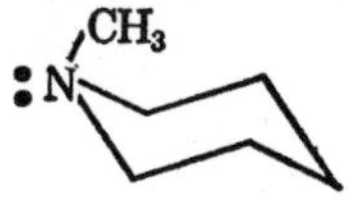   FIG. 4.

appears to be much larger in hydroxylic solvents by virtue of hydrogen bonding (E. L. Eliel, personal communication).

Interaction of the structure in Fig. 3 with an electrophilic center would be subjected to unfavorable 1,3-diaxial interference from the two axial hydrogen atoms located on C-3 and C-5 of the piperidine ring. Similar interaction of the structure in Fig. 4 would be free of such steric inhibition. This steric interference with the availability of the amino electron pair of the structure in Fig. 3 would decrease its nucleophilicity compared to quinuclidine. However, inasmuch as the inversion of substituents on nitrogen is extremely rapid, and since the structure in Fig. 4 is undoubtedly a much better nucleophile than that in Fig. 3, interaction with an electrophilic center may proceed almost completely by way of the Fig. 4 structure.

This mixture of structures 3 and 4 which constitutes 1-methylpiperidine may, therefore, be expected under similar environmental conditions to exhibit almost the same nucleophilic character as quinuclidine. In conformity with this assumption is the finding that the BDI of the glycolate esters of 1-methyl-4-hydroxypiperidine (Fig. 1) is almost identical with the BDI for the quinuclidyl esters.

The observation that the esters of 1-methyl-3-piperidinol are generally less active than those of 1-methyl-4-piperidinol can be explained by considering the greater ease with which the 3-isomer can undergo intramolecular, electronic interactions of the type depicted by Fig. 5. Interaction of the carbonyl group of this ester with the non-bonded electron pair on nitrogen would not necessitate a "boat" form conformation (Fig. 6), as it would in the 4-isomer. Such intramolecular electronic interactions could markedly

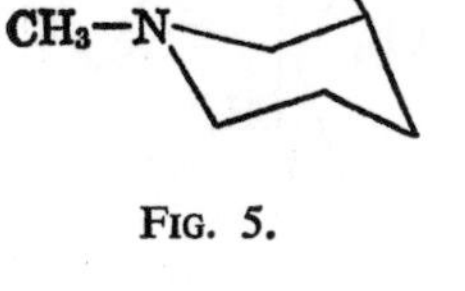

FIG. 5. 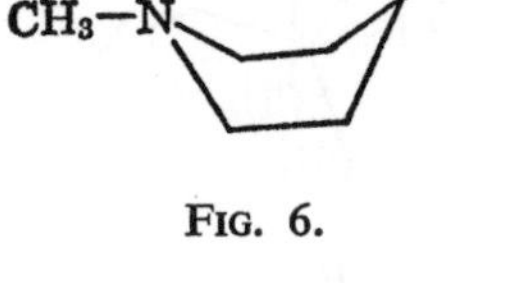   FIG. 6.

decrease the possibility for intermolecular interaction of the electron pair on nitrogen with an electrophilic center. An illustration of this effect is the facile migration of the benzoyl group from oxygen to nitrogen in the benzoyl derivative of norpseudotropine. The occurrence of intramolecular interaction would tend to diminish the probability of combination of the nitrogen with an electrophilic receptor (Fodor and Nador, 1953).

A similar type of conformational analysis was carried out with a variety of ring structures including tropanol and granatanol, as well as with ring substituents in the piperidinol series. The effect of substituents in the piperidinol on the availability of the non-bonded electron pair on nitrogen is illustrated by the examples in Figs. 7 and 8.

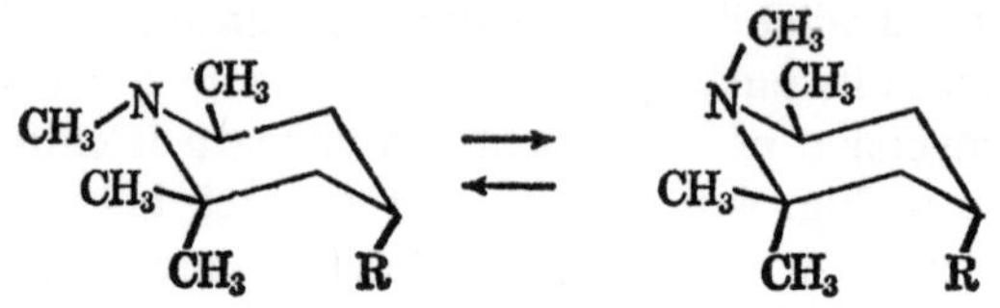

FIG. 7.   FIG. 8.

Methyl substituents in the 1 and 2 ring positions diminish potency. The N-methyl group should be equatorial in the conformers (Figs. 7 and 8); and it is apparent (from a construction of Dreiding models) that there are associated with the N-electron pair of conformer (Fig. 5) four 1,3-diaxial non-bonded interactions due to the hydrogens on C-3 and C-5 and the methyl substituents in the 2- and 6-positions. Since there are only three such interactions attributable to methyl groups in the structure shown in Fig. 8, interaction with an electrophilic center may occur primarily in this somewhat less hindered configuration.

With an additional methyl substituent, as in 1,2,2,6,6-pentamethyl 4-piperidinol (Figs. 9 and 10), the esters of which are virtually devoid of

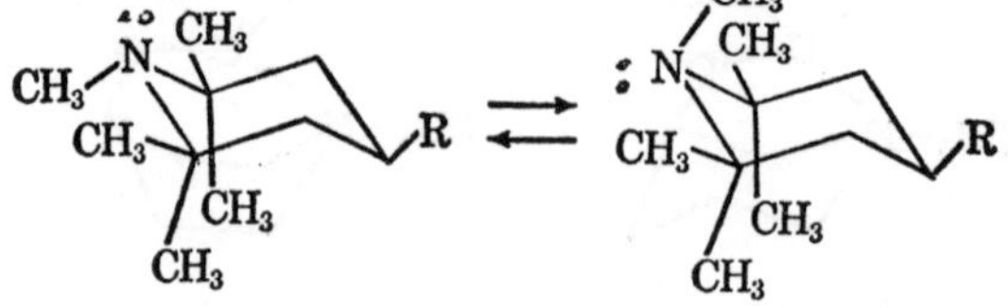

FIG. 9.   FIG. 10.

psychotomimetic activity, the imino nitrogen is severely hindered. An electrophilic center would be subjected to four 1,3-diaxial non-bonded interactions. As corroboration for the inaccessibility of the imino group, the 1,2,2,6-tetramethylpiperidine is alkylated in an extremely low yield even after prolonged heating (Hall, 1957).

Recently, Nogrady and Algieri (1968) subjected this hypothesis to a more crucial test by determining the correlation of BDI with specific chemical interactions dependent upon the availability of the non-bonded electron pair on the ring nitrogen. Working with a series of benzoyl esters of the various heterocyclic imino alcohols utilized in the studies of Gabel and Abood (1965), they showed that the rate of quaternization (with methyl iodide) and formation of a charge-transfer stability complex (with chloranil) correlated well with BDI. The separate comparison of charge-transfer stability and quaternization rate constants with BDI also permitted one to determine if binding forces were involved other than those due to non-bonding electrons (*e.g.*, π complexes of the phenyl groups in the acidic moiety). Their studies clearly established the validity of the hypothesis that the availability of the non-bonded electron pair on the ring nitrogen is correlated with the psychotomimetic potency of the glycolate esters.

DRUG INTERACTION WITH MEMBRANES

The other part of this discussion is concerned with the possible mechanism of action of the esters at the level of the excitatory (synaptic) membrane. With the use of tritiated glycolates it can be shown that the administered drug is localized in the nerve endings, axonal-dendritic processes and other membranous components of rat brain (Abood and Biel, 1962). The drug appears to be primarily associated with the lipid components of the membranes, where it is held by both electrostatic and hydrophobic bonding. From electrophysiological studies it can be shown that the glycolates substitute and interfere with the regulatory action of calcium on the excitatory membrane. For example, the decrease in the intracellular resting potential of frog sartorius muscle fibers following Ca^{2+} removal can be restored by the addition of a glycolate ester at 1/10 the concentration of Ca^{2+} needed for restoration.

It was inferred that the drug was replacing the Ca^{2+} which was bound mainly to the phosphate groups of the membranous phospholipid. To test this hypothesis, studies were carried out with surface films of brain and purified lipids, measuring such parameters as surface potential, pressure, viscosity and adsorption (Rogeness *et al.,* 1966; Abood and Rushmer, 1968). The results clearly demonstrated that the drug was capable of substituting for Ca^{2+} and exerted similar as well as dissimilar physical effects upon the lipid monolayers.

A molecular model of the surface interaction of the drug and the lipid is presented in Fig. 11. The phospholipid is represented by the bent lines extending into the air or lipophilic region, with the phosphoryl-amino portion projecting into the aqueous or hydrophilic region. A molecule of cholesterol is interspersed between two adjacent phospholipids to simulate more correctly the biological membranes. The drug (N-methyl-4-piperidyl-benzilate) is inserted between the cholesterol and a phospholipid molecule, with the lipophilic aromatic groups in the lipid region and the piperidyl nitrogen projecting into

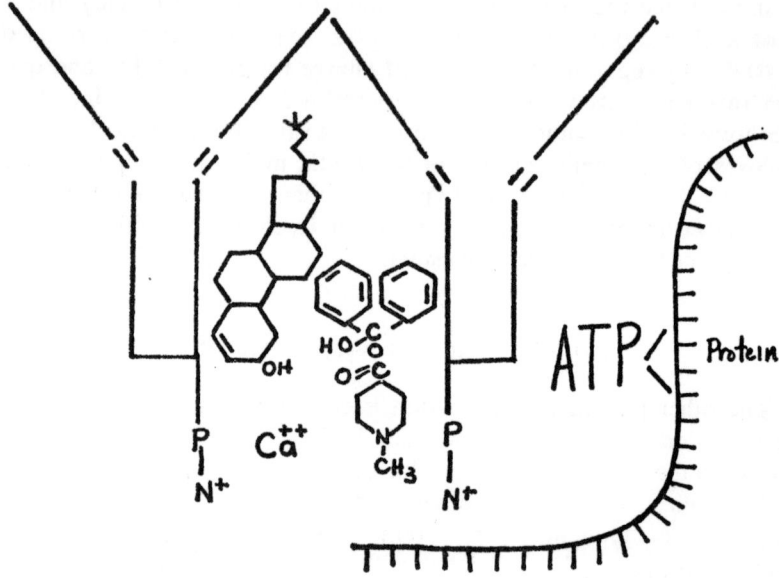

FIG. 11. A membrane model depicting the interaction of a glycolate ester (see text for description).

the aqueous phase. Normally, Ca^{2+} would be associated with the phosphate groups, so that the phospholipid molecules are closer together (*i.e.*, the surface film is condensed in contrast to the expanded state prevailing with the drug). With closer proximity of the phospholipid molecules, the Ca^{2+} can combine with two adjacent phospholipid molecules to form an even more condensed film which is more impermeable, viscous, and lipophilic. The presence of the drug in the surface layer, although contributing to a more expanded film, imparts properties to the film resembling those contributed by

Ca^{2+}. A structural protein which binds ATP is also capable of interacting with the surface complex. It is represented by a hydrophobic portion projecting into the lipophilic region and a hydrophilic one extending into the aqueous phase. The ATP interacts with a cationic site on the protein, and through weaker van der Waals and other bonds (Abood and Matsubara, 1968).

Another type of interaction involving the drugs and ATP is also of significance from the standpoint of membrane excitability. ATP, a strong chelating agent which is concentrated in synaptic and other membranous components, is presumed to regulate the Ca^{2+} association-dissociation processes occurring in the membrane during excitation. It has been possible to show that ATP can form a surface complex with a phospholipid, either in the presence of Ca^{2+} or of the drug. An interaction of ATP and drug near the membrane surface could conceivably influence the Ca^{2+}-ATP interaction critical for the regulation of bioelectric events.

Admittedly, the applicability of such data from studies with lipid films to an excitable membrane is somewhat tenuous, but it does afford a reasonable working hypothesis. It has recently been possible to construct membranes from Ca^{2+} and lipids which resemble normal biological membranes in their ultrastructural characteristics (Abood and Rushmer, 1968). Without the presence of Ca^{2+}, the lipid membranes assume an amorphous hexagonal configuration, in contrast to the lamellar structure characteristic of normal biological membranes. When the drugs are used in place of Ca^{2+}, similar lamellar structures are obtainable.

More recent findings, however, suggest that a high molecular weight structural protein is the site of ATP binding in the synaptic membrane (Abood and Matsubara, 1968). This protein, which has a strong lipophilic character, can interact with Ca^{2+}-phospholipid complexes in the membrane. It undoubtedly plays an important role in the structural and functional properties of the excitatory membrane. To date, it has been shown that the glycolates can interact with this protein and modify the ability of the protein to interact with ATP. This interaction is now being investigated. Obviously, the membrane is a far more complex system than initially imagined; however, methods for investigating its chemical and physical properties are now available.

REFERENCES

Abood, L. G.: The psychotomimetic glycolate esters. In: *Medicinal Research Series, Vol. 2: Drugs Affecting the Central Nervous System,* edited by A. Burger, pp. 127–167. Marcel Dekker, New York (1968).

Abood, L. G. and Biel, J. H.: Anticholinergic psychotomimetic agents. *Intern. Rev. Neurobiol.* 4: 217–273 (1962).

Abood, L. G. and Matsubara, A.: Properties of an ATP-binding protein isolated from membranes of nerve endings. *Biochim. Biophys. Acta 163:* 539–549 (1968).

Abood, L. G. and Rushmer, D.: Surface interaction of calcium and ATP with phospholipids and other surfactants. In: *Molecular Association in Biological and Related Systems,* edited by E. Goddard, pp. 169–188. American Chemical Society, Washington (1968).

Abood, L. G., Ostfeld, A. M., and Biel, J. H.: Structure activity relationships of 3-piperidyl benzilates with psychotogenic properties. *Arch. Intern. Pharmacodyn. 120:* 186–200 (1959).

Adamski, R. J. and Cannon, J. G.: Synthesis of compounds with potential psychotomimetic activity. III. *J. Med. Chem. 8:* 444–446 (1965).

Buehler, C. A., Thames, S. T., Abood, L. G., and Biel, J. H.: Physiologically active compounds. VI. Cyclic amino thiolesters of substituted chloroacetic, benzilic and glycolic acids. *J. Med. Chem. 8:* 643–647 (1965).

Fodor, G. and Nador, K.: The stereochemistry of tropane alkaloids. I. The configuration of tropine and ψ-tropine. *J. Chem. Soc.* 721–727 (1953).

Freiter, E. R., Cannon, J. G., Milne, L. D., and Abood, L. G.: Synthesis of compounds with potential psychotomimetic activity. IV. *J. Med. Chem. 11:* 1041–1045 (1968).

Gabel, N. and Abood, L. G.: Stereochemical factors related to the potency of anticholinergic psychotomimetic drugs. *J. Med. Chem. 8:* 616–619 (1965).

Hall, H. K., Jr.: Steric effects on the base strengths of cyclic amines. *J. Amer. Chem. Soc. 79:* 5444–5447 (1957).

Nogrady, T. and Algieri, A. A.: Charge transfer complexes in medicinal chemistry. I. Correlations with the psychotropic activity of piperidinol esters and related compounds. *J. Med. Chem. 11:* 212–213 (1968).

Rogeness, G. C., Krugman, L. G., and Abood, L. G.: The interaction of the psychotomimetic glycolate esters with calcium, APT, and lecithin monolayers. *Biochem. Biophys. Acta 125:* 319–327 (1966).

DISCUSSION

DR. LATIES: Dr. Abood, are the curves that you get with the various components of the BDI similar to the average curve you have shown? It strikes me as a poor policy to use this conglomeration of three very different types of behavior. This implies that "behavior" is some sort of unitary concept, with the peep test, the ability to swim and general activity all measures of something called "behavior."

DR. ABOOD: Actually, hyperactivity as measured by us (Abood and Biel, 1962) takes into account the head movements peculiar to the drug, and so does the "peep" test. The latter, however, also measures a behavioral deficit. The swim maze measures the ability of the mouse to perform in a learning situation and tests the animal's ability to remember. Confusion and disorientation are among the striking effects of the drugs in humans. The fact remains that all three tests alone or in combination correlate with the drug's psychotomimetic action in humans.

DR. LATIES: Why not break them out and present three curves?

DR. ABOOD: You get much the same results. Where one score is high, usually the other two are also high, and likewise for the low scores. There are some differences with certain classes of the glycolates, for example, in the case of the piperizinio glycolates (Abood and Biel, 1962).

DR. LATIES: Well, it may be wise to pay attention to the differences. It would be very interesting, for instance, if some compound produced no change in activity but produced a great change in the ability of an animal to swim through a maze.

DR. KORNETSKY: Dr. Abood, how do you know that the animal doesn't have bellyache causing all this?

DR. ABOOD: To what test are you referring?

DR. Kornetsky: You say they are highly correlated in terms of the effects. Maybe if you gave the animal a good bellyache you would also find high correlation between structure, a bellyache and the behavior under study.

PROFESSOR ABOOD: Only low doses of these compounds are required, to a tenth of a milligram per kilogram level or less on some of these tests.

DR. FREEDMAN: Leo, you could try a Pepto-Bismol!

DR. BIEL: I'd like to probe a little more into this concept of membrane stabilization.

Would you say that these esters would stabilize the membranes to a greater extent than calcium, and that one could relate this fact possibly to an inhibition of neurotransmitter release?

DR. ABOOD: Yes, it's possible. Undoubtedly their ability to stabilize the excitatory membrane may be one of the factors involved in their action. In the membrane of sartorious muscle they are a few hundred times more potent as membrane stabilizers than is calcium. Also, calcium is believed to be involved along with ATP in the binding of amines within the synapse, and possibly in their transport. The drugs could interfere with the storage, release, and transmitter action of the biogenic amines. Amines and even acetylcholine might be involved.

DR. BIEL: The latest theory is that calcium has to be traveling into the synaptic zone to expel a packet of norepinephrine, so to speak. So if you stabilize the membrane too much, you might prevent the release of dopamine or norepinephrine.

DR. LEHRER: You brought in the question of the sodium-potassium activated ATPase. This enzyme is thought to be more concerned with the sodium pump than with synaptic function.

DR. ABOOD: That was an old slide. I put that in because we could show there is both a hydrophilic and a lipophilic center on the enzyme, the lipophilic center being the potassium-activated one, and the hydrophilic center the sodium activated one. I would rather substitute the ATP-structural protein into this scheme; but the arrangement of the structural protein with respect to phospholipids and cholesterol may be much the same as in the case of the ATPase. Incidentally, the ATP-binding protein is not an ATPase.

DR. WASER: We have been interested in synaptosomes for some years now. We isolate them in a manner similar to yours, probably, and we work with shocked and nonshocked synaptosomes.

We thought it would be worthwhile to investigate the action of different psychotomimetics, neuroleptics or thymoleptics on the enzyme system of the membrane: on the ATPase, cholinesterase, and so forth. And we found some very interesting actions. For instance, LSD has a very strong action on ATPase, but hyoscyamine has not. I don't know why.

DR. ABOOD: LSD inhibits ATPase?

DR. WASER: Yes. One thing I dislike about it is that the concentration of LSD must be rather high. It doesn't look very nice and specific because you would suspect the concentration of drug in the brain *in vivo* to be very low, although I do not know what the concentration at the membrane in the animal really is. Also, chlorpromazine inhibits the action of ATPase, but one does not find any inhibition with barbiturates.

DR. ABOOD: Blei (*Arch. Biochem. Biophys., 109:* 321, 1965) has shown that chlorpromazine interacts with ATP under certain conditions. A number of psychoactive drugs can interact with ATP, and my guess is that they particularly interact with membranous ATP. It's quite conceivable that LSD does too.

DR. HOLMSTEDT: Could you explain to me how you shock the synaptosomes?

DR. WASER: We shock them with distilled water. You can also use a detergent.

DR. ABOOD: They swell in hypertonic solutions and rupture.

DR. WASER: Can you close them again?

DR. ABOOD: Yes, you can.

DR. WASER: And they regain their elasticity and organized activity?

DR. ABOOD: Yes. We have not looked too carefully though.

DR. WASER: This is the sign of an intact membrane.

DR. ABOOD: The filamentous membranes tend to become joined at the ends as if by fusion. One can actually prepare membranes from dispersions of the synaptic membranes (by sonication or detergents) or by solubilizing them in chloroform-methanol or butanol-water mixtures. Electron micrographs of such artificial membranes show striking similarities to the original membranes (Abood and Rushmer, 1968).

DR. DOMINO. Dr. Abood, I need you to straighten me out on my pharmacology in this area. I always thought of these compounds as acting like an overdose of atropine. I know this area is controversial. What about atropine and scopolamine? Do they show a similar index as Ditran®? What about the action of anticholinesterase agents such as DFP[1] or eserine? Do they antagonize your compounds? In other words, are we really talking about atropine derivatives that are especially hallucinogenic, or are we talking about something entirely different?

DR. ABOOD: No. Many of the esters are potent anticholinergics, but some of them are 10 to 100 times more potent than atropine or scopolamine in their action on the central nervous system. My personal feeling, however, is that they do not act in the central nervous system merely by cholinergic blockade, if that is what you mean. Cholinergic blockade might be a criterion of predictability for psychotomimetic potency but is not the mechanism of action.

The BDI score for atropine and scopolamine is comparatively low. Incidentally, from our conformational analysis and the studies on charge-transfer stability and quaternization rate constants (Nogrady and Algieri, 1968) one can predict the lower central action of scopolamine and atropine.

DR. BIEL: As a corollary to this, the correlation with oxotremorine is much better than with acetylcholine, probably because of the central effects of oxotremorine. So, if you are talking in terms of central muscarinic activity, you get a much better correlation with acetylcholine where you have to take peripheral tissue to establish a correlation.

DR. AGHAJANIAN: The atropine-like compounds are effective in blocking effects of acetylcholine applied iontophoretically to certain single units in the central nervous system. This work certainly demonstrates that cholinergic blockade may be a mechanism for the action of these drugs in the central nervous system. So, I'm not sure why you would want to reject this possibility at this point.

Another comment: When you postulate a membrane stabilizing action of the glycolates, and I assume atropine and scopolamine would have a similar action, you are thinking of this as generally applying to all membranes. And yet, going to the peripheral cholinergic systems, we know that certain membrane systems are exquisitely sensitive to atropine, scopolamine, and to the glycolates, and others are not. The distinction between nicotinic and muscarinic sites is an example of such selective action. Now, why shouldn't some specific and very sensitive site be responsible for the action of these drugs in the central nervous system rather than some generalized membrane effects?

DR. ABOOD: I think that is a valid statement. I can't answer that but

---

[1] Di-isopropyl fluorophosphate (Ed.).

can only speculate. I don't think membrane stabilization alone explains what is happening. It is conceivable that the sensitivity of a given membrane or synapse to calcium may be a factor in its level of excitability. The more susceptible the membrane is to calcium depletion, the more excitable it may be. Those membranes which are more sensitive to calcium depletion may be more susceptible to drug action. So, in other words, differential excitability within the central nervous system may be due simply to a variance in calcium sensitivity.

DR. AGHAJANIAN: In regard to a question raised earlier, it is interesting that physostigmine is very effective in reversing the effects of atropine-like drugs in man.

DR. ABOOD: It is not very effective. I shall defer that question to Dr. Sim who is here and who has had much experience in this type of study.

DR. SIM: It is interesting that these compounds are effective; there is a definite lapse of time, depending on the drug and its concentration, before effects with compounds like physostigmine are noted. The antidotal effect of physostigmine in glycolate intoxication is short lived. It must be repeated every 2 to 4 hours for as long as 24 hours in order to alleviate signs of relapse into unresponsive behavior.

The easiest method by which to differentiate the central-peripheral potency of the atropine-like compounds is the use of the isolated rat iris preparation.[1] For rapid assessment of relative potency, we have found this method to have high correlation with human studies.

DR. ABOOD: Yes, we found that too.

DR. DOMINO: Dr. Efron talked about possible therapeutic use. I have been interested in atropine toxicity therapy for psychotics since it was started by Gorden Forrer in Michigan many years ago. I wonder whether your most potent derivative wouldn't make a very interesting agent for chemical shock therapy.

DR. ABOOD: Well, Ditran, you know, has been used for that purpose quite effectively for some time. It has proven to be quite effective in the treatment of some depressions (Meduna, J. and Abood, L. G., *J. Nerv. Ment. Dis.*, 127: 546–550, 1958). It is by no means the most potent drug of the series, however.

---

[1] This method is described by Wilson, K. M. and Corbett, W. R.: An isolated rat iris preparation for the bioassay of autonomic drugs. *Fed. Proc.* 21(2): 331, abstract No. 238, Mar.-Apr., 1966, and by Wilson, K. M.: Some pharmacodynamic properties of iris muscle. *Army Science Conference Proceedings*, 2: 523–537, June 14–17, 1966. See especially paragraph 2, page 525 of the latter reference, which is obtainable from the Clearinghouse for Federal Scientific and Technical Information, Department of Commerce, Springfield, Virginia 22151. (Ed.)

DR. DOMINO: What is your most potent compound?

DR. ABOOD: Well, I can't go into that, but they are probably too dangerous to work with.

DR. GESSNER: As I hear the discussion, the simplest hypothesis would be that these glycolic acid esters are psychotomimetic by virtue of being anticholinergic compounds. Since this is the simplest hypothesis, I would want to have strong grounds before rejecting it. I don't know quite what you are saying in this respect.

DR. ABOOD: Well, it is a difficult point, and the reason is that we do not know what the action of an anticholinergic drug is on the central nervous system simply because we don't know too much about cholinergic transmission itself in the central nervous system. It's a very complicated and confused topic, and until such time as these mechanisms are elucidated and better understood at the electrophysiological level, I don't think one can really say very much. All I can say is that there is a correlation between anticholinergic and hallucinatory activities, but this does not mean that the mechanism of action of the drug is related to cholinergic blockade.

DR. LEHRER: In your elegant presentation of steric effects, it appears clear that there is a degree of three-dimensional fit involved on the receptor site, which has been part of the main subject of your talk; am I correct?

DR. ABOOD: Yes.

DR. LEHRER: In that case, I wonder if you explored either of two possibilities. In the amino alcohol there is one center of asymmetry, and in the glycic acid there is another. Now if in fact you specified a degree of three-dimensional fit on the amino alcohol site, this must involve an asymmetric membrane site and, therefore, three dimensions rather than two.

It would seem that there should be a strong possibility that if the acid and the amino alcohol were tested by examining both optical isomers you should then find a remarkable difference in those made from the isomers of the two asymmetric alcohols, but if the acid isomers were resolved, you should find no degree of difference whatsoever between the esters made from the two different acids. If, however, both sites are involved, then you could predict that, and you would find a four-fold or eight-fold enhancement. Has this kind of thing been looked at?

DR. ABOOD: We thought about it for many years, and Biel and others have attempted to resolve these isomers, with no degree of reasonable success.

DR. BIEL: You don't need to worry too much about the acid portion because the benzilate, the esters, are quite potent. You have no asymmetric carbon there.

DR. LEHRER: This would rather tend to suggest that there is no effect involved from that portion of the molecule. Of course, this could be put to the test. But, according to your theory, there should be none, and Dr. Biel's point would be a valid one.

DR. BURGER: Ladies and gentlemen, this has been a very satisfactory session. It is gratifying to see that so many of you who are actually not chemists have become chemists for the occasion and are interested in molecular and sub-molecular phenomena.

On the other hand, most of my colleagues are quantitative scientists who work with either reaction rates in mathematical terms or with quantum mechanical and submolecular calculations, and I have learned to be extremely careful in making statements about qualitative relations concerning structure and activity.

What we have heard here this morning are attempts to describe structure-activity relationships of the psychotomimetic agents discussed, but I have missed to a great extent the electronic accuracy which is involved in carefully calculating effects, let's say, of all groups in a molecule together influencing each other, and so on. Such efforts, especially those of Hanson and Fujita, have not been mentioned this morning. I think Dr. Shulgin's long series would lend itself beautifully to regression analysis.

I want to thank all the speakers, and I hope I will be around 20 years from now when such a discussion can be sharpened up and focused much more clearly.

SESSION II

PHARMACOLOGY

Daniel H. Efron, M.D., Ph.D. and Peter Waser, M.D., Ph.D.,
Co-Chairmen

BIOCHEMICAL AND METABOLIC CONSIDERATIONS CONCERNING THE MECHANISM OF ACTION OF AMPHETAMINE AND RELATED COMPOUNDS

Fridolin Sulser, M.D. and Elaine Sanders-Bush, Ph.D.

Psychopharmacology Research Center, Department of Pharmacology, Vanderbilt University School of Medicine, Nashville, Tennessee 37203

The past few years have been marked by extensive efforts to correlate neurochemical variables with pharmacological changes evoked by amphetamine-like drugs. Attention has focused mainly on adrenergic mechanisms which mediate the pharmacological actions of amphetamine, methamphetamine and of certain ring substituted aralkylamines. The various theories on the central stimulatory action of amphetamine have been extensively reviewed by Stein (1964). It is the aim of the present paper to discuss some specific biochemical and metabolic problems pertinent to the mode of action of amphetamine-like drugs in relation to recent experimental data.

DIRECT VERSUS INDIRECT CENTRAL ACTION OF AMPHETAMINE

The peripheral sympathomimetic action of amphetamine is generally thought to be mediated through the liberation of norepinephrine (Burn and Rand, 1958; Burn, 1960; Trendelenburg et al., 1962). This hypothesis is based on the observation that amphetamine fails to elicit its cardiovascular effects or its effects on the nictitating membrane in animals whose norepinephrine stores have been depleted by reserpine. Several studies have shown, however, that amphetamine still exerts its behavioral effects in reserpinized animals (van Rossum et al., 1962; Smith, 1963). In fact, some of the central actions of amphetamine, e.g., psychomotor stimulation, are strikingly enhanced in animals treated acutely or chronically with reserpine (Stolk and Rech, 1967; 1968). Since pretreatment with reserpine does not impair the synthesis of catecholamines in brain (Glowinski et al., 1966a; Rutledge and Weiner,

1967), the persistence of the central action of amphetamine in reserpinized animals can, however, no longer be interpreted to indicate that amphetamine is a directly acting sympathomimetic. Moreover, since prolonged treatment of rats with reserpine causes a more pronounced increase in the response to amphetamine than does treatment with single doses (Stolk and Rech, 1968), the possibility of an enhanced receptor sensitivity after extended reserpine treatment (Dahlström et al., 1967) must also be considered. Recent studies (Glowinski and Axelrod, 1965) have provided evidence that amphetamine may both release physiologically active norepinephrine from adrenergic neurons and prevent its reuptake into the cell. Following the intraventricular administration of ^{3}H-norepinephrine, Glowinski et al. (1966b) have observed that amphetamine causes a marked increase in ^{3}H-normetanephrine which is associated with a decrease in ^{3}H-catechol deaminated metabolites. Although these data are consistent with other proposed actions of amphetamine (e.g., monoamine oxidase inhibition and blockade of reuptake of norepinephrine), it is pertinent that only very high doses of amphetamine (> 5 mg/kg) will elicit these biochemical effects, whereas marked pharmacological responses occur with doses as low as 0.5 mg/kg.

Recent studies with tyrosine hydroxylase inhibitors have suggested that amphetamine is an indirectly acting sympathomimetic amine whose central action requires an uninterrupted synthesis of norepinephrine (Weissman et al., 1966; Hanson, 1967; Dingell et al., 1967). For example, pretreatment of rats with the tyrosine hydroxylase inhibitor α-methyl-tyrosine (α-MT) prevents the psychomotor stimulation elicited by amphetamine (Fig. 1). Since α-MT can exert considerable toxicity (Moore et al., 1967), it is noteworthy that the stimulatory action of amphetamine is blocked by doses of α-MT which do not alter the locomotor activity of control animals and do not exert central adrenergic blocking properties (Weissman et al., 1966). Moreover, α-MT in the doses used does not interfere with either the metabolism of amphetamine or its entry into the brain (Table I). Other anti-amphetamine actions of α-MT include antagonism of stereotyped behavior and anorexigenic effects, as well as blockade of the stimulation of nondiscriminated avoidance behavior (Weissman et al., 1966). In keeping with the proposed hypothesis of selective release of newly synthesized norepinephrine, doses of amphetamine as low as 0.1 mg/kg have been found to displace norepinephrine from extragranular cytoplasmic sites in the heart (Carlsson and Waldeck, 1966), whereas very high doses (more than 20 mg/kg) are required to lower significantly the levels of norepinephrine in brain (Moore, 1963). However, it remains to be demonstrated that these sites correspond to the sites of intraneuronal synthesis of norepinephrine. Moreover, the storage of norepinephrine does not appear to be essential for the central stimulant action of amphetamine, as long as catecholamine synthesis is maintained (Sulser et al., 1968). It is noteworthy in

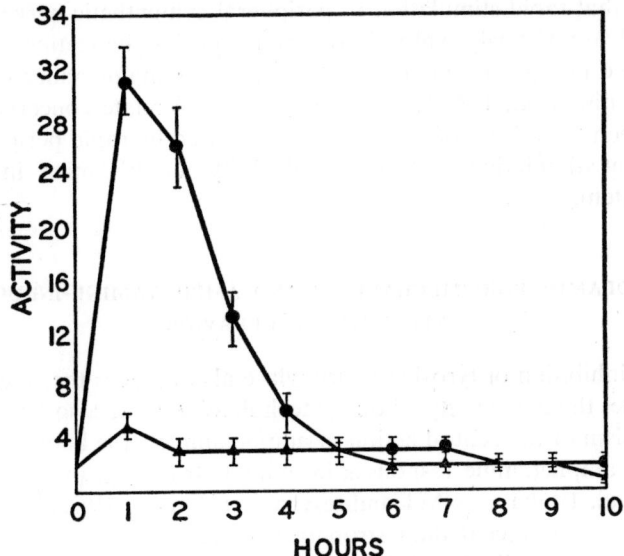

FIG. 1. Effect of α-methyltyrosine (α-MT) on psychomotor stimulation elicited by d-amphetamine.

●────● = d-amphetamine
▲────▲ = α-MT + d-amphetamine

Activity is expressed as integrated counts per hour. Each value represents the mean of 6 to 20 animals. Vertical bars indicate the standard error of the mean. α-MT (50 mg/kg) was given intraperitoneally 2½ hours before d-amphetamine sulfate (4.1 mg/kg i.p.). From Dingell et al. (1967).

TABLE I

Effect of α-methyl tyrosine (α-MT) pretreatment on the levels of ^3H-d-amphetamine in brain

	d-amphetamine μg/g		
	1 hour	3 hours	6 hours
Controls	2.51 ± 0.41	0.55 ± 0.11	0.12 ± 0.01
α-methyl tyrosine	2.58 ± 0.58	0.70 ± 0.10	0.18 ± 0.04

Rats were given α-MT (50 mg/kg i.p.) or its solvent (controls) 2½ hours before the intraperitoneal administration of ^3H-d-amphetamine (3 mg/kg). Results are reported as the mean values obtained with six rats ± standard deviation. From Sulser et al. (1968).

this regard that rapid stimulation of peripheral sympathetic nerves results in a selective release of newly synthesized norepinephrine, indicating that mobilization of stored norepinephrine plays a minor role in maintenance of transmitter release (Kopin et al., 1968). It is tempting to speculate concerning the similarity between the release of norepinephrine caused by rapid peripheral sympathetic nerve stimulation and that evoked by amphetamine in the central nervous system.

DOPAMINERGIC MECHANISMS AND AMPHETAMINE-INDUCED STEREOTYPED BEHAVIOR

Since inhibition of tyrosine hydroxylase also reduces the rate of synthesis of dopamine, the availability of this catecholamine must also be considered in the mechanism of the central action of amphetamine. It is known that *l*-DOPA can restore amphetamine responses in animals treated with α-MT (Randrup and Munkvad, 1966) or α-MT and reserpine (Hanson, 1967; Weissman et al., 1966). Moreover, recent data strongly suggest that the stereotyped activity (continuous sniffing, licking, biting, etc.) elicited by amphetamine depends on the availability of dopamine, whereas norepinephrine appears to be required for other forms of activity, e.g., locomotor activity and aggression. For example, diethyldithiocarbamate, an inhibitor of dopamine β-hydroxylase, decreases both spontaneous and amphetamine-induced locomotor activity, but does not inhibit the amphetamine-induced stereotyped activity (Randrup and Scheel-Krüger, 1966). Results obtained in rats after selective depletion of dopamine in the caudate nucleus by destruction of the zona compacta of the substantia nigra are also compatible with the above view. Thus, the administration of amphetamine to such animals still caused psychomotor stimulation, even though the stereotyped behavior was no longer observed (Janssen, 1968). Although preliminary, these studies shed some light on a possible action of amphetamine on the nigro-neostriatal dopamine neurons.

MODIFICATION OF THE CENTRAL ACTION OF AMPHETAMINE BY TRICYCLIC ANTIDEPRESSANTS AND CHLORPROMAZINE

Imipramine-like antidepressants enhance and prolong various behavioral effects of amphetamine in a variety of experimental situations (Carlton, 1961; Hill et al., 1961; Stein and Seifter, 1961; Scheckel and Boff, 1964; Halliwell et al., 1964; Sulser et al., 1964; Bernstein and Latimer, 1968). These properties of imipramine-like drugs have been used to formulate various hypotheses on the mode of their antidepressant action. Moreover, the enhancement of various effects of amphetamine has been utilized as a tool to screen for antidepressants which are devoid of stimulatory activity in normal animals. However, this action of tricyclic antidepressants has recently been shown to be the consequence of an inhibition of the metabolism of amphetamine (Sulser *et al.*, 1966; Valzelli *et al.*, 1967; Consolo *et al.*, 1967). Such studies emphasize the importance of metabolic considerations in the proper interpretation of drug interaction studies.

Small doses of chlorpromazine have also been reported to intensify or prolong the amphetamine-induced locomotor stimulation (Babbini *et al.*, 1960), stereotyped behavior (Halliwell *et al.*, 1964), self-stimulation (Stein, 1962) and anorexigenic activity (Spengler and Waser, 1959). Since these effects are similar to the potentiating actions of tricyclic antidepressants, studies were undertaken to determine if these actions of chlorpromazine might also be the consequence of a change in the distribution or metabolism of amphetamine. Like the tricyclic antidepressants, chlorpromazine, in low doses, enhanced the central stimulatory action of amphetamine (Fig. 2). A temporal

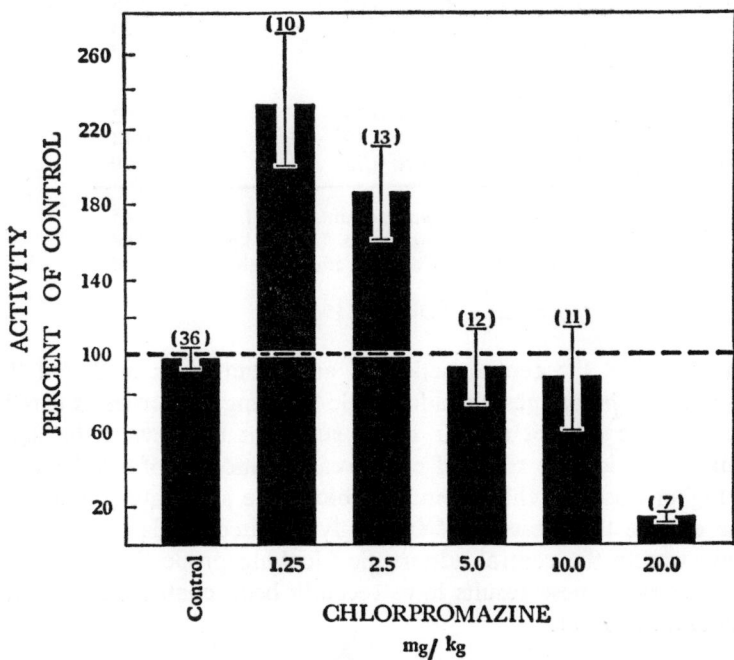

FIG. 2. The effect of various doses of chlorpromazine on the psychomotor stimulation elicited by *d*-amphetamine. The activity was measured over a period of 10 hr and is expressed as a percentage of the activity of the rats receiving amphetamine alone. The number of animals is in parentheses. Vertical bars indicate the S.E.M. From Sulser and Dingell (1968*a*).

analysis of these data revealed that the enhancement is due to a striking prolongation of the drug's action. Unlike desipramine (Sulser and Dingell, 1968b), chlorpromazine, in higher doses, blocked the action of amphetamine. An analysis of the concentration of amphetamine in brain revealed that both low and high doses of chlorpromazine caused a marked and prolonged elevation of the levels of amphetamine (Table II).

TABLE II

The effect of various doses of chlorpromazine on the level of ^{3}H-d-amphetamine in brain

Chlorpromazine (mg/kg)	^{3}H-d-amphetamine in brain (μg/g)	
	1 hour	6 hours
Experiment 1		
none	2.32 ± 0.20	0.10 ± 0.02
1.25	4.04 ± 0.62	0.49 ± 0.13
2.50	3.86 ± 0.68	0.92 ± 0.23
10.0	5.35 ± 0.42	1.17 ± 0.25
Experiment 2		
none	2.20 ± 0.29	0.06 ± 0.02
10.0	5.40 ± 0.39	1.56 ± 0.14
20.0	5.26 ± 0.73	2.12 ± 0.70

Chlorpromazine was administered i.p. to rats 45 min before ^{3}H-d-amphetamine (3 mg/kg, i.p.). The results are expressed as the mean values obtained with 6 rats ± S.D.

From Sulser and Dingell (1968a).

Assuming that the central action of amphetamine is mediated through the release of catecholamines, the adrenergic blocking properties of small doses of chlorpromazine do not appear to be sufficient to prevent the action of catecholamines which are released by increased amounts of amphetamine. In contrast, higher doses of chlorpromazine block the stimulatory action of amphetamine despite the presence of strikingly elevated levels of amphetamine, thus demonstrating the central adrenergic blocking properties of this phenothiazine derivative. These results have recently been confirmed and extended by Borella et al. (1969).

METABOLIC ASPECTS OF AMPHETAMINE

The major pathways for the metabolism of amphetamine are oxidative deamination and p-hydroxylation with subsequent conjugation (Axelrod,

1954; Ellison et al., 1966; Dring, 1966). Dingell and Bass (1969) attempted to investigate the inhibitory action of tricyclic antidepressants on the parahydroxylation of amphetamine. They found that neither d- nor l-amphetamine was metabolized by microsomal preparations of rat liver, whereas amphetamine was rapidly metabolized in the isolated perfused liver. These results suggest the interesting possibility that either the amphetamine-hydroxylase is not a microsomal enzyme or that it requires cofactors other than NADPH and oxygen.

The para-hydroxylation pathway is of particular interest because this reaction is a prerequisite for β-hydroxylation to form p-hydroxynorephedrine in vivo (Goldstein and Anagnoste, 1965). It appears that p-hydroxynorephedrine, but not p-hydroxyamphetamine, meets the generally accepted criteria of a "false transmitter" in the peripheral adrenergic system (Kopin, 1968). Thus, after the administration of amphetamine, p-hydroxynorephedrine could be detected in splenic perfusates during sympathetic nerve stimulation (Thoenen et al., 1966). Moreover, the same investigators found no β-hydroxylated metabolites of amphetamine in chronically denervated spleens. It thus appears likely that the peripheral sympathetic effects of amphetamine are mediated through displacement of norepinphrine by p-hydroxynorephedrine. Since the hydroxylation of amphetamine in the para position must occur prior to β-hydroxylation, blockade of the aromatic hydroxylation by imipramine-like drugs would prevent the formation of p-hydroxynorephedrine and the displacement of norepinephrine in adrenergic neurons. This action could explain the well known blockade of the peripheral effects of amphetamine by tricyclic antidepressants (Sigg, 1959). Since the central effects of amphetamine are enhanced and prolonged by imipramine-like drugs, the pharmacological action of amphetamine on the peripheral adrenergic system does not reflect its action at central adrenergic neurons.

PARA-CHLORINATED AMPHETAMINE DERIVATIVES

Para-chlorinated amphetamines exert pharmacological effects which are qualitatively similar to those of the unsubstituted parent compounds. Quantitatively, the chlorinated derivatives have been reported to elicit a more potent anorexigenic action than their parent compounds, whereas other pharmacological effects, such as central stimulation and peripheral sympathomimetic properties, appear to be weaker (Nielsen et al., 1967; Frey and Magnussen 1968). The specific biochemical effects elicited by the chlorinated compounds were first described by Pletscher et al. (1963). Unlike amphetamine, p-chloroamphetamine causes a prolonged lowering of cerebral 5-hydroxytryptamine (5-HT) and 5-hydroxyindole acetic acid (5-HIAA) in rats and guinea pigs, without altering the concentration of norepinephrine and dopamine in the brain. Investigations by Jouvet and his coworkers (Jouvet, 1969) suggest a correlation between the lowering of brain 5-HT and the prolonged insomnia caused by p-chloroamphetamine.

The mechanism by which the p-chlorinated amphetamines lower 5-HT and 5-HIAA in brain is not clear. The similarity in structure and biochemical effects of p-chloroamphetamine and p-chlorophenylalanine would suggest a common mechanism of action. Koe and Weissman (1966) have demonstrated that p-chlorophenylalanine inhibits the synthesis of 5-HT at the tryptophan hydroxylase step. However, the failure of p-chloromethamphetamine to inhibit hepatic tryptophan hydroxylase or to block the increase in cerebral 5-HT following subcutaneous administration of large doses of tryptophan lead to the conclusion that an inhibition of tryptophan hydroxylase was not involved in the action of the chlorinated amphetamines. As an alternative explanation, several investigators suggest a unique mechanism for the release of 5-HT (Pletscher et al., 1964; 1966; Fuller et al., 1965; Fuller, 1966).

Recent observations from our laboratory suggest that p-chloroamphetamine is a specific inhibitor of cerebral tryptophan hydroxylase. The inability of p-chloroamphetamine to decrease cerebral 5-HT-^{14}C after its intraventricular administration provided the first indication that a releasing mechanism could probably not explain the decrease in endogenous 5-HT. However, the failure of reserpine and RO4-1284 to release 5-HT-^{14}C after its intraventricular administration indicated that intraventricular 5-HT-^{14}C cannot be used as a reliable tool for the study of 5-HT metabolism in brain (Sanders-Bush and Sulser, in preparation). Further studies revealed that p-chloroamphetamine failed to decrease 5-HT-^{14}C derived from 5-hydroxytryptophan-^{14}C (5-HTP-^{14}C), while reserpine and RO4-1284 caused a marked depletion of the labelled amine. These data lead us to reevaluate the possibility that the chlorinated amphetamine could block the synthesis of 5-HT.

The increase in the levels of 5-HT resulting from an inhibition of monoamine oxidase provides an indication of the rate of synthesis of 5-HT. Pretreatment of rats with p-chloroamphetamine partially blocked the increase in cerebral 5-HT caused by pargyline administration (Table III). The use of labelled precursors of 5-HT has indicated that the site of this inhibition occurs at the hydroxylation step. Thus, pretreatment of rats with p-chloroamphetamine prior to the intraventricular administration of the labelled amino acids increased the amount of 5-HT-^{14}C in brain formed from 5-HTP-^{14}C, whereas it decreased that formed from tryptophan-^{14}C (Table IV). The decrease in the *in vivo* synthesis of 5-HT-^{14}C from tryptophan-^{14}C, but not from 5-HTP-^{14}C, and the report that p-chloromethamphetamine exerted no effect on hepatic tryptophan hydroxylase (Pletscher et al., 1964; Fuller et al., 1965), indicates

TABLE III

Effect of p-chloroamphetamine pretreatment on the pargyline induced increase in brain serotonin

	5-HT, ng/g ± S.E.	
	2 hours	4 hours
Control	369 ± 74	589 ± 29
p-Chloroamphetamine	153 ± 14	147 ± 23

p-Chloroamphetamine (5 mg/kg i.p.) was administered 21 and 5 hours prior to pargyline (40 mg/kg i.p.). From Sanders-Bush and Sulser (1969).

TABLE IV

Effect of p-chloroamphetamine on the synthesis of serotonin from 5-hydroxytryptophan and tryptophan

	Precursor	5-HT-^{14}C nc/g ± S.E.	% Control
Control	d, l-5-HTP-^{14}C	1.61 ± 0.20	100
p-Chloroamphetamine	d, l-5-HTP-^{14}C	3.06 ± 0.35	190
Control	l-TRYPT-^{14}C	1.79 ± 0.10	100
p-Chloroamphetamine	l-TRYPT-^{14}C	0.99 ± 0.09	55

Three μc of d, l-5-hydroxytryptophan-^{14}C (d, l-5-HTP-^{14}C) or l-tryptophan-^{14}C (l-TRYPT-^{14}C) were administered intraventricularly 16 hours after p-chloroamphetamine (5 mg/kg i.p.). The animals were sacrificed 6 hours after d, l-5-HTP and 30 minutes after l-TRYPT. From Sanders-Bush and Sulser (1969).

that the chlorinated amphetamines are specific inhibitors of cerebral tryptophan hydroxylase. This conclusion is in agreement with the observation that p-chloromethamphetamine and p-chloroamphetamine do not reduce the level of 5-HT in the intestine. *In vitro* studies of cerebral tryptophan hydroxylase are in progress and should clarify the mechanism of inhibition.

From the pharmacologic point of view, it is noteworthy that amphetamine and p-chloroamphetamine differ not only in their effects on 5-HT metabolism but also in the potentiation or blockade of their CNS stimulatory activity. For example, tricyclic antidepressants potentiate and prolong the central action of amphetamine but not of p-chloroamphetamine; low doses of α-MT block the psychomotor stimulation elicited by amphetamine, but relatively high doses of α-MT are required to block that caused by p-chloroamphetamine (Frey and Magnussen, 1968; and unpublished results from this laboratory). Since it has been found that tricyclic antidepressants prolong the action of amphetamine by inhibiting its metabolism (p-hydroxylation), the failure of imipramine-like drugs to prolong the action of p-chloroamphetamine is not surprising. However, the failure of α-MT to antagonize the central action of p-chloroamphetamine in doses which clearly block the CNS stimulation evoked by amphetamine remains unexplained.

CONCLUDING REMARKS

Evidence derived from biochemical and pharmacological studies supports the view that the central stimulatory action of amphetamine and its peripheral sympathomimetic effects are mediated through the release of catecholamines. Moreover, the storage of catecholamines does not appear to be essential for the central action of amphetamine as long as synthesis remains unimpaired. In the peripheral adrenergic system, the sympathomimetic effects of amphetamine probably result from the displacement of norepinephrine by p-hydroxynorephedrine. Studies with tyrosine hydroxylase inhibitors and with inhibitors of amphetamine hydroxylation are consistent with these views. The fundamental question, however, remains: How are changes in availability of catecholamines translated into the various behavioral responses? The task of identifying specific cellular material (adrenergic receptor sites) with which catecholamines interact to evoke particular effects in the central nervous system is formidable. Since many actions of catecholamines appear to be mediated through cyclic 3'5'-AMP (Robison et al., 1968), it has been suggested that the adrenergic receptor could be a component of the adenyl cyclase system (Robison et al., 1967). As far as brain tissue is concerned, subcellular distribution studies of adenyl cyclase are compatible with a synaptic localization (de Robertis et al., 1967), and extrapolation from studies with pineal gland homogenates suggests a postsynaptic localization (Weiss and Costa, 1967). Preliminary results obtained by Dr. E. Palmer in our laboratory showed an increased sensitivity of the adenyl cyclase system to norepinephrine in specific functional areas in the brain of animals chronically treated with reserpine. These preliminary data parallel the increased sensitivity of reserpinized animals to the amphetamine-induced release of catecholamines, and are consistent with the receptor hypothesis proposed by Robison et al. (1967).

Acknowledgment: The original studies reported in this publication have been supported by USPHS Grants MH-11468 and 1-F2-MH-281T8.

REFERENCES

Axelrod, J.: *J. Pharmacol. Exp. Therap. 110:* 315 (1954).
Babbini, M., Missere, G. and Tonini, G.: In: *Acta of the International Meeting on Techniques for the Study of Psychotropic Drugs,* p. 88. Societa Tipografica Modenese, Modena (1961).
Bernstein, B. M. and Latimer, C. N.: *Psychopharmacologia 12:* 338 (1968).
Borella, L., Herr, F. and Wojdan, A.: *Canad. J. Physiol. Pharmacol. 47:* 7 (1969).
Burn, J. H. and Rand, M. J.: *J. Physiol. 144:* 314 (1958).
Burn, J. H.: In: *Adrenergic Mechanisms,* edited by J. R. Vane, G. E. W. Welstenholme and M. O'Connor, p. 326. Churchill, London (1960).
Carlsson, A. and Waldeck, B.: *J. Pharm. Pharmacol. 18:* 252 (1966).
Carlton, P. L.: *Psychopharmacologia 2:* 364 (1961).
Consolo, S., Dolfini, E., Garattini, S. and Valzelli, L.: *J. Pharm. Pharmacol. 19:* 253 (1967).
Dahlström, A., Fuxe, K., Hamberger, B. and Hokfelt, T.: *J. Pharm. Pharmacol. 19:* 345 (1967).
de Robertis, E., Arnaiz, G. R. D. L., Alberici, M., Butcher, R. W. and Sutherland, E. W.: *J. Biol. Chem. 242:* 3487 (1967).
Dingell, J. V., Owens, M. L., Norvich, M. R. and Sulser, F.: *Life Sci. 6:* 1155 (1967).
Dingell, J. V. and Bass, A. D.: *Biochem. Pharmacol.* (1969, in press).
Dring, L. G., Smith, R. L. and Williams, R. T.: *J. Pharm. Pharmacol. 19:* 402 (1966).
Ellison, T., Gutzait, L. and van Loom, E. J.: *J. Pharmacol. Exp. Therap. 152:* 383 (1966).
Frey, H. H. and Magnussen, M. P.: *Biochem. Pharmacol. 17:* 1299 (1968).
Fuller, R. W., Hines, C. W. and Mills, J.: *Biochem. Pharmacol. 14:* 483 (1965).
Fuller, R. W.: *Life Sci. 5:* 2247 (1966).
Glowinski, J. and Axelrod, J.: *J. Pharmacol. Exp. Therap. 149:* 43 (1965).
Glowinski, J., Iversen, L. L. and Axelrod, J.: *J. Pharmacol. Exp. Therap. 151:* 385 (1966a).
Glowinski, J, Axelrod, J. and Iversen, L. L.: *J. Pharmacol. Exp. Therap. 153:* 30 (1966b).
Goldstein, M. and Anagnosti, B.: *Biochim. Biophys. Acta. 107:* 166 (1965).
Halliwell, G., Quinton, R. M. and Williams, F. E.: *Brit. J. Pharmacol. 23:* 330 (1964).
Hanson, L. C. F.: *Psychopharmacologia 10:* 289 (1967).
Hill, R. T., Koosis, I., Minor, N. W. and Sigg, E. B.: *Pharmacologist 3:* 75 (1961).
Janssen, P. A. J.: Discussion on adrenergic mechanisms in the central actions of tricyclic antidepressants and substituted phenothiazines. *Agressologie 9:* 286 (1968).
Jouvet, M.: In: *Psychopharmacology: A Review of Progress,* edited by D. Efron, p. 523. U.S. Dept. of Health, Education and Welfare (1968).
Koe, B. K. and Weissman, A.: *J. Pharmacol. Exp. Therap. 154:* 499 (1966).
Kopin, I. J., Breese, G. R., Krauss, K. R. and Weise, V. K.: *J. Pharmacol. Exp. Therap. 161:* 271 (1968).
Kopin, I. J.: *Ann. Rev. Pharmacol. 8:* 377 (1968).
Moore, K. E.: *J. Pharmacol. Exp. Therap. 142:* 6 (1963).
Moore, K. E., Wright, P. E. and Bert, J. K.: *J. Pharmacol. Exp. Therap. 155:* 506 (1967).
Nielsen, C. K., Magnussen, M. P., Kampmann, E. and Frey, H. H.: *Arch. Int. Pharmacodyn. Therap. 170:* 428 (1967).
Pletscher, A., Burkard, W. P., Bruderer, H. and Gey, K. F.: *Life Sci. 11:* 828 (1963).

Pletscher, A., Bartholini, G., Bruderer, H., Burkard, W. P. and Gey, K. F.: *J Pharmacol. Exp. Therap. 145:* 344 (1964).
Pletscher, A., daPrada, M., Burkard, W. P., Bartholini, G., Steiner, F. A., Bruderer, H. and Bigler, F.: *J. Pharmacol Exp. Therap. 154:* 64 (1966).
Randrup, A. and Munkvad, J.: *Nature 211:* 540 (1966).
Randrup, A. and Scheel-Krüger, J.: *J. Pharm. Pharmacol. 18:* 752 (1966).
Robison, G. A., Butcher, R. W. and Sutherland, E. W.: *Ann. N.Y. Acad. Sci. 139:* 703 (1967).
Robison, G. A., Butcher, R. W. and Sutherland, E. W.: *Ann. Rev. Biochem. 37:* 149 (1968).
Rutledge, C. O. and Weiner, N.: *J. Pharmacol. Exp. Therap. 157:* 290 (1967).
Sanders-Bush, E. and Sulser, F.: In: *International Symposium on Amphetamines and Related Compounds,* edited by S. Garattini and E. Costa. Raven Press, New York (1969).
Scheckel, C. L. and Boff, E.: *Psychopharmacologia 5:* 198 (1964).
Sigg, E. B.: *Canad. Psychiat. Assoc. J. 4:* Suppl. S75 (1959).
Smith, C. B.: *J. Pharmacol. Exp. Therap. 142:* 335 (1963).
Spengler, J. and Waser, P.: *Arch. Exp. Pathol. Pharmakol. 237:* 171 (1959).
Stein, L. and Seifter, T.: *Science 134:* 286 (1961).
Stein, L.: In: *Psychosomatic Medicine,* p. 297. Lea and Febiger, Philadelphia (1962).
Stein, L.: *Fed. Proc. 23:* 836 (1964).
Stolk, J. M. and Rech, R. H.: *J. Pharmacol. Exp. Therap. 158:* 140 (1967).
Stolk, J. M. and Rech, R. H.: *J. Pharmacol. Exp. Therap. 163:* 75 (1968).
Sulser, F., Bickel, M. H. and Brodie, B. B.: *J. Pharmacol. Exp. Therap. 144:* 321 (1964).
Sulser, F., Owens, M. L. and Dingell, J. V.: *Life Sci. 5:* 2005 (1966).
Sulser, F. and Dingell, J. V.: *Biochem. Pharmacol. 17:* 634 (1968a).
Sulser, F. and Dingell, J. V.: *Agressologie 9:* 281 (1968b).
Sulser, F., Owens, M. L., Norvich, M. R. and Dingell, J. V.: *Psychopharmacologia 12:* 322 (1968).
Thoenen, H., Hürlimann, A., Gey, K. F. and Haefely, W.: *Life Sci. 5:* 1715 (1966).
Trendelenburg, U., Muskus, A., Fleming, W. W. and Gomez Alonso de la Sierra, B.: *J. Pharmacol. Exp. Therap. 138:* 181 (1962).
Valzelli, L., Consolo, S. and Morpurgo, C.: In: *Proceedings of the First International Symposium on Antidepressant Drugs,* edited by S. Garattini and M. N. G. Dukes, p. 61. Excerpta Medica Foundation, Amsterdam (1967).
Van Rossum, J. M., van der Schoot, J. B. and Hurkmans, J. A. T. M.: *Experientia 18:* 229 (1962).
Weiss, B. and Costa, E.: *Science 156:* 1750 (1967).
Weissman, A., Koe, B. K. and Tenen, St. S.: *J. Pharmacol. Exp. Therap. 151:* 339 (1966).

DISCUSSION

DR. EFRON: Thank you very much, Dr. Sulser, for your very interesting report on the various aspects of the pharmacology and biochemistry of amphetamines.

DR. SNYDER: I wonder if you could say a few words more about the effects of norepinephrine on cyclic AMP levels in different brain regions?

DR. SULSER: Preliminary data obtained by Dr. E. Palmer in our laboratory demonstrate that biogenic amines such as norepinephrine cause a many-fold increase in the level of cyclic 3′,5′-AMP in the hypothalamus, hippocampus and cerebral cortex. These effects are consistently obtained if chopped tissue preparations are used, but are not as obvious when brain homogenates are employed. Interestingly, chronic reserpinization of rats appears to increase the sensitivity of the adenyl cyclase system to norepinephrine in specific functional areas in the brain (*e.g.,* hypothalamus).

DR. SNYDER: One other question. You said that desmethylimipramine (DMI) slows the disappearance of radioactive amphetamine. I know that it also slows the disappearance of radioactive norepinephrine in the brain. Do you feel there is any relationship?

DR. SULSER: I don't think so. The effect of DMI on the half-life of amphetamine appears to be the consequence of an impaired metabolism of amphetamine; that is, DMI blocks the hydroxylation of amphetamine by liver microsomal enzymes.

DR. FREEDMAN: Did either DMI or any of the tricyclic antidepressants alter the effects of amphetamine in the mouse?

DR. SULSER: DMI does not potentiate the action of amphetamine in the mouse.

DR. FREEDMAN: It does not?

DR. SULSER: To be more specific, DMI does not prolong the action of amphetamine in the mouse as it does in the rat. This is presumably due to the fact that *p*-hydroxylation is not as predominant a pathway in the mouse as it is in the rat. Moreover, DMI and other tricyclic antidepressants do not enhance and prolong the action of *p*-chloroamphetamine in the rat.

DR. LEHRER: Are you measuring intraneuronal nucleotide?

DR. SULSER: Since cyclic AMP is generated intracellularly, we are measuring with our method the endogenous intracellular nucleotide.

DR. LEHRER: In reference to the experiments you quoted with the subsequent degeneration of the dopaminergic system, in man we have such a model in Parkinson's disease. We have long been giving amphetamine to Parkinson's disease patients, especially to counteract the depressant effect of diphenhydramine (Benadryl®). Clinically, I was never struck with any difference in the effects of amphetamine in Parkinson's disease patients and in normals. I wonder if you have any comments on that?

DR. SULSER: If one assumes that a deficiency of dopamine in the extrapyramidal system is partially responsible for some of the symptoms seen in patients with Parkinson's disease, one might expect clinical improvement with amphetamine, provided of course that the doses are large enough and do or can release dopamine.

DR. FREEDMAN: In other words, if you go along with the people who say the disease is related to a deficiency of dopamine, then with amphetamines you should see the same effect you see with DOPA, shouldn't you?

DR. AGHAJANIAN: However, this fits into the theory in another way. If amphetamine acts indirectly, the presence of intact nerves would be required from which dopamine could be released. I don't know if there is any evidence that amphetamine actually does release dopamine, but if such were the case, one might expect amphetamine not to be effective in Parkinson's disease because the nerves aren't there from which the dopamine could be released. Thus, it seems to fit.

I had another question about the relative cleanliness of *p*-chloroamphetamine as a tool for studying serotonin (5-HT). As I recall Pletscher's data, *p*-chloroamphetamine has an early excitatory effect which isn't correlated with depletion of 5-HT.

DR. MANDELL: *p*-Chloroamphetamine has an excitatory effect during the initial hours.

DR. SULSER: Yes, this is correct.

DR. MANDELL: And after 24 hours, when the depletion of 5-HT is maintained, the excitatory effect has disappeared.

DR. SULSER: The excitatory effects of *p*-chloroamphetamine are transient and disappear after three to four hours.

DR. MANDELL: Well, I think that has to be seen as a complication in the use of *p*-chloroamphetamine, since it may have multiple effects on brain chemistry. I think the new "clean" drugs which are described as having one effect may turn into "dirty" drugs with many actions as research with them continues.

DR. SULSER: This is undoubtedly true. In the case of *p*-chloroamphetamine, it is possible, however, to distinguish between initial and late effects; the initial excitatory action elicited by *p*-chloroamphetamine is similar to the one caused by amphetamine. It has been shown by S. Strada in our laboratory to be temporarily related to its effect on the metabolism of brain norepinephrine and not to that of brain serotonin. The reported long-lasting insomnia produced by *p*-chloroamphetamine could, however, be associated with the decrease in availability of serotonin caused by blockade of its synthesis at the rate limiting step.

DR. EFRON: I would like to ask a question. Why does amphetamine act completely differently in adults than in children? How do you interpret this difference in action of amphetamine? Is there a difference in metabolism between children and adults?

A VOICE: Your argument that there is no relationship between the catecholamine levels and the central action of amphetamine is based on one behavioral indicator, psychomotor activity. You should not say then that you demonstrated the independence of these two things with respect to all central effects, but just with respect to psychomotor activity.

DR. SULSER: I agree with you.

DR. LUDWIG: I would like to come back to Dr. Efron's question, since it is interesting from a clinical point of view. I believe it is more accurate to say that it does have similar effects in adults and children. However, it is the hyperactive child in whom you get these paradoxical calming effects. I would be very interested in hearing how you might somehow put together some of the things you theorized about and how amphetamine might block hyperactivity in a child, for example.

DR. BENDER: I would contradict the statement that only hyperactive children react differently to the amphetamines from adults. All prepuberty children react differently to it. But it is possible, as I analyze our material more carefully, that the first dose or two given to the children produces actions similar to those seen in adults, but children may gain tolerance much more quickly, and thus we get the paradoxical effect. This seems to be a possible way of explaining what happens.

DR. SULSER: This is very interesting. Though the mechanism of this paradoxical action of amphetamine is presently unknown, it is possible that it might involve a difference in the metabolism of the drug in these individuals. For example, amphetamine might be more readily metabolized to *p*-hydroxyamphetamine in liver and then converted to *p*-hydroxynorephedrine in brain. The accumulation of *p*-hydroxynorephedrine in central adrenergic neurons and its release as a false transmitter might explain the paradoxical calming action of amphetamine. Although only hypothetical, this mechanism could be investigated by examination of the urinary excretion pattern of amphetamine and its metabolites in appropriate individuals. In this regard it is noteworthy that *p*-hydroxynorephedrine not only is formed in man after the administration of amphetamine but can actually cause hypotension in hypertensive patients. If these findings in the periphery accurately reflect the action of *p*-hydroxynorephedrine in adrenergic neurons in the CNS, it is reasonable to expect that accumulation of *p*-hydroxynorephedrin in brain after the administration of amphetamine could result in decreased central adrenergic function.

DR. MANDELL: The amphetamine-induced sedation of children first reported by Dr. Bender may be a norepinephrine-involved phenomenon analogous to the reported norepinephrine behavioral depression that we see in the baby chick. We have recently demonstrated a dose-response antagonism between norepinephrine and imipramine using motor activity in this animal. This antagonism is associated with a relative *decrease* in normetanephrine, suggesting that in this animal imipramine decreases or impedes synaptically active norepinephrine. These chemical findings are opposite to those reported by Schildkraut and others in rats following tricyclic antidepressant treatment. Perhaps the pertinent discriminating observation here is that whereas tricyclic drugs behaviorally activate the chick (like man), the rat is not behaviorally altered by these drugs. Perhaps, therefore, the rat is not the appropriate animal to work out the neurochemical mechanisms underlying tricyclic antidepressant drug action.

We have recently been attempting to elucidate neurochemical mechanisms underlying the post-amphetamine behavioral depression which lasts a variable length of time, depending on species and dose. Our chicks manifest post-chronic amphetamine "down" for several hours. "Speed freaks" are behaviorally depressed from weeks to months following "binges." Since (1) norepinephrine in the chick is a behavioral depressant, (2) amphetamine both releases and blocks reuptake of norepinephrine, and (3) norepinephrine is probably a feedback inhibitor of its own biosynthesis, we speculated that amphetamine increased the biosynthesis of norepinephrine. This, in turn, if outlasting the stimulatory effects of amphetamine, would lead to a norepinephrine-induced behavioral depression. Consistent with this general hypothesis is our recent finding that amphetamine induces an increase in brain tyrosine hydroxylase. This increase can be inhibited by cycloheximide. It is of interest that this enzyme appears to have a half-life of about 3 hours, which would not account for the prolonged behavioral depression in our chicks. Another argument against our proposed mechanism for the post-amphetamine depression is our recent finding that the instantaneous activation by imipramine of chicks treated chronically with amphetamine (rather than the 90–120 minute depressed period latency following imipramine in saline pretreated controls) can be seen *five weeks* following the last amphetamine administration. This suggests some very long term effect probably outlasting the half-life of brain enzymes. In addition, if this imipramine activation is related to the post-amphetamine depression, it would seem equally difficult to speculate that a *p*-hydroxy-pseudotransmitter would be stored and active that long.

DR. SULSER: If I were confronted with this problem, I would first find out how the chick handles amphetamine, how the chick handles imipramine and how the two drugs interfere with each other. It is impossible to draw meaningful conclusions on the mechanism of action of a particular drug from drug interaction studies, unless it is first established that one drug does not interfere with the distribution or metabolism of the other.

Generally, we agree that it is dangerous to extrapolate from one species to another. I don't know if you are familiar with our work on the metabolism of imipramine and desipramine in different species. What is true for the rat is not true for the mouse. Although demethylation and hydroxylation are the major pathways of imipramine metabolism, the relative contribution of each varies greatly from one species to another. For example, rat liver preparations metabolize imipramine mainly by N-demethylation to form DMI, which is slowly oxidized to other products. In contrast, mouse and rabbit liver microsomes oxidize imipramine mainly to 2-hydroxyimipramine.

A VOICE: We just finished a pilot study in which one μg of norepinephrine was given to rats via chronically implanted cannulas into the ventricles, and it antagonized one mg/kg of peripherally administered amphetamine in a simple avoidance task.

DR. BIEL: There are some scattered clinical reports that p-chloromethamphetamine is an antidepressant. Is there any substance to this, and, if there is, can you tie this in with your theory?

DR. SULSER: The only study I recall is the one by Van Praag et al. (*Psychopharmacologia 13:* 145, 1968). These authors reported that p-chloromethamphetamine behaved in depressed patients like an antidepressant drug, not like a simple stimulant of the amphetamine type. It has to be seen, however, if this difference in clinical activity can be attributed to its action on 5-HT metabolism.

DR. STEIN: You attributed the insomnia produced by p-chloroamphetamine possibly to an effect on 5-HT. How would you explain the insomnia-producing effects of amphetamine?

DR. SULSER: If one assumes that 5-HT is an antagonist to norepinephrine at central effector or receptor sites (there are data in the literature that the activation of adenyl cyclase in the pineal gland by norepinephrine is diminished in the presence of 5-HT), one might speculate that the absence of 5-HT caused by blockade of its synthesis and the increased availability of norepinephrine caused by its release will have similar physiological consequences.

DR. LATIES: It is well known that amphetamine has different effects on animal behavior depending upon the underlying schedule supporting the behavior. Decreasing the rate of behavior, for instance, when the animal is working on a ratio schedule, perhaps increasing the rate when the animal is working on some other schedule, yields a lower rate of response in the first place. In light of the fact that the *particular* behavior is very, very important, it is really not paradoxical that you get a different effect in children who are hyperactive from that which you get in children who are less active, or in relatively inactive adults.

I would like to end with a question. Does anyone know what the effects of amphetamine are on hyperactive adults, on manic adults, and so on?

A VOICE: Amphetamine drugs are used in prisons among hyperactive juvenile delinquents, prisoners, etc. There have been some reports of improvement in behavior; they show less susceptibility to their own impulses, and have longer concentration spans.

My own work observing amphetamine addicts has led me to believe that although we think of amphetamine as a stimulant drug in adults, the stimulant effect is very, very short-lived in doses above 30 to 50 mg. It just doesn't exist at these dosages.

DR. FREEDMAN: Methamphetamine was used in the 1950's to relax patients with neuroses, and I made an attempt to use it in DT's. Had it not driven up blood pressure it would have been a fairly good treatment for DT's, because the patient became very tranquil and felt as if nothing was bothering him. Then, as the DT's wore off, they seemed anxious and agitated. But what these flip-flop mechanisms are, I don't know, and the first attempt I have seen to experimentally approach these problems is contained in a recent report by Dr. Kornetsky. Perhaps you would like to comment?

DR. KORNETSKY: We have given amphetamines in large single doses to schizophrenic patients. Twenty mg of d-amphetamine given at 8:00 P.M. every night for a week caused no significant change in sleep time during the night. Of the nine patients we studied, three slept slightly more, three slightly less, and three showed no change. Modell has reported that d-amphetamine has an attenuated effect on the appetite of schizophrenics when compared to normal controls.

Thus it is clear that the effects of amphetamine will depend a great deal upon the state of the organism. We have postulated that the attenuated effects of amphetamine for even a reversal in the classic stimulating effect is due to a state of central hyperactivation in some schizophrenic patients. Also, Dr. Laties has already pointed out that the effect observed is often a function of dose and the particular behavior under study.

DR. WEST: I wonder if anyone could comment about thyroid activity during post-amphetamine depression. Perhaps Dr. Mandell has looked into that.

DR. MANDELL: We haven't studied thyroid activity. I think it is a very interesting possibility in terms of the relationship between thyroid activity and monoamine oxidase (MAO) inhibition, which is pretty complicated. Dr. Lipton's imipramine and thyroid hormone work may be pertinent.

DR. LIPTON: MAO inhibition in hyperthyroidism has been shown by Zile and Lardy in animals and in biopsy specimens from the human gut by Sjoerdsma's group. It took very severe hyperthyroidism for prolonged periods of time to produce MAO inhibition in the rat tissues. In the human studies hyperthyroidism was quite severe, though probably less so than in the rat, and the changes found were significant but small compared to what can be produced by a pharmacological MAO inhibitor. The reverse side of the question, *i.e.*, what is the effect of MAO inhibition upon thyroid function, has not been answered as far as I know. I doubt that there would be a direct effect because MAO is not used in the synthesis or degradation of thyroid hormones. But there might be indirect effects through mechanisms affecting releasing factors for TSH, for example.

DR. WEST: I was thinking of the contrary question, Dr. Lipton. I wonder whether there might be some inhibitory effect upon thyroid activity that occurs during the period of amphetamine stimulation which then leads to an inhibition of the output of thyroxine. This might persist for a time. Perhaps at least a component of the post-amphetamine depressive situation (which sometimes seems to last for so long that it is obviously not pharmacological any more) is related to thyroid function.

DR. MANDELL: At your suggestion, Dr. West, we did run PBI's on patients in post-amphetamine depression. We had only two patients, but the change was not something you would look at and be impressed by. The post-amphetamine depression certainly does not have the signs that one might expect in the hypothyroid. It is a mood depression, but there is certainly no somatic depression through cardiac activity, etc. So I would doubt that there is a depression of thyroid activity, but I would also agree that it would be well worth taking a look at.

DR. STEIN: I would like to comment further on the hypothesis that amphetamine is a rate-normalizing drug, *i.e.*, that its action is to facilitate low-rate behaviors and to inhibit high-rate behaviors. I do not agree with this hypothesis. I think that amphetamine has both rate-augmenting effects and rate-decreasing effects, and that these effects come in at different doses. In general, amphetamine facilitates operant behavior at moderate doses and suppresses behavior at high doses. The importance of the baseline rate is that it (among other factors) determines the point on the dose-effect curve at which facilitation shifts to inhibition. An experiment by Dr. Barry Berger and myself nicely demonstrates this, I think. Two groups of rats were trained to press a lever for an electrical brain stimulation reward. In one group, a very high rate of response was produced by a fixed-ratio schedule (70 lever presses produced one reward). In the second group, a moderate response rate was produced by a variable-interval schedule (rewards were aperiodically programmed every 18 seconds). In the case of the high-rate, fixed-ratio behavior, facilitation was observed at the very low dose of 0.1 mg/kg and was maintained up to a dose of 1 mg/kg. A dose of 2 mg/kg, however, completely suppressed the rate of self-stimulation. In the case of the moderate-rate, variable-interval behavior, facilitation was first observed at 1 mg/kg and inhibition at 8 mg/kg. The high-rate behavior thus was more sensitive than the low-rate behavior to both effects of amphetamine. Berger and I conclude from these results that it is not the baseline rate which determines the direction of the amphetamine effect, but rather the threshold dose at which each effect occurs. Specifically, we suggest that high baseline rates of response lower the threshold of both the facilitatory and inhibitory effects of amphetamine.

DR. BENDER: There is evidence in my own experience with children (and this is also true with adults) that amphetamine specifically inhibits sexual drives, attitudes, and preoccupations. That might contribute very much to the changes in behavior seen, *e.g.,* in the young prisoners that were spoken of. It certainly has such an effect in children who have been sexually stimulated. This seems to be another action of the drug which could be thoroughly investigated. I haven't heard whether it has been.

DR. GRIFFITH: Bell (*Arch. Gen. Psychiat. 4:* 100, 1961) has reviewed the literature pertaining to the effect of amphetamine on human sexual behavior and has reported on the sexual behavior of 14 amphetamine addicts. He found that some subjects reported loss of sexual interests while others stated that their sexual activity was either unchanged or enhanced. I am of the opinion that large, chronic doses of amphetamine inhibit sexual activity, perhaps by depressing the secretion of human pituitary gonadotropins. At Vanderbilt university we are studying the effect of amphetamine on this endocrine function.

DR. DEMENT: Some more strange things that amphetamine does: We have given *p*-chlorophenylalanine (PCPA) chronically, as Dr. Michel Jouvet and others have reported. There is a pronounced insomnia which develops over several days, and accompanying this is what we call a release of the phasic events of REM sleep, in particular, the ponto-geniculate-occipital (PGO) spikes that are characteristically seen in REM periods. They appear in the waking stage, and during bursts of this activity the animal either hallucinates or behaves as if he expects to see something but doesn't actually see it. A very low dose of 5-hydroxytryptophan will immediately suppress PGO spike activity and put the animal to sleep with normal REM sleep EEG patterns.

Interestingly enough, a very low dose of amphetamine, 5 mg/kg, will also immediately suppress PGO activity, but will not put the animal to sleep.

Theobald and Morpurgo showed that amphetamine elicited mounting behavior and aggressive posturing in groups of rats who were pretreated with reserpine. We found that amphetamine had the same action in animals who were merely REM deprived for a few days prior to giving amphetamine, so that reserpine and deprivation of REM sleep have some kind of commonality with respect to amphetamines.

DR. SULSER: Dr. Koella has also shown that intraventricular 5-HTP, but not 5-HT, can restore slow wave sleep which had been reduced close to zero levels by *p*-chlorophenylalanine. Moreover, Dr. Schlesinger at Boulder demonstrated that 5-HTP, but not intraventricular 5-HT, restores the decreased threshold to seizures after 5-HT had been depleted in brain. The lack of effect of large intraventricular doses of 5-HT can be explained by studies conducted by Dr. Sanders-Bush in our laboratory. She demonstrated that after intraventricular administration of large doses of ^{14}C-5-HT, the amine appears to be bound predominantly at sites which differ from those for the endogenous amine, whereas ^{14}C-5-HT formed from ^{14}C-5-HTP behaved like the endogenous amine.

DR. DOMINO: I would like to ask Dr. Freedman if he studied the influence of introducing a halogen on the amphetamine molecule?

DR. FREEDMAN: No, we didn't.

DR. DOMINO: I raise that question because there is an amphetamine derivative that has been used clinically in Europe called fenfluramine (Laboratoires Servier, Paris and A. H. Robins, Richmond). It has a trifluoromethyl group in the 3-position, that is, in the *meta* rather than the *para* position. Oswald has pointed out that this compound (*Pharmacol. Rev.* 20: 273–303, 1968) depresses slow wave sleep. This is extremely important because it suggests that it as well as *p*-chloroamphetamine is a tryptophan hydroxylase inhibitor.

PHARMACOLOGICAL STUDIES OF 5-METHOXY-N,N-DIMETHYLTRYPTAMINE, LSD AND OTHER HALLUCINOGENS

Peter K. Gessner, Ph.D.

Department of Pharmacology, State University of New York at Buffalo, Buffalo, N.Y. 14214

My interest in hallucinogens, and particularly hallucinogenic tryptamines, dates back to 1958, at which time I joined Irving Page and his research group at the Cleveland Clinic. This group had earlier isolated serotonin from blood (Rapport *et al.*, 1948), and this was shown by Rapport (1948) to be 5-hydroxytryptamine. Page and his group showed serotonin to be also a component of brain tissue (Twarog and Page, 1953), and therefore they were understandably excited by a report by Stromberg (1954) that bufotenine, the N,N-dimethyl derivative of 5-hydroxytryptamine, was a component of the seeds of *Piptadenia peregrina* Benth from which the South American Indians prepared a psychotropic snuff called cahoba. It was decided therefore that we should study the metabolic fate of bufotenine (Gessner *et al.*, 1960). However, upon review of the literature, the hallucinogenic effects of bufotenine did not appear to be very impressive (Fabing, 1956; Fabing and Hawkins, 1956; Turner and Merlis, 1959). Considering the structure of bufotenine and the presence of a rather hydrophilic hydroxy group in the molecule, it appeared rather likely that this compound would have poor lipid solubility, and hence would experience difficulty in crossing the blood-brain barrier. One way of rendering the compound more lipophilic while still retaining the oxygen moiety in the 5 position of the indole ring was to synthesize the 5-methoxy-N,N-dimethyltryptamine, and this we did. Using as a test system the conditioned avoidance response of trained rats, we obtained a measure of the potency of 5-methoxy-N,N-dimethyltryptamine (Gessner and Page, 1962). We found it to be somewhat more active in this test system than either N,N-diethyltryptamine or N,N-dimethyltryptamine, tryptamines shown to be hallucinogenic in man by Szara (1957), and somewhat less active than LSD. Bufotenine, in this test system, appeared to have only marginal activity. These experiments provided us with quantitative data; they did not, however, provide a measure of the significance of the observed potency differences. Accordingly, after moving to Buffalo, I proceeded to design experiments that would yield this information. Again, the conditioned avoidance response of trained rats was used as the test system, but the design followed was that of a Latin square, such that in a group of, say, five rats, each rat would receive each of the drugs over a period of time. I also embarked at this time, together with Dr. Domodar D. Godse, on a synthetic program. We synthesized, in addition to the 5-methoxy, the 4-, 6- and 7-methoxy-N,N-dimethyltryptamines, and tryptamines with substituents other than dimethyl on the side chain nitrogen. On testing the relative potency of these compounds on our behavioral test system, we found (Gessner et al., 1968) the 5-methoxy-N-methyl-N-ethyltryptamine to be significantly more potent than the 5-methoxy-N,N-dimethyltryptamine or the 4-methoxy-N,N-dimethyltryptamine, the activity of the latter compound approaching that of 5-methoxy-N,N-dimethyltryptamine. The 6- and 7-methoxy-N,N-dimethyltryptamines, on the other hand, proved to be significantly less potent than 4-methoxy-N,N-dimethyltryptamine. 5-Methoxy-N,N-dimethyltrpytamine proved significantly more potent than psylocin (4-hydroxy-N,N-dimethyltryptamine) or N,N-diethyltryptamine.

The similarity in the structure of the various tryptamines and 5-hydroxytryptamine leads to a working hypothesis that the observed effects of the various tryptamines are mediated by their acting on, or interfering with, the 5-hydroxytryptamine receptor. Accordingly, it appeared reasonable to Dr. Jerrold C. Winter and me to continue these structure-activity studies utilizing a tissue preparation in which the effects of these agents could be studied *in vitro*. To this end we selected Vane's (1957) rat stomach fundus preparation, a tissue which is contracted by 5-hydroxytryptamine but relaxed by catecholamines. Using this preparation, we compared not only a number of substituted tryptamines, but also compounds isosteric to these, in which the ring nitrogen of the indole moiety was substituted for by a methylene bridge or by a sulfur atom. We found that in terms of contracting the rat stomach fundus, these isosteric compounds were about as active as the tryptamines (Winter et al., 1967). While doing this work, however, we made some observations which suggested to us that the tryptamines could perhaps contract the rat stomach fundus by acting on more than one type of receptor. Therefore, we undertook a pharmacological analysis using agents blocking the tryptamine sensitive receptors in the rat stomach fundus (Winter and Gessner, 1968). 5-Hydroxytryptamine itself contracts the rat stomach fundus by action on a receptor which can be completely blocked by pretreatment with phenoxybenzamine. No matter how much phenoxybenzamine is used, however, other tryptamines still retain, in varying degrees, an ability to contract this tissue. This leads therefore to the conclusion that they must contract the rat stomach fundus by acting, at least in part, on a receptor other than that for 5-hydroxytryptamine. Furthermore, we found that these tryptamines, when present in bath concentrations necessary to obtain a maximal response, also occupied the 5-hydroxytryptamine receptor and are able to protect it against phenoxybenzamine block. Interesting as these observations were, they did indicate the complexity involved in using the rat stomach fundus for the investigation of the mechanism of action of tryptamines.

As Drs. Laties and Kornetsky have pointed out earlier in this meeting, one cannot expect a direct correlation between the psychic action of a hallucinogen in man and its effect on the randomly chosen behavioral parameter in animals. By definition, hallucinations are subjective phenomena and can be studied only in men. Nonetheless, hallucinogens do exert marked pharmacological effects in animals, be these behavioral or otherwise. These may be mediated by the same mechanism of action as the hallucinations in men. The likelihood of this being so is enhanced if a clear correlation can be empirically established between the known hallucinogenic potency of these compounds and their potency in bringing about certain effects in animals. One of the pharmacological parameters that Drs. Richard T. La Rosa, William J. Fiden and I became interested in was the ability of hallucinogens to alter body temperature. Jacob and Lafille (1963) in France have shown that there is a high degree of correlation between the hyperthermic effects of a variety of hallucinogens in animals and the hallucinogenic activity of these agents in man. Using mice at an ambient temperature of 29° centigrade, we were able to show (Fig. 1) that 5-methoxy-N,N-dimethyltryptamine does indeed cause a hyperthermia, the duration and extent of which are proportional to dose, but that this is followed by a hypothermic effect which is quite prolonged.

Another pharmacological parameter that Dr. Richard La Rosa and I became interested in was the ability of a number of hallucinogens to cause tremor. We had noticed in the behavioral work described above that rats, given various hallucinogens, exhibited a fine tremor. Investigation of the literature showed that a number of other hallucinogens have also been observed to cause tremor in small mammals (Lessin *et al.*, 1965; Jarvik, 1965; Cohen, 1967). We moved therefore to utilize this property, and did so by measuring the ballistographic activity of severely restricted mice.

Mice were placed in a cage such that their freedom of movement was rather limited (they could not scratch), and the mouse and its cage were hung from a force displacement transducer. The voltage output from the

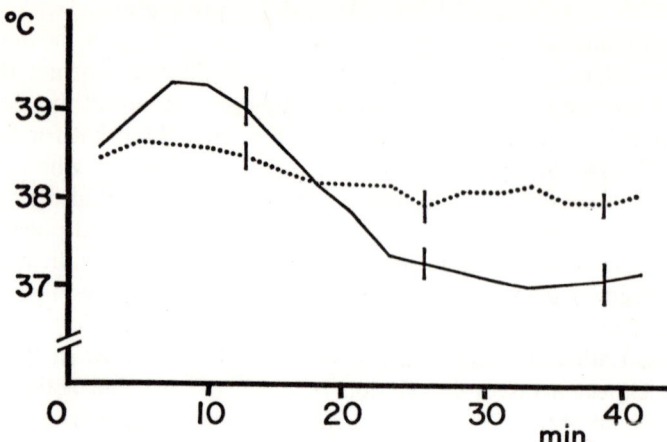

FIG. 1. Body temperature of mice kept at 29°C at various times following injection of 10 μmoles/kg of 5-methoxy-N,N-dimethyltryptamine (———) as compared to mice injected with saline (......). Vertical lines are standard errors of the mean (N = 7).

transducer was fed into a Grass polygraph equipped with a unit integrator. In this manner it became possible to obtain a quantitative measure of the ballistic movements of the mouse in its restraining cage. By determining the amount of activity in the six minutes following intraperitoneal injection of various doses of a hallucinogen, we were able to obtain dose-response curves for a number of these compounds. These showed, for instance, that 5-methoxy-N,N-dimethyltryptamine was less potent in this system than LSD and more potent than N,N-dimethyltryptamine, which in turn was more potent than N,N-diethyltryptamine (Fig. 2).

Using this system Dr. La Rosa and I undertook a pharmacological investigation designed to cast some light on the possible mechanism of action of these compounds in producing this type of activity. The experimental design used was to select three groups of five mice, each chosen at random, and to pretreat two of these groups with a drug designed to alter monoamine function in the CNS. Then, after an appropriate lapse of time, one of the pretreated groups and the group given no pretreatment would be dosed with the hallucinogen, and the ballistographic activity of each animal would be recorded. An analysis of variances was applied to activity observed during the first six minutes following injection of the hallucinogen to determine whether the pretreatment had any significantly synergistic or inhibitory effect upon the action of the hallucinogen. In this manner it was possible to show (Table I), for instance, that pretreatment with p-chlorophenylalanine brings

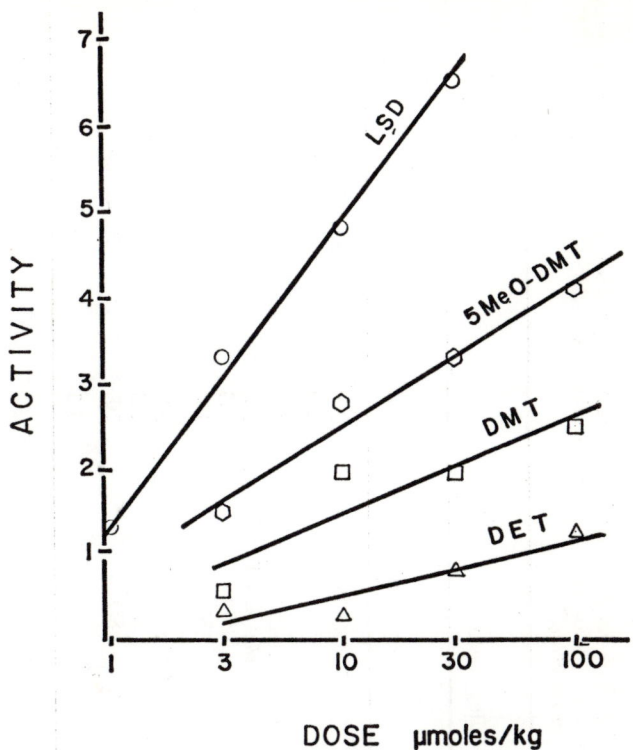

Fig. 2. Ballistographic activity (see text) of mice injected with various doses of LSD, 5-methoxy-N,N-dimethyltryptamine (5 MeO-DMT), dimethyltryptamine (DMT) and diethyltryptamine (DET).

about a significant increase in the activity observed following administration of 5-methoxy-N,N-dimethyltryptamine (Fig. 3) or LSD. A distinction should be drawn between the results of our interaction experiments and the conclusions that can be drawn from them. Thus, there is little doubt of the statistical significance of our findings and the high degree of correlation between the results obtained with two different hallucinogens. On the other hand, only one pretreatment time interval and, in most instances, a fixed dose of the pretreatment agent was employed. These times and doses were arrived at by review of the effects of these agents on monoamine function in the CNS as reported in the literature. It is possible that the use of different pretreatment times or doses would have led to somewhat different results. For instance, p-chlorophenylalanine in the pretreatment schedule used by us has been

TABLE I

The effect of pretreatment with various agents, considered to have an effect on brain 5-hydroxytryptamine function, on the increase in ballistographic activity (see text) is observed following administration of either LSD or 5-methoxy-N,N-dimethyltryptamine (5 MeO-DMT) to restrained mice.

Pretreatment			Hallucinogen			Effect of pretreatment on observed activity	
Agent	Dose mg/kg	Time hours	Compound	Dose μmoles/kg		Direction	Percent
p-Chlorophenylalanine	100	24, 48, 72	5 MeODMT	30		Potentiation	+67.0*
			LSD	3.3		Potentiation	+15.8*
5-Hydroxytryptophan	100	1	5 MeODMT	3		Inhibition	−32.6*
			5 MeODMT	30		Inhibition	−3.2
			LSD	3.3		Inhibition	−25.4*
			LSD	10		Inhibition	−24.3*
Reserpine	2	4	5 MeODMT	30		Inhibition	−27.5*
			LSD	3.3		Inhibition	−60.0*
			LSD	10		Inhibition	−28.5*
Morphine	0.5	4	LSD	3.3		Inhibition	−24.02*

* $P < 0.05$

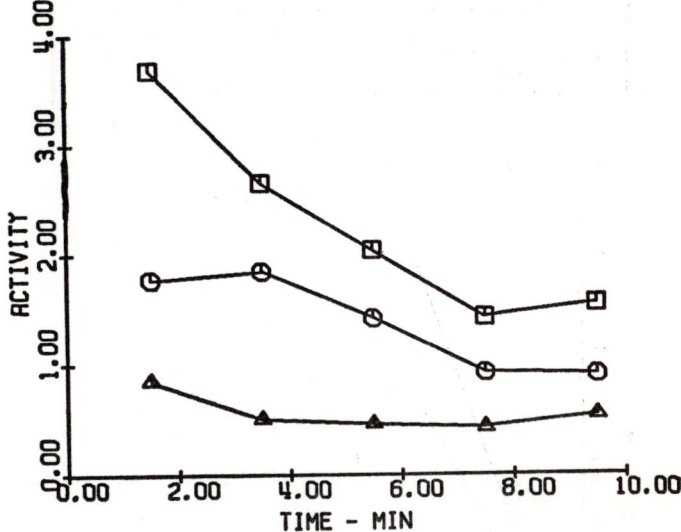

Fig. 3. Effect of pretreatment with *p*-chlorophenylalanine (100 μg/kg 24, 48 and 72 hours prior) on the ballistographic activity (see text) of mice injected with 5-methoxy-N,N-dimethyltryptamine (5 MeO-DMT).

shown by Koe and Weissman (1966) to deplete significantly brain 5-hydroxytryptamine in mice. This depletion results from a block of tryptophan hydroxylase, and thus an inhibition of 5-hydroxytryptamine synthesis (Jequier, 1967). It could therefore be postulated that *p*-chlorophenylalanine reduces the amount of 5-hydroxytryptamine reaching the receptor. Accordingly, the synergistic effect of this pretreatment on the action of the two hallucinogens could be considered to suggest that these may also act to reduce the amount of 5-hydroxytryptamine reaching its receptor. This possibility is enhanced by the results we obtained (Table I) upon pretreating animals with 5-hydroxytryptophan. Mice were pretreated with 100 mg/kg of 5-hydroxytryptophan one hour prior to the administration of the hallucinogen. This pretreatment brings about an increase in brain 5-hydroxytryptamine (Prockop *et al.*, 1959), while the activity exhibited by mice thus pretreated was significantly lower than that of controls. This pretreatment resulted in a significant reduction in the activity seen following administration of 5-methoxy-N,N-dimethyltryptamine or LSD (Fig. 4). Here it could be argued that 5-hydroxytryptophan, by in-

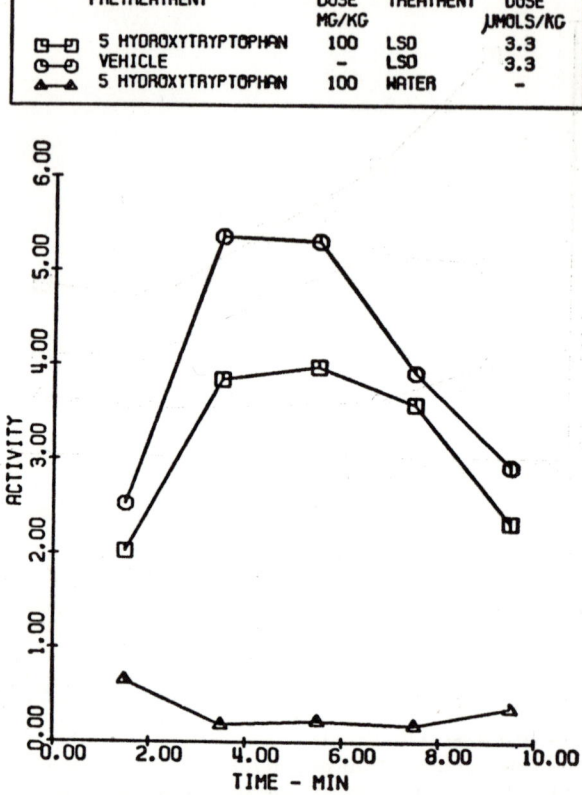

FIG. 4. Effect of a 1 hour pretreatment with 5-hydroxytryptophan on the ballistographic activity (see text) of mice injected with LSD.

creasing the local concentration of 5-hydroxytryptamine, may counteract an ability of the hallucinogen to reduce the amount of 5-hydroxytryptamine reaching the receptor. Similar arguments could be used to explain the ability of reserpine pretreatment to reduce the activity observed following administration of the hallucinogens (Fig. 5), since it has been postulated that reserpine acts

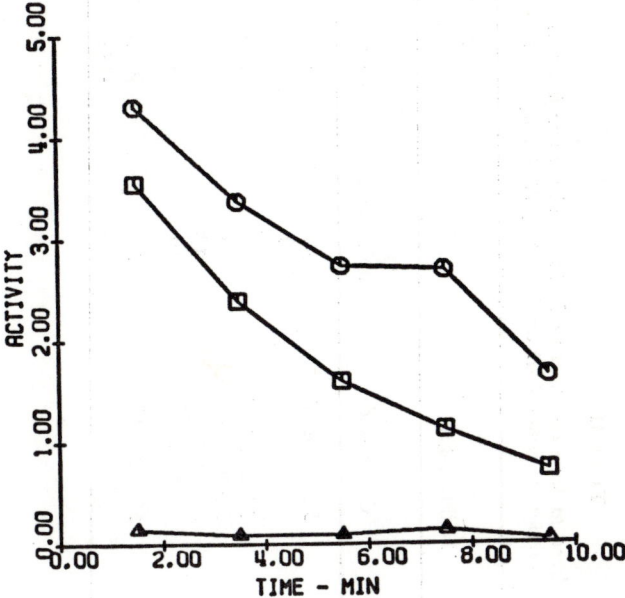

FIG. 5. Effect of a 4 hour pretreatment with reserpine on the ballistographic activity (see text) of mice injected with 5-methoxy-N,N-dimethyltryptamine (5 MeO-DMT).

by increasing the turnover of 5-hydroxytryptamine at its receptor (Brodie et al., 1966). Finally, in view of a report by Way et al. (1968) that morphine enhances the turnover rate of brain 5-hydroxytryptamine, it is of interest that pretreatment with this agent also decreases significantly the activity seen following LSD administration (Table I).

We have also investigated the effect of pretreatment with agents known to influence brain catecholamine function. Thus disulfiram, a drug shown to inhibit dopamine-β-hydroxylase (Goldstein et al., 1964; Musacchio et al., 1964) and to cause an elevation in brain dopamine levels and a decrease in brain norepinephrine level (Goldstein and Nakajima, 1967), was also shown (Table II) by us to decrease significantly the activity observed following

TABLE II

The effect of pretreatment with various agents, considered to have an effect on brain catecholamine function, on the increase in ballistographic activity (see text) observed following administration of either LSD or 5-methoxy-N,N-dimethyltryptamine to restrained mice.

Pretreatment		Hallucinogen			Effect of pretreatment on observed activity	
Agent	Dose mg/kg	Time hours	Compound	Dose μmoles/kg	Direction	Percent
Disulfiram	400	12	5 MeODMT	30	Inhibition	−24.4*
			LSD	10	Inhibition (trend)	−11.4
Dihydroxyphenylalanine	200	0.25	5 MeODMT	30	Inhibition	−30.1*
	600	0.25	5 MeODMT	30	Inhibition	−83.4*
			LSD	3.3	Inhibition	−71.2*
			LSD	10	Inhibition	−70.0*
Dihydroxyphenylserine	1000	1	5 MeODMT	30	Potentiation	+52.6*
			LSD	3.3	N.S.	

* $P < 0.05$

5-methoxy-N,N-dimethyltryptamine administration. Fifteen minute pretreatment with *l*-dihydroxyphenylalanine (*l*-DOPA) also leads to a significant decrease in the activity observed following administration of either 5-methoxy-N,N-dimethyltryptamine (Fig. 6) or LSD. Everett and Wiegand (1962) have

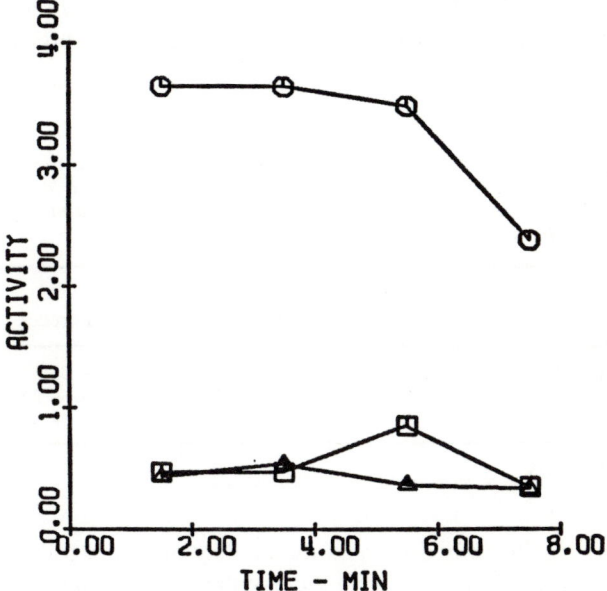

FIG. 6. Effect of a 15 minute pretreatment with dihydroxyphenylalanine on the ballistographic activity (see text) of mice injected with 5-methoxy-N,N-dimethyltryptamine (5 MeO-DMT).

shown that 30 minutes after *l*-DOPA administration there is a three-fold increase in brain dopamine in mice, while brain norepinephrine levels are but slightly increased. It appears reasonable, therefore, to attribute these effects of pretreatment with *l*-DOPA to the dopamine formed from it by decarboxylation, rather than to any norepinephrine that might be formed by the subsequent β-hydroxylation. To test this further, we pretreated the animals with threo-3,4-dihydroxyphenylserine (DOPS) which on decarboxylation yields norepinephrine directly, and which in the dose and time of pretreatment used by us has been shown (Carlsson, 1964) to increase brain norepinephrine levels. In contrast to pretreatment with l-DOPA, pretreatment with DOPS did not bring about any decrease in the activity observed following the administration of either hallucinogen, but instead actually significantly increased the activity observed following 5-methoxy-N,N-dimethyltryptamine administration (Table II).

The one agent which has been shown conclusively to counteract the psychic effects of LSD in man is chlorpromazine (Isbell *et al.*, 1957). It was of interest to us therefore to determine whether it would have a similar effect in our test system. We find (Table III) that a one hour pretreatment with

TABLE III

Effect of pretreatment with p-chlorophenylalanine on the increase in ballistographic activity (see text) observed following administration of either LSD or 5-methoxy-N,N-dimethyltryptamine (5 MeO-DMT to restrained mice.

Hallucinogen	Dose μmoles/kg	Direction	Percent
5 MeODMT	30	Inhibition	-38.3*
LSD	3.3	Inhibition	-69.2*
LSD	10	Inhibition	-18.9*

* $P < 0.05$

chlorpromazine significantly decreases the activity observed following administration of either 5-methoxy-N,N-dimethyltryptamine or LSD.

Finally, we have explored the effect of pretreatment with 2-bromo-LSD (BOL). The antagonism exhibited by BOL towards 5-hydroxtryptamine in isolated tissues, coupled with its inability to mimic the central effects of LSD (Cerletti and Rothlin, 1955), constitutes a major objection to the hypothesis (Gaddum, 1953) that the central effects of LSD are related to its ability to antagonize 5-hydroxytryptamine. In our test system, BOL by itself causes a significant decrease in activity over saline treated controls. Furthermore, pretreatment with BOL significantly diminishes the activity observed following LSD administration (Table IV). Although the dose of BOL was ten times as large as that of LSD, these results are nonetheless rather striking, and suggest that it may be worthwhile to reevaluate the central pharmacology of BOL.

TABLE IV

The effect of pretreatment with 2-bromo-LSD (BOL) on the increase in ballistographic activity (see text) observed following administration of LSD to restrained mice.

Dose µmoles/kg	Hallucinogen	Effect of pretreatment on tremor activity	
		Direction	Percent
3	LSD	inhibition	-80.6*

* $P < 0.05$

REFERENCES

Brodie, B. B., Comer, M. S., Costa, E. and Dalbac, A.: The role of brain serotonin in the mechanism of the central action of reserpine. *J. Pharmacol. Exp. Therap.* 152: 340–349 (1966).

Carlsson, A.: Functional significance of drug-induced changes in brain monoamine levels. *Prog. Brain Res.* 8: 9–27 (1964).

Cerletti, A., and Rothlin, E.: Role of 5-hydroxytryptamine in mental diseases and its antagonism to lysergic acid derivatives. *Nature* 176: 785–786 (1955).

Cohen, S.: Psychotomimetic agents. *Ann Rev. Pharm.* 7: 301–318 (1967).

Everett, G. M., and Wiegand, R. G.: Central amines and behavioral states. A critique and new data. In: *Proceedings of the First International Pharmacology Meeting*, Vol. 8, pp. 85–92. Pergamon Press, Oxford (1962).

Fabing, H. D.: On going berserk: a neurochemical inquiry. *Amer. J. Psychiat.* 113: 409–415 (1956).

Fabing, H. D. and Hawkins, J. R.: Intravenous injection of bufotenine in man. *Science* 123: 886 (1956).

Gaddum, J. H.: Tryptamine receptors. *J. Physiol.* 119: 363–368 (1953).

Gessner, P. K., Khairallah, P. A., McIsaac, W. M., and Page, I. H.: The relationship between the metabolic fate and pharmacological activity of serotonin, bufotenine and psilocybin. *J. Pharmacol. Exp. Therap.* 130: 126–133 (1960).

Gessner, P. K. and Page, I. H.: Behavioral effects of 5-methoxy-N,N-dimethyltryptamine, other tryptamines and LSD. *Amer. J. Physiol.* 203: 167–172 (1962).

Gessner, P. K., Godse, D. D., Krull, A. H. and McMullan, J. M.: Structure-activity relationships among 5-methoxy-N,N-dimethyltryptamine, 4-hydroxy-N,N-dimethyltryptamine (psilocin) and other substituted tryptamines. *Life Sci.* 7: 267–277 (1968).

Goldstein, M., Anagnosta, B., Lauber, E., and McKerghan, M. R.: Inhibition of dopamine-β-hydroxylase by disulfiram. *Life Sci.* 3: 763–767 (1964).

Goldstein, M. and Nakajima, K.: The effect of disulfiram on catecholamine levels in the brain. *J. Pharmacol. Exp. Therap.* 157: 96–102 (1967).

Isbell, H. and Logan, C. R.: Studies on the diethylamide of lysergic acid (LSD-25). *Arch. Neurol. Psych.* 77: 350–358 (1957).

Jacob, J. and Lafille, C.: Caractérisation et détection pharmacologiques des substances hallucinogénes. I. Activités hyperthermisantes chez le lapin. *Arch. Int. Pharmacodyn.* 145: 528–545 (1963).

Jarvik, M. E.: Drugs used in the treatment of psychiatric disorders. In: *The Pharmacological Basis of Therapeutics*, edited by L. S. Goodman and A. Gilman, p. 205. MacMillan, New York (1965).
Jequier, E.: Tryptophan hydroxylase inhibition: the mechanism by which p-chlorophenylalanine depletes rat brain serotonin. *Molec. Pharm. 3:* 274–278 (1967).
Koe, B. K. and Weissman, A.: p-Chlorophenylalanine: A specific depletor of brain serotonin. *J. Pharmacol. Exp. Therap. 154:* 499–516 (1966).
Lessin, A. W., Long, R. F., and Parkes, M. W.: Central stimulant actions of α-alkyl substituted tryptamines in mice. *Brit. J. Pharmacol. 24:* 49–67 (1965).
Musacchio, J., Kopin, I. J. and Snyder, S.: Effect of disulfiram on tissue norepinephrine content and subcellular distribution of dopamine tyramine and their β-hydroxylated metabolites. *Life Sci. 3:* 769–775 (1964).
Prockop, D. J., Shore, P. A. and Brodie, B. B.: Anticonvulsant properties of monoamine oxidase inhibitors. *Ann. N.Y. Acad. Sci. 80:* 643–650 (1959).
Rapport, M. M.: Serum vasoconstrictor (serotonin). V. Presence of creatinine in complex. Proposed structure of vasconstrictor principle. *J. Biol. Chem. 180:* 961–969 (1948).
Rapport, M. M., Green, A. A. and Page, I. H.: Serum vasoconstrictor (serotonin). Isolation and characterisation. *J. Biol. Chem. 176:* 1243–1251 (1948).
Stromberg, V. L.: The isolation of bufotenine from *Piptadenia peregrina*. *J. Amer. Chem. Soc. 76:* 1707 (1954).
Szara, S.: In: *Proceedings of the International Symposium on Psychotropic Drugs*, edited by S. Garattini and V. Ghetti, pp. 460–467. Elsevier, New York (1957).
Turner, W. J. and Merlis, S.: Effect of some indolealkylamines on man. *Arch. Neurol. Psychiat. (Chicago.) 81:* 121–129 (1959).
Twarog, B. M. and Page, I. H.: Serotonin content of some mammalian tissues and urine. *Amer. J. Physiol. 175:* 157–161 (1953).
Vane, J. R.: A sensitive method for the assay of 5-hydroxytryptamine. *Brit. J. Pharmacol. 12:* 344–349 (1957).
Way, E. L., Loh, H. H. and Shen, F. H.: Morphine tolerance, physical dependence and synthesis of brain 5-hydroxytryptamine. *Science 162:* 1290–1292 (1968).
Winter, J. C., Gessner, P. K. and Godse, D. D.: Synthesis of some 3-indenealkylamines. Comparison of the biological activity of 3-indenealkylamines and 3-benzo [b] thiophenealkylamines with their tryptamine isosteres. *J. Med. Chem. 10,* 856–859 (1967).
Winter, J. D. and Gessner, P. K.: Phenoxybenzamine antagonism of tryptamines, their indene isosteres and 5-hydroxytryptamine in the rat stomach fundus preparation. *J. Pharmacol. Exp. Therap. 162:* 286–293 (1968).

DISCUSSION

DR. LEHRER: I wonder if anyone could tell me what an effective dose of LSD for the mouse would be. The doses used in these experiments were 1 to 3 mg/kg; in terms of man they seem enormous.

DR. AGHAJANIAN: In rats 50 to 100 µg/kg i.v. is an effective dose in terms of the electrophysiological activity.

A VOICE: You have to consider what dose for what effect, and what systematic data you get thereby. The half-life of a drug varies so vastly among animals that this is also significant.

DR. GESSNER: I might bring your attention to the fact that in 1962 a paper was published in *Science* stating that a dose which, on the basis of its effects in monkeys and cats wasn't all that large, when administered to an elephant proved rapidly fatal. As the size of the animal decreases the doses you have to give to observe similar effects are larger and larger.

DR. OSMOND: That was extrapolated on the basis of body weight. Not on the basis of body size.

DR. GESSNER: You mean body surface. If you extrapolate down to the mouse in terms of body surface, I don't think these doses are so high.

DR. DOMINO: I think Dr. Gessner's work emphasizes the fact that in addition to dose-effect and dose-duration problems, another important aspect is the end-point of hallucinogenic effects in animals. Thus, depression of tremor may not be a good end-point. I wonder if in some of these drug interactions we wouldn't be better off to ask clinical pharmacologists to try these things in man. I don't know how to interpret your DOPA experiment since we do know that DOPA when given to animals produces a reduction in motor activity which in itself would antagonize the tremor.

DR. GESSNER: In our mice the doses of DOPA we gave were not sedative. With respect to your other remarks, I am with you 100 percent. To determine by what mechanism these compounds cause hallucinations in man their study in man will be necessary. The question remains as to who will undertake this work. For instance, we have synthesized a number of bufotenine esters. Knowledge of their structure-activity relationships in man would be extremely informative. Yet they are just sitting in our safe; we can't do this work ourselves.

Incidentally, while I am on the subject, after Dr. Holmstedt showed that 5-methoxy-N,N-dimethyltryptamine was a major component of the hallucinogenic *epéna* snuff, there have been various statements in the literature that it is hallucinogenic in man. I wonder if anybody knows whether it has actually been given as the pure compound to man and whether under those conditions it proves hallucinogenic. If so, it would be interesting to put it on the record.

DR. SHULGIN: We have it in clinical trial now. It is much more active than dimethyltryptamine. It is much less active than LSD and it is only active parenterally, as is the case with DMT. This is about all I can say.

DR. SNYDER: How does it compare with psilocin?

DR. SHULGIN: It is more active than psilocin, but I can't say how much more with any confidence.

DR. GESSNER: This is all in accord with our data.

DR. SHULGIN: We used 5 to 10 mg of 5-methoxy-N,N-dimethyltryptamine; perhaps even a lower dose can be used.

DR. HOLMSTEDT: I have not tested the pure compound, but I have tested in the field the *epéna* the South American Indians use, and that takes effect very quickly, within 30 seconds if you inhale it. I took back with me the same material and analyzed it. It contained 11 percent alkaloids, out of which about 10 percent were 5-methoxy-N,N-dimethyltryptamine.

DR. GESSNER: May I ask another question of those who are knowledgeable? Dr. Richard Alpert has told me that people who use dimethyltryptamine repeatedly over a short period of time do show tremor. Has anybody else seen this?

DR. HOLMSTEDT: This is not something you see when the Indians take this. The somatic symptoms are: staggering gait, characteristic facial expression, and profuse sweating. Not tremor. I have not seen that.

DR. DIAMOND: I have seen tremor with 100 μg of LSD in an experienced user, someone who has taken over 1500 doses. It has to be amplified to be seen. It was very rapid, very fine, and it came at about the same time as pupillary dilatation and an increase in pulse rate.

DR. DOMINO: I would like to raise the question whether 5-methoxy-N,N-dimethyltryptamine acts like two different types of receptors: the receptors D and M, as described by Gaddum, in the intestine. In his experiment, both morphine and dibenzylene blocked the actions of 5-HT. Your data would suggest that both receptors are involved because morphine, as well as dibenzylene, were antagonistic to tremorogenic effect of 5-methoxy-N,N-dimethyltryptamine.

DR. GESSNER: You refer to the D and M receptors in the guinea pig ileum. One cannot extend those concepts to other tissues. It does not work.

DR. DOMINO: Can one extend this concept to rat stomach fundus?

DR. GESSNER: No, one cannot. The rat stomach fundus is different, it has no M receptors.

DR. DOMINO: You mean morphine does not block the action of 5-HT on the gut?

DR. GESSNER: I do not know, but the M receptors in the guinea pig ileum are blocked by atropine. Atropine, however, is without effect on the ability of 5-HT and other tryptamines to contract the rat stomach fundus.

DR. KOPIN: I would like to ask you about the interpretations of the results of the experiments you reported. Can you tell me if you could distinguish between an animal that is struggling and an animal with tremor, and can you distinguish the various types of tremor? Clinically there are certainly many types of tremors that one sees in patients, and conceivably tremors could be of different types in animals as well.

In interpretation of drug effects, especially with something like brom-LSD (BOL) and LSD, where the structures are very closely related, one need not assume that they interact at the same receptor. They might react with a transport system.

DR. GESSNER: We thought of that.

DR. KOPIN: There is a whole series of variables in drug distribution and metabolism and interference with access that should be considered when you are dealing with the action of one drug on another. I am sure you have thought of them, but these have not yet entered the discussion. I thought that this might be an appropriate time to bring them up.

DR. GESSNER: I think the first point to make clear is that the interpretations which are given are obviously given with the thought of trying to piece the thing together somehow. They are not more than informed guesses or working hypotheses. The first and simplest hypothesis, in terms of the interaction of drugs, is that they interact at the same receptor. However, with BOL, this appears to be a low probability hypothesis because we know that both 5-methoxy-N,N-dimethyltryptamine and BOL can act on a 5-HT receptor by inhibiting it. So the possibility that pretreatment with BOL somehow blocks the access of LSD to whatever receptor it acts on appears to be a more reasonable hypothesis. To test it we administered LSD first and BOL afterwards. BOL reversed the effects of LSD. It does not appear therefore that this interaction is due to BOL blocking the passage of LSD to its site of action. I don't have an explanation.

DR. WEST: Dr. Holmstedt, can you explain the metabolism of our compound?

DR. HOLMSTEDT: Yes, but I would like to discuss this last question first. I don't think, Dr. Kopin, there are too many clinical kinds of tremor. I would appreciate the opinion of the clinicians present here, but as I have read, tremor is very constant among various animal species. Actually one should not speak of tremor because Dr. Gessner is not recording tremor, and he said so. I hope he does not write "tremor" in his paper. One can isolate tremor frequencies. In most cases and in most animals, tremor has a frequency between approximately 15 to 30 cycles per second; one could insert a filter in the recording machine and largely remove the spontaneous movements of the animals, *i.e.,* the excitation which isn't due to tremor. It has been said that tremor is the oldest primitive kind of movement. You find it in jellyfish and throughout the animal species, but there is one notable exception, and this is the tremor in Parkinson's disease, which can go below five cycles per second, unluckily for the experiments of pharmacologists.

DR. GESSNER: Well, I wanted to get to the term "tremor." I will say that there are certainly different types of tremors. For instance, carbachol causes a tremor which is blocked by atropine and is inhibited by norepinephrine. I believe Dr. Holmstedt tried blocking the "tremor" from 5-methoxy-

N,N-dimethyltryptamine with atropine and it didn't work. But you can block it.

DR. HOLMSTEDT: You can block it with chlorpromazine.

Since I probably shall not have time to go into this during my own presentation, perhaps you would now like to hear what happens to this compound in the metabolism of the rat.

We gave 5-methoxy-N,N-dimethyltryptamine to rats in doses of five, ten, and 70 mg/kg, which are huge doses. Now, several things happened here. It becomes converted to 5-methoxyindoleacetic acid. There is a portion of it which goes to bufotenine by O-demethylation. This bufotenine is then metabolized, either to 5-hydroxyindoleacetic acid or to the corresponding alcohol. A certain amount of the compound, between six and twelve percent, is excreted unchanged. There is a slight amount of bufotenine, but the interesting thing is that when you step up the dose, much more is converted to the 5-methoxyindoleacetic acid than to these other compounds, relatively speaking. No 5-methoxy-6-hydroxy compound is formed.

A VOICE: This is in reference to tremor that one can see. One kind of tremor is the shivering that one sees with the onset of hyperthermia, and particularly since it is correlated with the rising phase of temperature. I wonder whether it is that kind of shivering that is seen here. Of course, there are other kinds of tremors in man. I don't know about animals. You have the epinephrine-type tremor of outstretched extremities. It is very different from the kind of thing you see in Parkinson's disease, of course, and the kind of tremors one sees with muscle fatigue, for example, or those initiated at the cord level. So there are many different modes of producing tremor from central mechanisms.

DR. GESSNER: It is still a way of measuring the effect of these drugs, and if it is due to hyperthermia and that is correlated with the hallucinogenic properties of these agents in man, we are still on similar ground.

MECHANISM OF THE FACILITATING EFFECTS OF AMPHETAMINE ON BEHAVIOR*

Larry Stein, Ph.D. and C. David Wise, Ph.D.

Wyeth Laboratories, Philadelphia, Pennsylvania 19101

INTRODUCTION

Many biochemical hypotheses have been offered to explain the behavior-facilitating effects of amphetamine. Early theories assumed that amphetamine acted on the central nervous system by inhibiting monoamine oxidase, thereby reducing the rate of formation of inhibitory aldehydes (Mann and Quastel, 1940), or by retarding the destruction of catecholamines (Burn, 1957). More recently, it has been proposed that amphetamine mimics norepinephrine and combines directly with norepinephrine receptors in the brain (Brodie and Shore, 1957; Smith, 1963; van Rossum, van der Schoot, and Hurkmans, 1962). Later, it also was suggested that amphetamine acts centrally by combining with serotonin or tryptamine receptors in the brain (Vane, 1960). The evidence against these theories has been summarized elsewhere (Stein, 1964b).

In the same paper, Stein (1964b) proposed for the first time that the behavioral-facilitating action of amphetamine, like its peripheral sympathomimetic action, is mediated indirectly by the liberation of norepinephrine. This theory was based mainly on evidence from psychopharmacological studies (Stein and Seifter, 1961; Stein, 1964b). In 1965 the theory was independently validated by the biochemical studies of Glowinski and Axelrod. Further pharmacological support for the theory was reported by Weissman,

---

* This material was presented by Dr. C. David Wise in similar form at the *International Symposium on Amphetamines and Related Compounds* in Milan, Italy, March, 1969. (*Proceedings of the Mario Negri Institute for Pharmacological Research,* edited by E. Costa and S. Garattini. Raven Press, New York.)

Koe and Tenen (1966); in addition, these investigators elaborated the theory by suggesting that the central action of amphetamine depends on the *de novo* synthesis of norepinephrine.

New studies described in this paper indicate that the Weissman *et al.* (1966) proposal is not precisely correct. Our studies suggest instead that the behavior-facilitating action of amphetamine depends on the availability of norepinephrine in functional or physiologically active pools,[1] rather than on the *de novo* synthesis of norepinephrine *per se*. We also report here new experimental results which indicate that amphetamine releases norepinephrine from synapses of the medial forebrain bundle in the amygdala and other forebrain sites (Stein, 1967a; 1967b; Stein and Wise, 1969). Finally, we present evidence which suggests that the norepinephrine released by amphetamine acts mainly as an inhibitory transmitter at the cellular level and depresses the activity of behaviorally-suppressive cell groups in the forebrain (Stein and Wise, 1969). In other words, we assume that amphetamine facilitates goal directed behavior by disinhibition rather than by direct excitation.

EFFECTS OF AMPHETAMINE ON SELF-STIMULATION OF THE BRAIN

The noradrenergic theory of amphetamine action was suggested initially by the observation that amphetamine markedly facilitates the rate of self-stimulation of the medial forebrain bundle and other reward areas of the brain (Stein and Seifter, 1961) (Fig. 1). In the self-stimulation method (Olds and Milner, 1954), an animal performs a predesignated response to deliver electrical stimulation to its own brain through permanently implanted electrodes. In addition to amphetamine, other substances that release norepinephrine rapidly from stores in the brain (α-methyl-*meta*-tyrosine, tetrabenazine in combination with monoamine oxidase inhibitor) also facilitate self-stimulation (Table I). Conversely, drugs that deplete the brain of norepinephrine (reserpine, α-methyl-*para*-tyrosine), or drugs that block noradrenergic transmission (chlorpromazine) suppress self-stimulation. Furthermore, if brain levels of norepinephrine are increased by administration of a monoamine oxidase inhibitor, or if the rebinding of released norepinephrine is retarded by cocaine, the facilitatory action of amphetamine on self-stimula-

---

[1] By "functional pools" we mean a small store or supply of norepinephrine from which nerve impulses release transmitter into the synapse. Functional pools should be distinguished from the relatively large "reserve pools" which normally appear to participate minimally or not at all in synaptic transmission. The precise cellular location of the two pools is presently unknown. It is commonly believed that the reserve pool is contained mainly in granular vesicles; the functional pool may be granular or extragranular.

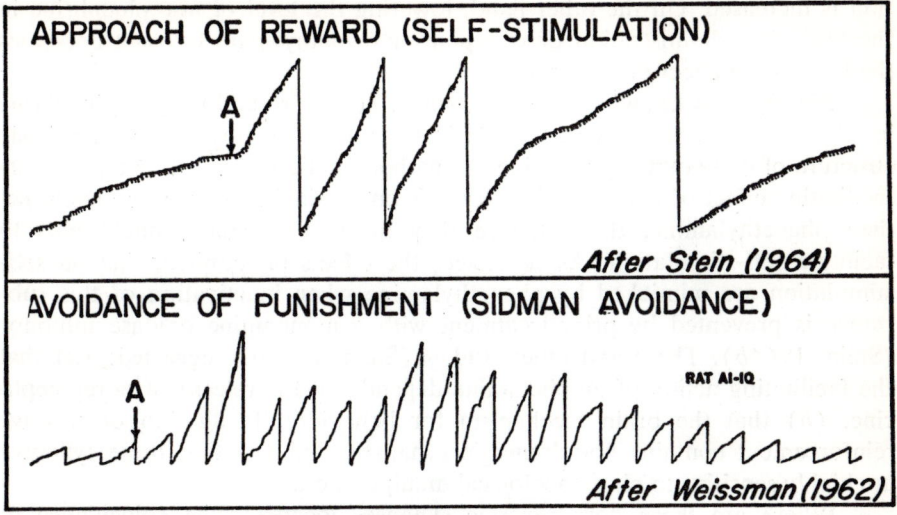

FIG. 1. Facilitating effects of amphetamine on two types of goal-directed behavior. Injections were made at A 30 minutes after start of the test in both cases. Curves are drawn by cumulating responses over time; the slope of the curve at any point is proportional to the rate of response. *Upper:* approach of reward or positively reinforced behavior. Lever-pressing responses deliver electrical stimulation to the medial forebrain bundle through permanently implanted electrodes on a 30 second variable interval schedule of reinforcement. Pen resets automatically after 500 responses. After Stein (1964b). *Lower:* active avoidance or negatively reinforced behavior. Lever pressing responses postpone the presentation of painful electric shocks to the feet for 20 seconds. Pen resets automatically after 10 minutes. After Weissman (1962).

TABLE I

Potentiators and antagonists of amphetamine stimulation

Drug	Effect on noradrenergic transmission
Potentiators	
Iproniazid	Inhibits norepinephrine catabolism
Cocaine	Blocks norepinephrine reuptake
Imipramine	Blocks norepinephrine reuptake, retards amphetamine metabolism
Antagonists	
Reserpine, tetrabenazine	Depletes norepinephrine
Chlorpromazine	Blocks norepinephrine transmission
α-Methyl-*p*-tyrosine, disulfiram, diethyldithiocarbamate	Inhibits norepinephrine biosynthesis

tion is increased. On the other hand, lowering the level of norepinephrine in the brain by administration of reserpine or α-methyl-*para*-tyrosine decreases the facilitating effect of amphetamine.

Finally, it is known that amphetamine closely resembles norepinephrine in chemical structure; both are derivatives of phenethylamine, the basic structure of compounds possessing sympathomimetic activity. If the behavior-facilitating effect of amphetamine depends on its similarity to norepinephrine, then phenethylamine, the structure they have in common, ought also to facilitate self-stimulation. As predicted, the effects of amphetamine on self-stimulation are mimicked by phenethylamine when inactivation of this substance is prevented by prior treatment with a monoamine oxidase inhibitor (Stein, 1964*b*). These and other studies (Stein, 1967*b*) suggested: (*a*) that the facilitating action of amphetamine depends on the release of norepinephrine, (*b*) that the brain mechanism for behavioral facilitation or positive reinforcement contains noradrenergic synapses, and (*c*) that these synapses are highly sensitive to pharmacological manipulation.

Where are these noradrenergic synapses located? The coincidence of behavioral and histochemical studies suggests that these synapses are formed by terminals of the medial forebrain bundle in forebrain and diencephalon. The behavioral work shows that the most intensely positively reinforcing or facilitating points in the brain are distributed along the medial forebrain bundle (Olds, 1962). The histochemical work shows that the medial forebrain bundle is the principal diencephalic pathway of ascending noradrenergic fibers (Hillarp, Dahlström and Fuxe, 1966). Thus the medial forebrain bundle is both the main pathway of norepinephrine containing neurons and the main focus of behavioral facilitation in the brain.

It therefore appears that electrical stimulation of the medial forebrain bundle produces at least part of its positively reinforcing effects by activating noradrenergic synapses in the diencephalon and forebrain. Amphetamine, like medial forebrain bundle stimulation, also facilitates operant behavior by releasing (or facilitating the release of) norepinephrine at these synapses, while chlorpromazine inhibits operant behavior by blocking adrenergic transmission at these sites.

INTERACTIONS OF AMPHETAMINE AND DOPAMINE-β-HYDROXYLASE INHIBITORS

Recent experiments with dopamine-β-hydroxylase inhibitors permit a direct test of the idea that the behavior facilitating effects of amphetamine are mediated by the release of norepinephrine from functional pools. These studies also indicate that the central action of amphetamine does not depend on the *de novo* synthesis of norepinephrine *per se*. In initial experiments (Wise and Stein, 1969), we found that systemic injections of disulfiram or intraventricular injections of diethyldithiocarbamate (DEDTC) suppressed self-stimulation (Fig. 2). Because intraventricular administration of *l*-norepinephrine selectively and rapidly reinstated the suppressed behavior, we concluded that disulfiram and DEDTC suppress self-stimulation by their inhibitory action on dopamine-β-hydroxylase, and not by some other action unrelated to the metabolism of norepinephrine. Furthermore, we ruled out an important role for serotonin and dopamine in these experiments, since neither substance was capable of reversing the effects of the drugs.

According to recent models of noradrenergic function (Axelrod, 1963; Sedvall, Weise and Kopin, 1968), norepinephrine in the nerve ending is contained in two pools—a small functional pool, and a larger, essentially nonfunctional, reserve pool. Because the norepinephrine in the reserve pool does not transfer readily to the functional pool (Weissman *et al.*, 1966), self-stimulation under normal conditions probably depends primarily on the synthesis *de novo* of norepinephrine in functional pools.

Consistent with this idea, inhibition of norepinephrine biosynthesis causes self-stimulation to fail after the small reserve of transmitter in the functional pool is exhausted (Wise and Stein, 1969). However, despite inhibition of norepinephrine biosynthesis, self-stimulation is reinstated by intraventricular administration of exogenous norepinephrine. Hence, *de novo* synthesis of norepinephrine is not essential for self-stimulation. It is more likely that self-stimulation depends rather on the availability of norepinephrine in functional pools.

In complementary experiments, the effects on self-stimulation of small doses of amphetamine were determined after inhibition of norepinephrine biosynthesis by DEDTC. Fifteen minutes after a 0.4 mg/kg dose of *d*-amphetamine sulfate, the rate of self-stimulation of otherwise untreated rats increased by 34%. In the same period of time after amphetamine, the rate of self-stimulation of rats pretreated with DEDTC decreased by 78% (Figs. 3 and 4). Thus, the behavior facilitating action of amphetamine may be blocked by prior administration of a dopamine-β-hydroxylase inhibitor. In two additional groups of DEDTC-treated rats, 5 μg of *l*-norepinephrine HCl was injected intraventricularly 10 minutes after DEDTC; five minutes later, one group received 0.4 mg/kg of *d*-amphetamine and one did not. Thirty minutes after the amphetamine injection in the DEDTC:*l*-norepinephrine:amphetamine group, the rate of self-stimulation was 131% of the predrug control rate Fig. 3). If *l*-norepinephrine was not given (DEDTC:amphetamine group), the self-stimulation rate was only 63% of control. The group that did not

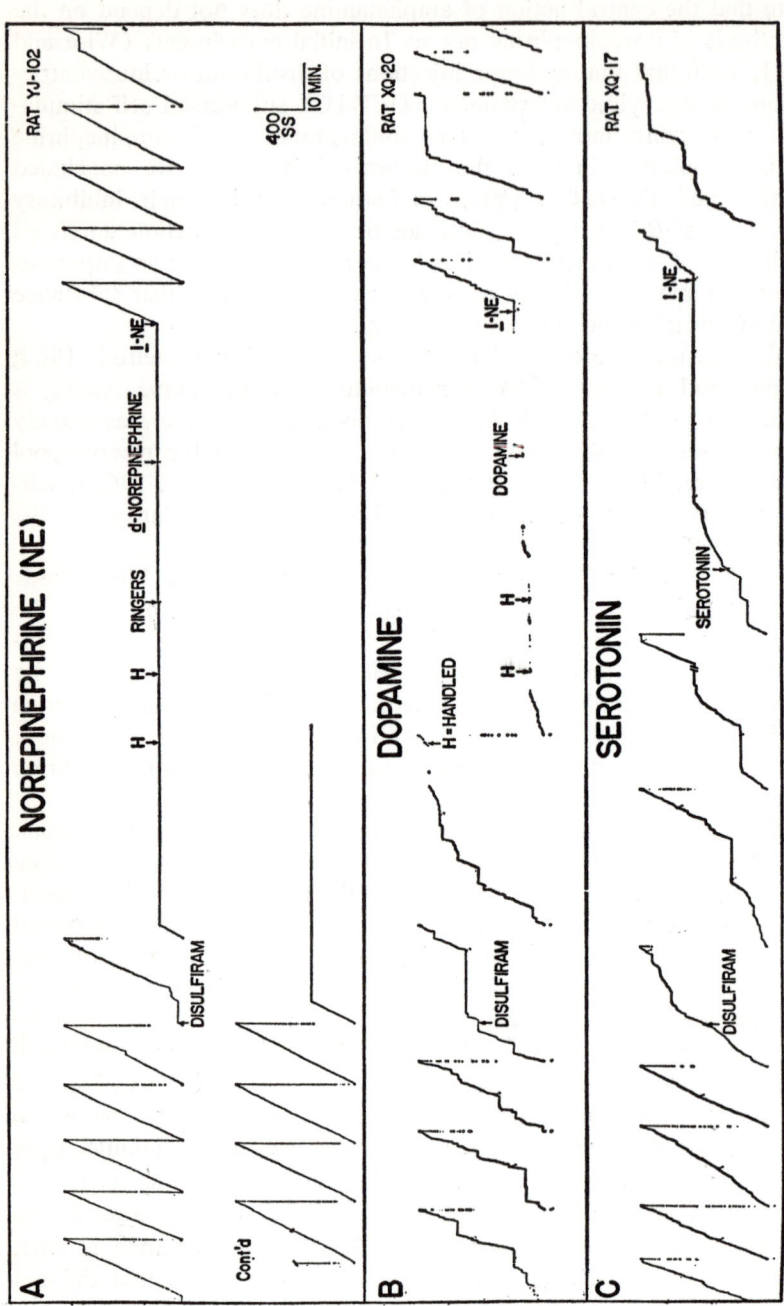

FIG. 2. Suppression of self-stimulation by disulfiram (200 mg/kg), and reversal of behavior suppression by intraventricular injection of *l*-norepinephrine (5 μg in *A* and *B*, 20 μg in *C*). Equivalent doses of *d*-norepinephrine, dopamine, or serotonin do not restore self-stimulation. The pen cumulates self-stimulations and resets automatically after 1000 responses. After Wise and Stein (1969).

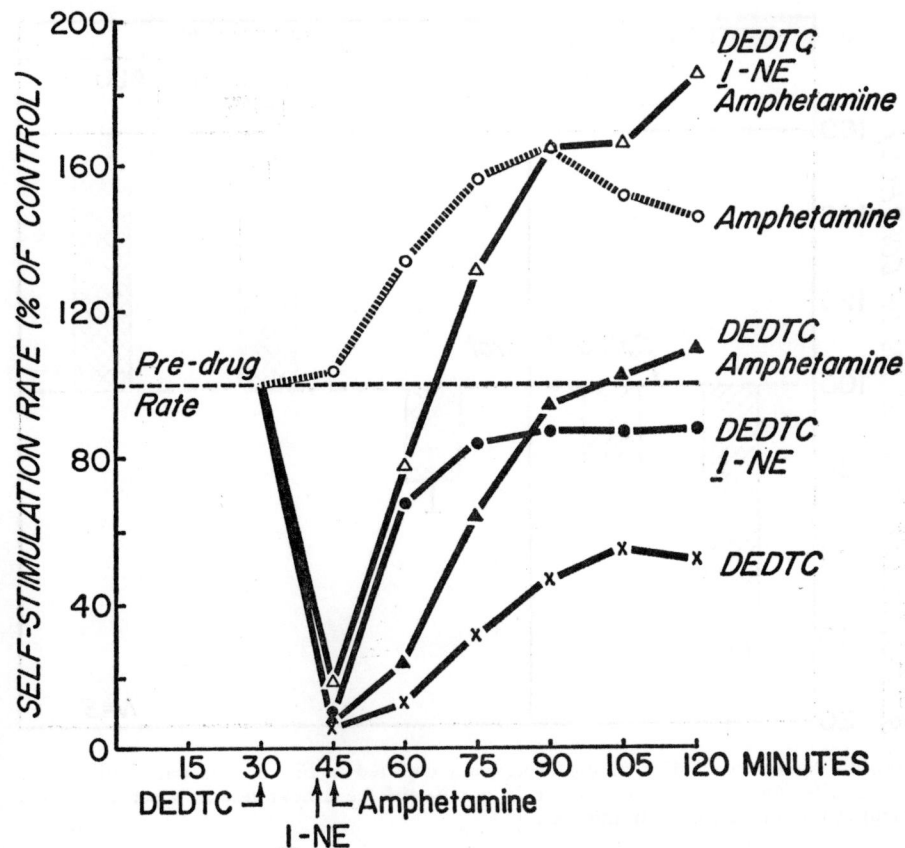

FIG. 3. Amphetamine-induced facilitation of self-stimulation is blocked after inhibition of norepinephrine biosynthesis, and is restored after intraventricular administration of *l*-norepinephrine. Curves show mean rate of self-stimulation of variously treated groups in successive 15 minute periods for the entire 2 hour test. The self-stimulation rate of each rat was calculated as a percentage of its predrug rate (in the first 30 minutes), and these percentages were averaged to generate the group curves. Drugs were administered as follows: diethyldithiocarbamate (DEDTC), 2 mg, intraventricularly, 30 minutes after start of the test; *l*-norepinephrine HCl, 5 μg intraventricularly, 40 minutes after start of test; *d*-amphetamine sulfate, 0.4 mg/kg intraperitoneally, 45 minutes after start of test.

receive amphetamine (DEDTC:*l*-norepinephrine group) had a rate of 84% of control. These results indicate that the facilitating action of amphetamine may be restored in DEDTC-treated animals by the intraventricular infusion of exogenous norepinephrine. The restoration is partial at 15 minutes after amphetamine; it is complete at 45 minutes, and at 75 minutes the facilitating effect of amphetamine is even augmented.

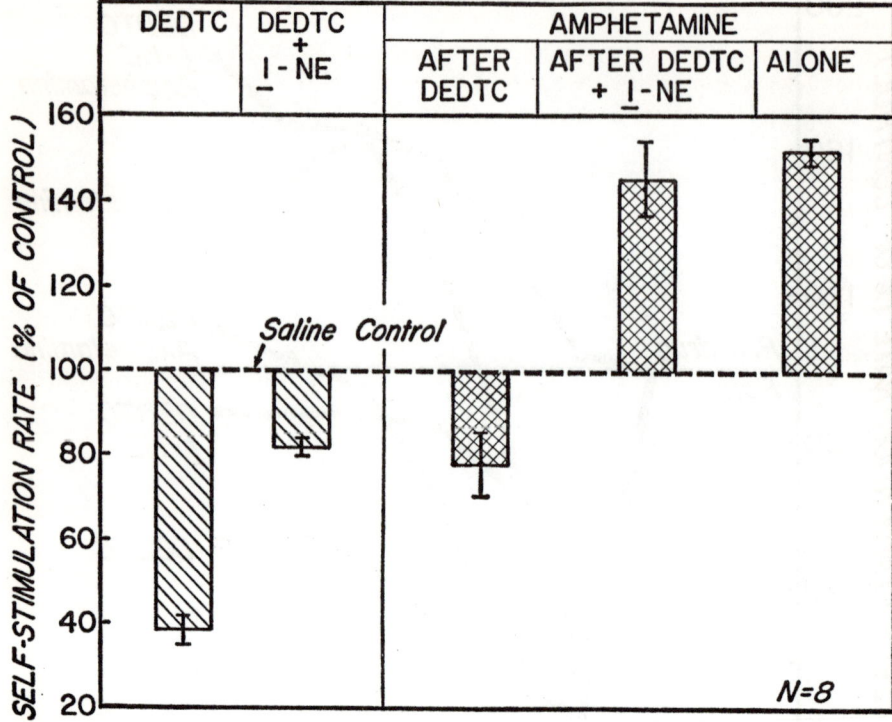

FIG. 4. Summary of data of the experiment depicted in Fig. 3. The bars indicate the mean self-stimulation rate in the last 75 minutes of the 2 hour test as a percent of the predrug rate in the initial 30 minutes.

In summary, these experiments indicate (*a*) that the effects of amphetamine are largely blocked at the peak of norepinephrine synthesis inhibition, and (*b*) that administration of exogenous *l*-norepinephrine largely reinstates the facilitating effect of amphetamine. These experiments thus support the idea that the behavior facilitating action of amphetamine depends on the availability of norepinephrine in functional pools rather than on the synthesis *de novo* of norepinephrine.

PERFUSION STUDIES

The next series of experiments permitted a direct test of the idea (Stein, 1964*a*; 1964*b*; 1968; Stein and Wise, in press) that the behavior facilitating effects of amphetamine are mediated by the release of norepinephrine from terminals of the medial forebrain bundle. These experiments derived from earlier work which demonstrated that norepinephrine could be released into a brain perfusate by rewarding electrical stimulation of the medial forebrain bundle. Using a permanently indwelling Gaddum push-pull cannula, Stein and Wise (1967, 1969) continuously perfused specific areas in the brains of unanesthetized rats with Ringer-Locke's solution for periods of up to six hours (Fig. 5). Among the areas perfused were the terminal sites of the

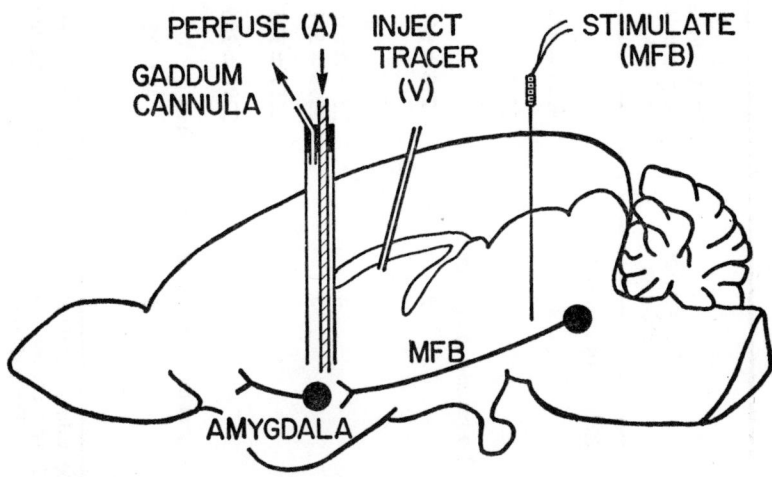

FIG. 5. Diagram of the perfusion experiment showing the relative locations of the stimulating electrode in the medial forebrain bundle (*MFB*), the perfusion cannula in the amygdala (*A*), and the needle for injection of radioisotopes into the lateral ventricle (*V*) on an outline of the rat brain.

medial forebrain bundle in rostral hypothalamus and amygdala. At intermittent periods, rewarding points in the medial forebrain bundle (as well as nonrewarding control points) were electrically stimulated in an attempt to release norepinephrine or its metabolites into the perfusate. In order to measure the small quantities of norepinephrine that might be released by rewarding stimulation, a sensitive radiotracer method was used (Glowinski, Kopin, and Axelrod, 1965). Forty-five minutes before the start of the perfusion experiment, ^{14}C-labeled (41 μg) or tritiated norepinephrine (0.3 μg) was injected into the lateral ventricle. Regional and subcellular distribution studies suggest that the labeled norepinephrine introduced into the brain in this way mixes with the endogenous store and can be used as a tracer.

TABLE II
Summary of results of perfusion experiments

Comment	Cannula location	Number of animals	Mean self-stimulation rate (responses/hr ± S.E.M.)	Radioactivity ratio (stimulation/control ± S.E.M.)
(A) Release of radioactivity				
Rewarding stimulation, adequate perfusion	Hypothalamus	20	4725 ± 495	2.45 ± 0.33
	Amygdala	4	3242 ± 315	3.02 ± 0.43
(B) No release of radioactivity				
Nonrewarding stimulation (includes 3 cortical electrodes)	Hypothalamus	9	210 ± 66	0.74 ± 0.07
Inadequate perfusion	Cortex and thalamus	4	2822 ± 816	0.77 ± 0.14
	Defective cannula	5	3390 ± 561	0.92 ± 0.08
Rewarding stimulation, adequate perfusion	Hypothalamus	8	2667 ± 385	0.95 ± 0.06
	Amygdala	2	2796 ± 286	0.72 ± 0.19
(C) Inhibition of spontaneous release of radioactivity				
Nonrewarding or punishing stimulation (thalamus and midbrain)	Hypothalamus	5	46 ± 32	0.17 ± 0.05

Radioactivity ratios were calculated from peak sample values obtained during stimulation and control periods, except that in the case of "inhibition of spontaneous release of radioactivity," the lowest control and stimulation values were used. All electrode tips were located in or near the medial forebrain bundle unless otherwise noted. From Stein and Wise (1969).

FACILITATION OF BEHAVIOR BY AMPHETAMINE

After a control period of 1 to 3 hours to allow the washout of radioactivity to stabilize, application of rewarding electrical stimulation caused substantial increases in the release of radioactivity in a large number of experiments (Figs. 6A-D; Table II.) Radioactivity levels peaked within several minutes and then declined after prolonged stimulation, due presumably to exhaustion of the reserve of radioactive material. When the current was turned off, the control baseline was rapidly recovered.

Releases of radioactivity were obtained only with highly rewarding electrodes that supported a self-stimulation rate of 1000 responses or more/hour (assessed in a self-stimulation test conducted before the perfusion

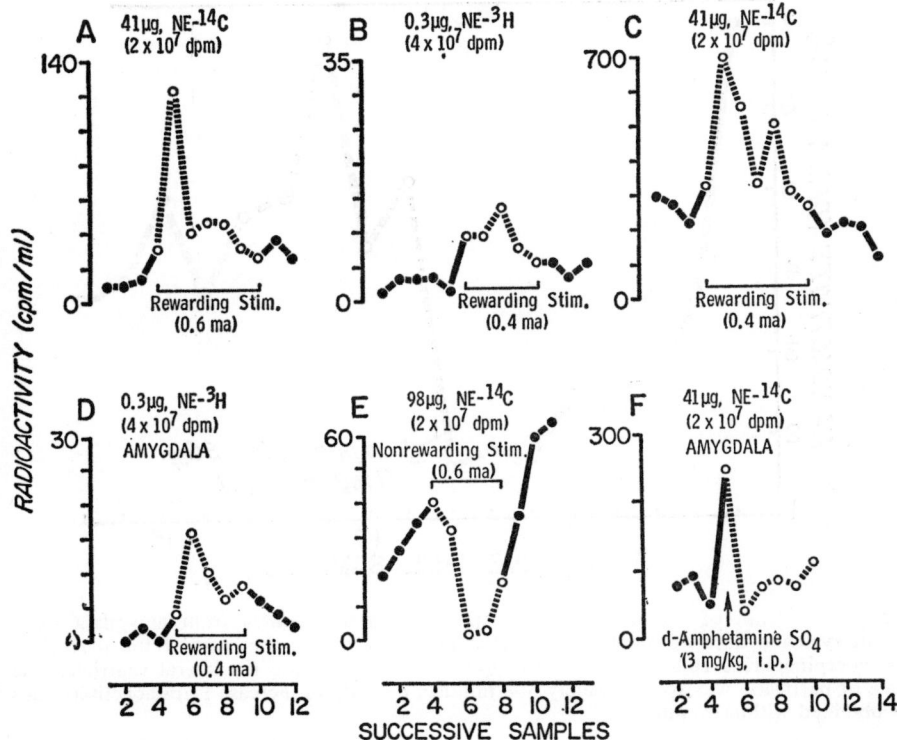

FIG. 6. Sample experiments illustrating the effects of rewarding brain stimulation, of nonrewarding stimulation, and of amphetamine on the release of radioactivity into hypothalamic (A-C, E) and amygdaloid (D, F) perfusates. In C, the monoamine oxidase inhibitor, pargyline (50 mg/kg, i.p.), was injected intraperitoneally 16 hr. before the start of perfusion. The radioisotope tracer and dose used in each experiment are indicated. Each sample contains 1 ml of perfusate. From Stein and Wise (1969).

experiment). Nonrewarding electrodes did not release radioactivity and, in some cases, if the stimulation was punishing or aversive, even inhibited its spontaneous release (Fig. 6E; Table II). In other control experiments, the radioactivity of cortical and thalamic perfusates did not increase during rewarding stimulation (Table II).

In parallel experiments, we used the same perfusion technique to demonstrate the release of norepinephrine into brain perfusates by small intraperitoneal doses of amphetamine. Three mg/kg of d-amphetamine sulfate substantially increased the radioactivity of amygdaloid perfusates in 13 out of 19 cases (Figs. 7 and 8). Doses of amphetamine as high as 5 mg/kg, how-

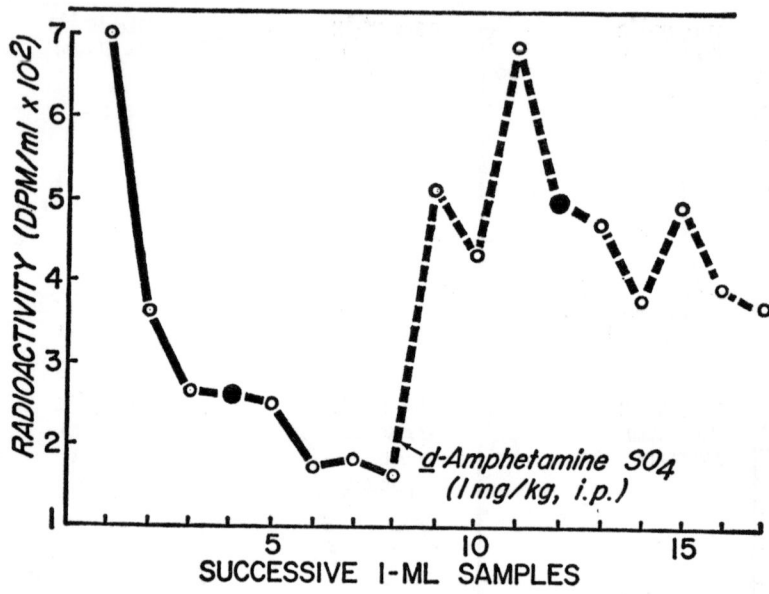

FIG. 7. Release of radioactive norepinephrine and metabolites from amygdala by a small systemic dose of amphetamine. One-half hour before the start of the perfusion, ^{3}H-norepinephrine (0.83 μg, 1.1×10^8 dpm) was injected into the lateral ventricle. The rate of perfusion was approximately 5–8 minutes per ml; an increase in radioactivity thus is obtained within minutes.

ever, did not increase the radioactivity of hypothalamic perfusates. In one experiment in which a DOPA-^{14}C tracer was used, amphetamine caused a three-fold increase in the radioactivity of a hypothalamic perfusate.

Preliminary chemical analyses of the radioactivity in perfusates of

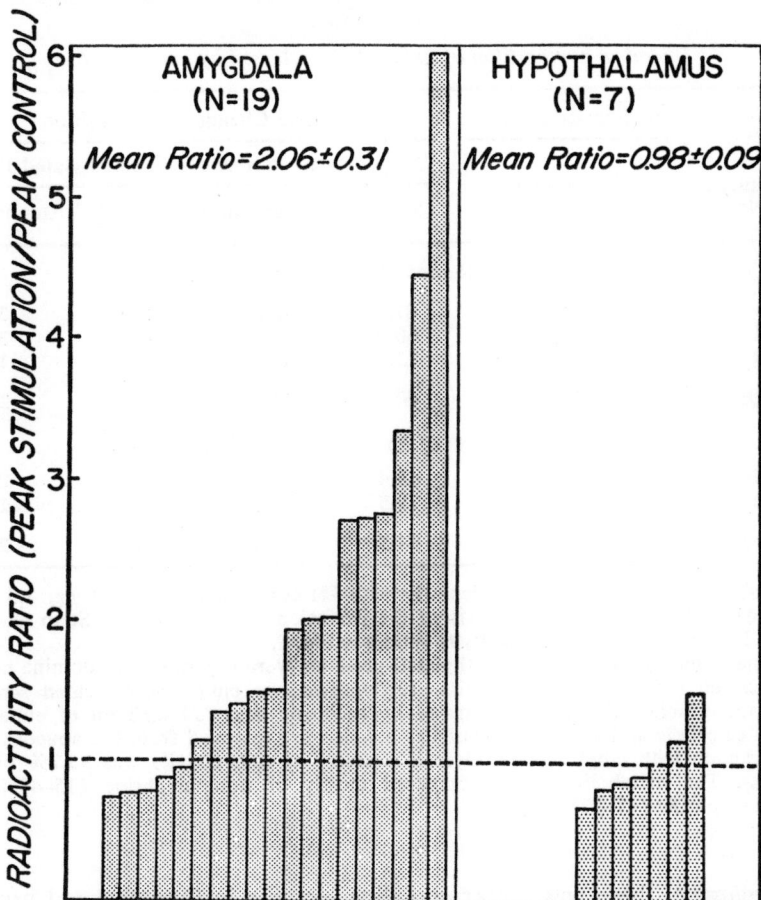

FIG. 8. Amphetamine-induced release of radioactive norepinephrine and metabolites from amygdala, but not from hypothalamus. One to 3 hr. after intraventricular injection of the radioisotope tracer, rats received 45 min. of rewarding electrical stimulation. After a 1 hr. rest period, 3–5 mg/kg of d-amphetamine sulfate was injected intraperitoneally. Radioactivity ratios were calculated from peak values of perfusate samples collected during the 45 min. periods before and after the amphetamine injection. Each bar stands for one experiment. From Stein and Wise (1969).

amygdala before and after the injection of amphetamine are summarized in Table III. In three cases, amphetamine substantially increased the radioactivity of the perfusates, and in two cases it failed to release radioactivity. Significantly, in the three cases in which radioactivity was increased by

Table III

Chemical composition of radioactivity released by amphetamine

Experiment (Rat No.)	Radioactivity Ratio Amphetamine /Control	Relative Chemical Composition			
		O-Methylated Products		Nonmethylated Products	
		Control	Amphetamine	Control	Amphetamine
Release of Radioactivity by Amphetamine					
XH-85	4.75	47.3	69.7	52.7	30.3
XJ-131	2.29	60.0	66.1	40.0	33.9
XJ-130	1.75	73.1	80.5	26.9	19.5
Average	2.93	60.1	72.1	40.0	27.9
Little or No Release of Radioactivity by Amphetamine					
XJ-145	0.94	69.4	72.0	32.5	28.0
XJ-130	1.02	79.5	81.3	20.4	18.8
Average	0.98	74.5	76.6	26.4	23.4

Rats were injected intraventricularly with ^{3}H-norepinephrine (0.94 μg, 1.3×10^8 dpm) one-half hour before the start of the perfusion experiment (See Stein and Wise, 1969). For explanation of radioactivity ratio, see Fig. 8.

The O-methylated and nonmethylated products were separated on alumina columns as described before (Stein and Wise, 1969). The two elutes were treated separately and strongly acidified with concentrated hydrochloric acid (50 μl/2 ml of elute). The neutral catechols and the O-methylated catechols were removed from the aqueous phases by extraction with ethyl acetate. Overall recovery of radioactivity was 95.7% on these columns. The metabolites were composed mostly of norepinephrine (15–49%) and normetanephrine (47–77%).

amphetamine, there was a corresponding increase in O-methylated products, principally normetanephrine. In contrast, in the two cases in which amphetamine failed to increase radioactivity, there was little change in the pattern of metabolites. Although these data are preliminary, it is worth noting that the shift toward O-methylated products is consistent with (a) our earlier observations of the pattern of metabolites after rewarding medial forebrain bundle stimulation (Stein and Wise, 1969), and (b) the biochemical studies of Glowinski and Axelrod (1965). The low amounts of deaminated products in our experiments suggest that amphetamine may release norepinephrine without exposure to intraneuronal monoamine oxidase. Furthermore, the increase in O-methylated products suggests that amphetamine releases norepinephrine into the synapse because the enzyme that forms these products, catechol-O-methyl-transferase, "is present mainly outside the neuron and is believed to be closely associated with the adrenergic receptor" (Axelrod, 1968, p. 66).

EVIDENCE THAT NOREPINEPHRINE IN THE AMYGDALA IS AN INHIBITORY TRANSMITTER

The perfusion work described above indicates that amphetamine releases norepinephrine from amygdala,[2] but not from hypothalamus. This finding of release from forebrain but not from diencephalic structures is consistent with the biochemical observations of Carlsson, Fuxe, Hamberger and Lindquist (1966) that the cortex and other forebrain areas are more sensitive than the brain stem to low doses of amphetamine. Results of both studies thus suggest that amphetamine may act selectively at forebrain sites to produce its facilitatory action on behavior.

What action does the norepinephrine released by amphetamine exert at the cellular level? Is the behavior facilitating effect of amphetamine wholly or partially dependent on the release of norepinephrine into the forebrain? If so, does the facilitating effect depend on the excitation of cells in the forebrain that facilitate behavior, or on the inhibition of cells that suppress behavior? These questions are taken up in more detail below; at this point it will suffice to indicate that a vast literature may be cited which demonstrates suppressor influences of the forebrain on behavior (Kaada, 1951; Hernández-Peón, Chávez-Ibarra, Morgane, and Timo-Iaria, 1963; Brutkowski, 1964; Clemente and Sterman, 1967). Hence, it is quite likely that the norepinephrine released by amphetamine acts mainly as an inhibitory transmitter which depresses the activity of behaviorally suppressant cell groups in the forebrain. In other words, amphetamine may facilitate behavior by a disinhibitory action.

An experiment by Margules (1968) provides somewhat more direct evidence that norepinephrine plays an inhibitory role in the amygdala. Animals were trained in a test in which a lever press response was both rewarded with milk and punished with a brief electrical shock to the feet (Geller and Seifter, 1960). The rate of lever pressing may be precisely regulated by the intensity of the shock, and any degree of behavioral suppression may be obtained by suitable adjustment of the shock level. After response rates

---

[2] Preliminary experiments indicate that self-stimulation of the medial forebrain bundle also causes rapid turnover of norepinephrine in the amygdala and other sites in the limbic system (Wise and Stein, unpublished experiments). In these experiments, tracer amounts of ^{14}C-tyrosine were injected intraventricularly 10 minutes before the start of self-stimulation. In 8 experiments, 15 to 20 minutes of self-stimulation caused an average increase in the specific activity of ^{14}C-norepinephrine of $28\% \pm 15.4$ (S.E.M.) in the limbic system.

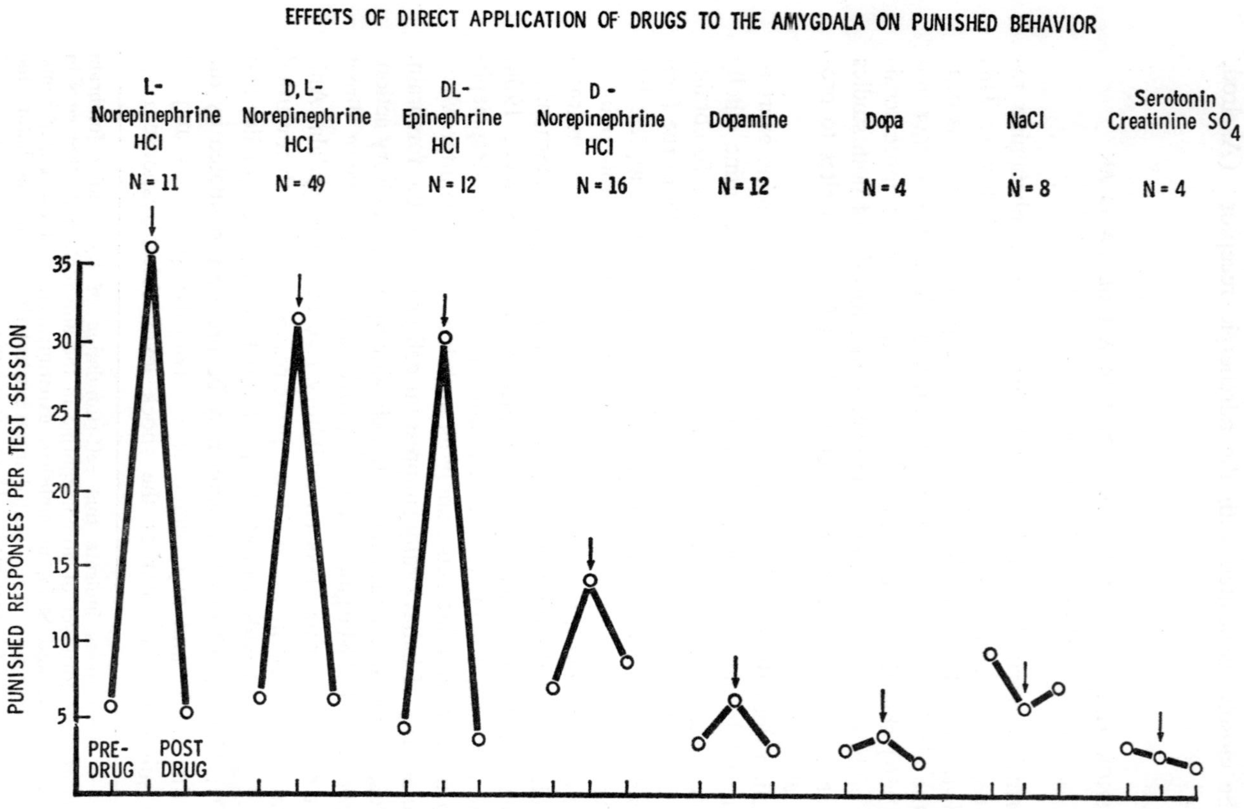

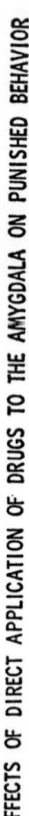

FIG. 9. Disinhibition of punishment suppressed behavior by direct bilateral applications of crystalline *l*- and *dl*-norepinephrine and *dl*-epinephrine to the amygdala. Similar applications of *d*-norepinephrine, dopamine, DOPA, sodium chloride, or serotonin had little or no effect. Animals were dosed twice, 15 minutes before and immediately before, the start of the test, with approximately 10 μg of crystalline material on each side. The mean number of responses in daily test sessions immediately preceding and following the drug

stabilized at a low level, cannulas were implanted bilaterally in the amygdala. Damage produced by penetration of the cannulas into the amygdala partially released the behavior from the suppression induced by punishment, in confirmation of earlier work of Ursin (1965) and Brutkowski (1965). The effects of amygdaloid lesions indicate that this structure normally functions to suppress behavior. Direct application of *l*-norepinephrine HCl crystals to the amygdala further decreased the suppressant effects of punishment very markedly, whereas application of *d*-norepinephrine HCl and sodium chloride had little or no effect. More recent studies (Stein, Margules, Wise and Morris, 1968) indicate that *l*-epinephrine is nearly as active as *l*-norepinephrine, but that dopamine and DOPA are almost inactive (Fig. 9.) Because direct applications of norepinephrine to the amygdala had the same effect as lesions, these noradrenergic synapses would appear to be inhibitory at the cellular level (Stein *et al.*, 1968; Margules, 1968). These behavior facilitating effects of norepinephrine in the punishment test, as well as those in the self-stimulation test reported by Wise and Stein (1969), thus may result from an inhibition of behavior suppressant cell groups in the amygdala and other forebrain structures.

BEHAVIORAL STUDIES

If amphetamine acts by enhancing the release of norepinephrine from terminals of the medial forebrain bundle, then electrical stimulation of the medial forebrain bundle ought to produce the same or similar behavioral effects as the drug. Such seems to be the case. Stimulation of the medial forebrain bundle and amphetamine both retard the extinction of food reinforced behavior and facilitate the performance of a shuttle-box avoidance response (Stein, 1964a; Fig. 10). It has also been demonstrated that rewarding brain stimulation, like amphetamine, speeds up low rates of response generated by a schedule in which only low rates are rewarded (Brady, 1958). Schuster and co-workers (personal communication) and Pickens and Harris (1968) have shown that monkeys and rats can be trained to perform a response for intravenous injection of amphetamine and related stimulant drugs in much the same way that they can be trained to work for electrical stimulation of the medial forebrain bundle; hence, both amphetamine and medial forebrain bundle stimulation have rewarding properties. These similarities in the behavioral effects of medial forebrain bundle stimulation and systemically administered amphetamine are paralleled by similarities in their biochemical effects. Both cause release of norepinephrine and its metabolites into per-

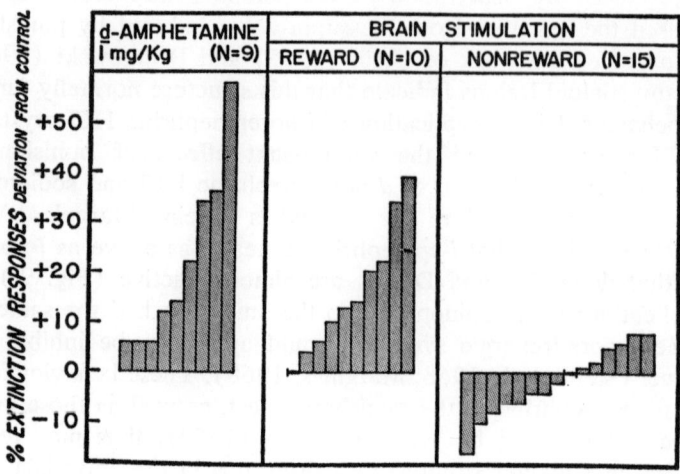
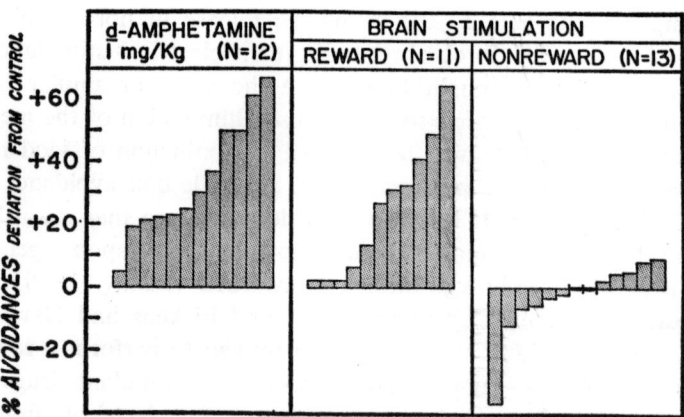

FIG. 10. Summary data showing the facilitating effects of amphetamine and rewarding brain stimulation on the tendency to respond in extinction (upper) or shuttle-box avoidance (lower). Each bar stands for one case and shows the absolute deviation from control induced by the drug or by brain stimulation.

fusates of the amygdala, and both cause shifts in the pattern of metabolites toward O-methylated products (Stein and Wise, 1967, 1969).

A theory of the mechanism of action of drugs should account for features that limit, as well as produce, the drug action. Amphetamine fails to facilitate behavior if the tendency to respond is extremely weak, either because of insufficient reinforcement or because of punishment (Stein, 1964b; Stein and Wise, in press). If the noradrenergic terminals of the medial forebrain bundle were in fact the major site of action of amphetamine, as assumed above, then it would be logical to ask how conditions of insufficient reinforcement or punishment might affect the medial forebrain bundle to limit its responsivity to the drug.

Evidence that the level of activity of the medial forebrain bundle is increased by rewarding stimulation or, more precisely, by the input of stimulation which signals that reward is forthcoming, has been reviewed elsewhere (Stein, 1968; Stein and Wise, in press). In addition, there is reason to believe that activity of the medial forebrain bundle is inhibited by punishment (Stein, 1964c; Stein and Wise, in press). Hence, the input of rewarding and punishing stimulation may jointly determine the level of activity of the medial forebrain bundle. The same factors also appear to determine whether or not amphetamine will be effective. It is therefore conceivable that the conditions of reward and punishment influence the action of amphetamine by regulating the level of activity of the medial forebrain bundle. According to this idea, amphetamine will facilitate behavior if the activity of the medial forebrain bundle exceeds some minimum level. Drug induced facilitation will not occur if the activity of the medial forebrain bundle is reduced below this level. Such reduction could be caused either by insufficient reinforcement or by punishment. A strong feature of this theory is that it nicely accounts for the intriguing observation of Hill (1967; 1969) that pipradol loses its facilitating effect on response rates in extinction if stimuli associated with reinforcement are removed. Presumably, such removal of stimuli that forecast reinforcement would deactivate the medial forebrain bundle and thus eliminate the facilitating effect of the drug.

One may speculate from the foregoing considerations that amphetamine influences the release of norepinephrine only if neurons are firing, and not if they are in the resting state. This suggests that amphetamine does not passively displace norepinephrine from its storage sites. Instead, amphetamine may potentiate the release of norepinephrine induced by nerve impulses. The mechanism of this potentiating action is presently unknown. Whatever the mechanism, however, it is clear that if the effects of amphetamine depend on a potentiation of nervous activity, the drug probably acts on the same functional pools of norepinephrine that mediate physiological function.

SUMMARY

On the basis of the evidence summarized below, we propose that amphetamine facilitates goal-directed or operant behavior by enhancing the release of norepinephrine from terminals of the medial forebrain bundle in the forebrain. We suggest further that the released norepinephrine acts mainly as an inhibitory transmitter at the cellular level, and depresses the activity of behaviorally suppressant cell groups in the forebrain. Thus we assume that amphetamine facilitates behavior by disinhibition rather than by direct excitation.

The theory was suggested initially (Stein, 1964b) by the observation that amphetamine markedly facilitates the rate of self-stimulation of the medial forebrain bundle and other reward areas in the brain. Phenethylamine, the chemical structure common to both amphetamine and norepinephrine, also facilitates self-stimulation in rats pretreated with monoamine oxidase inhibitors. Drugs that block noradrenergic transmission (chlorpromazine), or drugs that deplete the brain of norepinephrine (reserpine, α-methyl-p-tyrosine), decrease the facilitating effects of amphetamine. Conversely, drugs that prevent the reuptake of norepinephrine (cocaine) or block its catabolism (iproniazid) potentiate the action of amphetamine. These studies suggest indirectly that the behavior facilitating action of amphetamine depends on the release of norepinephrine.

In the second series of studies, inhibition by diethyldithiocarbamate of dopamine-β-hydroxylase, the enzyme responsible for the final step in the biosynthesis of norepinephrine, eliminated the facilitating effects of amphetamine on self-stimulation. Intraventricular administration of *l*-norepinephrine reinstated the action of amphetamine. These experiments demonstrate directly that the behavioral facilitating action of amphetamine depends on the availability of norepinephrine in functional pools, and not on *de novo* synthesis *per se*.

In a third series of experiments, terminal areas of the medial forebrain bundle of unanesthetized rats were perfused with Locke's solution via permanently indwelling Gaddum push-pull cannulas. Rewarding electrical stimulation of the medial forebrain bundle released norepinephrine and its metabolites into perfusates of hypothalamus and amygdala. *d*-Amphetamine sulfate (1-3 mg/kg, i.p.) also released norepinephrine and metabolites from amygdala, but not from hypothalamus. Both amphetamine and rewarding brain stimulation caused shifts in the pattern of metabolites toward O-methylated products.

In a fourth series of experiments, direct application of norepinephrine to the amygdala caused the same release of punishment-suppressed behavior as did lesions of amygdala. This and other evidence suggests that the facilitating effects of norepinephrine (whether directly applied or released by amphetamine) result from an inhibition of behaviorally suppressive cell groups in the amygdala and other forebrain structures.

Finally, behavioral studies indicated that rewarding medial forebrain bundle stimulation and amphetamine produced similar effects in a variety of different tests. Both serve as a reward for operant behavior, both retard the extinction of a nonreinforced response, and both facilitate the performance of a shuttle-box avoidance response.

ACKNOWLEDGEMENT

We thank Alfred T. Shropshire and John Monahan for excellent technical assistance in running the experiments, William J. Carmint who performed the histology and assisted in its interpretation, Dr. Barry Berger for useful discussions during various phases of the experiments and during the preparation of the manuscript, and Mrs. Eleanor Buckley for editorial assistance.

REFERENCES

Axelrod, J. (1963): *Clinical Chemistry of Monoamines*, p. 5. Elsevier, Amsterdam.
Axelrod, J. (1968): The fate of norepinephrine and the effect of drugs. *The Physiologist* 11: 63.
Brady, J. V. (1958): *Reticular Formation of the Brain*, p. 689. Little, Brown and Company, Boston.
Brodie, B. B. and Shore, P. A. (1957): A concept for a role of serotonin and norepinephrine as chemical mediators in the brain. *Annals of the New York Academy of Sciences 66:* 631.
Brutkowski, S. (1964): Prefrontal cortex and drive inhibition. In: *The Frontal Granular Cortex and Behavior*, edited by J. M. Warren and K. Akert. McGraw-Hill, New York.
Brutkowski, S. (1965): Functions of prefrontal cortex in animals. *Physiological Reviews 45:* 721.
Burn, J. H. (1957): *The Principles of Therapeutics*, p. 130. Charles C. Thomas, Springfield.
Carlsson, A., Fuxe, K., Hamberger, B. and Lindquist, M. (1966): Biochemical and histochemcal studies on the effects of imipramine-like drugs and (+)-amphetamine on central and peripheral catecholamine neurons. *Acta Physiologia Scandinavica 67:* 481.
Clemente, C. D., and Sterman, M. B. (1967): Basal forebrain mechanisms for internal inhibition and sleep. In: *Sleep and Altered States of Consciousness*, edited by S. S. Kety, E. V. Evarts, and H. L. Williams. Williams & Wilkins, Baltimore.
Geller, I. and Seifter, J. (1960): The effects of meprobamate, barbiturates, *d*-amphetamine and promazine on experimentally induced conflict in the rat. *Psychopharmacologia 1:* 482.
Glowinski, J. and Axelrod, J. (1965): Effect of drugs on the uptake, release, and metabolism of H^3-norepinephrine in the rat brain. *The Journal of Pharmacology and Experimental Therapeutics 149:* 43.

Glowinski, J., Kopin, I. J. and Axelrod, J. (1965): Metabolism of [^{3}H] norepinephrine in the rat brain. *Journal of Neurochemistry 12:* 25.

Hernández-Peón, R., Chávez-Ibarra, G., Morgane, P., and Timo-Iaria, C. (1963): Limbic cholinergic pathways involved in sleep and emotional behavior. *Experimental Neurology 8:* 93.

Hill, R. T. (1967): *A Behavioral Analysis of the Psychomotor Stimulant Effect of a Drug: The Interaction of Pipradol with Conditioned Reinforcers.* Ph.D. thesis, Columbia University, New York.

Hill, R. T. (1969): Facilitation of conditioned reinforcement as a mechanism of psychomotor stimulation. In: *International Symposium on Amphetamines and Related Compounds,* edited by E. Costa and S. Garattini. Raven Press, New York, in press.

Hillarp, N.-Å., Fuxe, K. and Dahlström, A. (1966): Demonstration and mapping of central neurons containing dopamine, noradrenaline, and 5-hydroxytryptamine and their reactions to psychopharmaca. *Pharmacological Reviews 18:* 727.

Kaada, B. R. (1951): Somato-motor, autonomic and electrocorticographic responses to electrical stimulation of rhinencephalic and other structures in primates, cat, and dog. *Acta Physiologica Scandinavica 24:* 1.

Mann, P. J. G. and Quastel, J. H. (1940): Benzedrine (β-phenylisopropylamine) and brain metabolism. *Biochemical Journal 34:* 414.

Margules, D. L. (1968): Noradrenergic basis of inhibition between reward and punishment in amygdala. *Journal of Comparative and Physiological Psychology 66:* 329.

Olds, J. and Milner, P. (1954): Positive reinforcement produced by electrical stimulation of septal area and other regions of rat brain. *Journal of Comparative and Physiological Psychology 47:* 419.

Pickens, R. and Harris, W. C. (1968): Self-administration of *d*-amphetamine by rats. *Psychopharmacologia (Berlin) 12:* 158.

Sedvall, G. C., Weise, V. K. and Kopin, I. J. (1968): The rate of norepinephrine synthesis measured *in vivo* during short intervals; influence of adrenergic nerve impulse activity. *Journal of Pharmacology and Experimental Therapeutics 159:* 274.

Smith, C. B. (1963): Enhancement by reserpine and α-methyl-DOPA of the effects of *d*-amphetamine upon the locomotor activity of mice. *Journal of Pharmacological and Experimental Therapeutics 142:* 343.

Stein, L. (1964a): Amphetamine and neural reward mechanisms. In: *Ciba Foundation Symposium on Animal Behavior and Drug Action,* edited by A. V. S. de Reuch and J. Knight, p. 91. Churchill, London.

Stein, L. (1964b): Self-stimulation of the brain and the central stimulant action of amphetamine. *Federation Proceedings 23:* 836.

Stein, L. (1964c): Reciprocal action of reward and punishment mechanisms. In: *The Role of Pleasure in Behavior,* edited by R. Heath, p. 113. Hoeber, New York.

Stein, L. (1967a): Noradrenergic substrates of positive reinforcement: site of motivational action of amphetamine and chlorpromazine. In: *Neuropsychopharmacology,* edited by H. Brill *et al.,* p. 765. Excerpta Medica Foundation, Amsterdam.

Stein, L. (1967b): Psychopharmacological substrates of mental depression. In: *Antidepressant Drugs,* edited by S. Garattini *et al.,* p. 130. Excerpta Medica Foundation, Amsterdam.

Stein, L. (1968): Chemistry of reward and punishment. In: *Psychopharmacology, A Review of Progress, 1957–1967,* edited by D. H. Efron, p. 105. U.S. Government Printing Office, Washington, D.C. P.H.S. Publication No. 1836.

Stein, L., Margules, D. L., Wise, C. D. and Morris, H. (1968): Noradrenergic inhibition of amygdala by the medial forebrain bundle (MFB) reward system. *Federation Proceedings 27:* 273.

Stein, L. and Seifter, J. (1961): Possible mode of antidepressive action of imipramine. *Science 134:* 286.

Stein, L. and Wise, C. D. (1967): Release of hypothalamic norepinephrine by rewarding electrical stimulation or amphetamine in the unanesthetized rat. *Federation Proceedings 26:* 651.

Stein, L. and Wise, C. D. (1969): Release of norepinephrine from hypothalamus and amygdala by rewarding medial forebrain bundle stimulation. *Journal of Comparative and Physiological Psychology 67:* 189.

Stein, L. and Wise, C. D. (in press): Central Action of Amphetamine. In: *Principles of Psychopharmacology,* edited by W. G. Clark *et al.* Academic Press, New York.

Ursin, H. (1965): The effect of amygdala lesions on flight and defense behavior in cats. *Experimental Neurology 11:* 61.

van Rossum, J. M., van der Schoot, J. B. and Hurkmans, J. A. T. M. (1962): Mechanism of action of cocaine and amphetamine in the brain. *Experientia 18:* 229.

Vane, J. R. (1960): *Adrenergic Mechanisms,* p. 356. Churchill, London.

Weissman, A., Koe, B. K. and Tenen, S. S. (1966): Antiamphetamine effects following inhibition of tyrosine hydroxylase. *Journal of Pharmacology and Experimental Therapeutics 151:* 339.

Wise, C. D. and Stein, L. (1969): Facilitation of brain self-stimulation by central administration of norepinephrine. *Science 163:* 299.

DISCUSSION

DR. MANDELL: I would like to present briefly some related results from our laboratory. We prepared rats with chronic intraventricular cannulas and gave a monoamine oxidase inhibitor four hours before doses of norepinephrine. Then they were run for eight consecutive 15-minute periods on a Sidman Avoidance Task test. The intraventricular norepinephrine (one, two, five and ten μg) did not change the response rate by much. One mg/kg of amphetamine sharply increased the number of responses. Now, when we did the same thing counting errors, that is, counting the number of shocks sustained instead of simply the response rate, we saw a progressive increase in the number of errors. Using the same criteria, we found that the number of errors was reduced after amphetamine. In similar studies, we found that thorazine decreased the response rate and increased the number of errors. A number of other drugs do this. The only drugs that do what norepinephrine appears to do are the ones that are commonly called "minor tranquilizers." Thus we have demonstrated behavioral depression, what we recently reviewed (*Science, 162:* 1442–1452, 1968) as the most common reported effect of norepinephrine when given in such a way that it gets into the brain. Dr. David Segal, in our laboratories, is currently engaged in a broad program involving multiple behavioral measures in rats with chronic, low rate, intraventricular infusions of norepinephrine.

The major objection I have to Dr. Stern's work is his failure to use a more obvious and less generally toxic inhibitor of norepinephrine synthesis, such as the tyrosine hydroxylase inhibitor, α-methyltyrosine, instead of the quite broadly acting disulfiram which affects energy metabolism, chelates trace metals, and does not drop norepinephrine levels in brain to the extent implied by Dr. Stein's discussion. Since dopamine-β-hydroxylase is not a rate-limiting step in the synthesis of norepinephrine, an inhibitor of this step seems less than ideal for the production of a significant decrease in brain norepinephrine levels.

DR. DOMINO: It seems to me we are discussing a very complicated drug. It has effects on self-stimulation which may in part involve norepinephrine release. I think we are going to have to accept Dr. Stein's data for that. Amphetamine effects are complex. It not only has facilitating effects, it has marked depressant effects as well. Some work we have done with Mrs. Olds on self-stimulation emphasizes the very complex effects of amphetamine. Behavioral base line rates, dose, time after injection, size of the operant chamber, etc., are all important parameters to control. There is no question, as Dr. Sulser pointed out, that psychomotor activity at least in reserpinized animals is still present after amphetamine. Clearly this cannot be due to norepinephrine release, but must be some sort of an agonistic action, as Dr. Sulser has pointed out. The comments of Dr. Laties with regard to high-rate or low-rate base lines are important. Amphetamine depresses high rates of behavior and stimulates low rates of behavior, as originally shown by Dews.

Amphetamine-induced repetitive behavior clearly involves the striatum. This means that a dopamine mechanism may be involved. We have studied the effects of amphetamine on EEG activation involving both neocortical and limbic systems. Amphetamine activation is reduced after reserpine. Amphetamine-serotonin interactions are present. As Dr. Sulser pointed out, brain serotonin levels are increased at the height of the psychomotor stimulant effect of amphetamine.

DR. STEIN: I didn't say that.

DR. DOMINO: Dr. Smith has shown this (*J. Pharmacol. Exp. Therap. 147:* 96–102, 1965). We also know that amphetamine releases acetylcholine from the neocortex. Thus amphetamine is a terribly complicated drug.

DR. STEIN: You left out its anorexic effects.

DR. DOMINO: Even if we assume that amphetamine acts through release of norepinephrine in the brain, we still have problems. We are in the habit of speaking about norepinephrine as having unitary behavioral significance. Yet, when one studies the distribution of norepinephrine-containing neurons in the brain, one cannot see a simple pattern. Amphetamine may be releasing norepinephrine at some brain sites and not at others.

DR. STEIN: Isn't it interesting though that you can, under very well-controlled circumstances, give amphetamine and get a graded physiological increase in the rate of behavior despite the complexity in neurochemistry that you correctly point out. This smooth physiological action suggested to Dr. Wise and myself that amphetamine does not simply displace norepinephrine from binding sites, but rather potentiates somehow the physiological release of the transmitter.

DR. DOMINO: I think that's because you are loading the dice in favor of that behavior.

DR. OSMOND: I sometimes wonder whether there are any "simple" drug effects in complex creatures. It might be easier for us if we recognized this more explicitly.

DR. KOPIN: That's close to what I was going to say, except I wanted to point out that if you have many things to explain, you can explain them all if you increase the number of variables. So that we can attempt to explain things, I would like to recall a paper by Eric Kandel in *Science* just about a year ago in which he showed that the frequency of nerve stimulation can have a bearing on the events that happen post-synaptically. At slow rates of stimulation of certain neurons in the abdominal ganglion of *Aplysia,* when there was a small amount of transmitter being transmitted per unit of time, there was a depolarizing effect; when the rate of stimulation was increased, the increased amount of transmitter released per unit of time had a hyperpolarizing effect. Kandel postulated that there were perhaps two receptors for the released transmitter on the same cell, one of which acted as a stimulant and the other as an inhibitor. Thus a low dose in the specific area of the receptor caused one effect; when a larger amount was released some could diffuse away from the immediate site of apposition of the afferent cell to react with more distant receptors of another type. This might help to explain the type of results that Dr. Mandell obtains when exogenous norepinephrine is administered. The exogenous norepinephrine may not be reaching the same receptor in the same specific way as norepinephrine released by a nerve stimulus and giving the type of result obtained by Dr. Stein.

DR. LATIES: I just wanted to make a comment on the use of shock with rats and mice in studying the effects of amphetamine.

Some years ago Dr. Bernard Weiss, Dr. Fred Blanton and I were working with the Sidman Avoidance Task test and, in order to get the animals to learn the task faster, we decided to give them amphetamine to increase their response rate. We postulated that they would avoid more shocks. Instead, we started killing the animals. And so we dropped the project we were studying and started studying how to kill rats. What we found was that rats being shocked have a much lower LD50 to amphetamine than rats not being shocked. We thus found an interaction between the simple reinforcer we were dealing with and the drug we were interested in (Weiss, Laties, and Blanton, *J. Pharmacol. Exp. Therap. 132:* 366–371, 1961).

DR. STEIN: Kety and Glowinski showed that the turnover of norepinephrine produced by shock stress is increased by amphetamine.

DR. LEHRER: Dr. Domino, your statement that you are loading the dice in favor of a particular response system may be interpreted by some people to imply some way of cheating. I think this kind of loading of the dice is precisely what is needed in scientific methodology for eliminating variables, and I am very impressed with Dr. Stein's experiments. I think the more variables you can eliminate in a system in order to look at one particular part of a system the more information and the less noise you are able to obtain.

DR. DOMINO: Obviously in science one should "load the dice." There was no implication of cheating.

I might add that I don't believe that only high rates of behavior are inhibited with amphetamine. In fact, Mrs. Olds and I have some data that even low rates of self-stimulation may also be inhibited by amphetamine.

DR. STEIN: Yes. I tried to indicate before that the high rate-low rate question is not a normalization of response rates, but may have something to do with the fact that amphetamine has opposing effects on behavior. At low doses it produces facilitation and at high doses it disrupts behavior. The base line rate affects the threshold dose of both actions—the higher the baseline rate, the lower the dose that is required for either effect. One explanation of this interaction could be that high rates of behavior are associated with high levels of activity of the median forebrain bundle, and consequently, high rates of release of norepinephrine. If to this high release rate you add the release of norepinephrine caused by amphetamine, then in effect you shift the dose-effect curve of the drug to the left. Thus, you produce facilitation at a lower absolute dose of amphetamine, but also disruption at a lower dose.

DR. KORNETSKY: I have two questions and one comment. You used reserpine, and I don't think you told us what reserpine alone does to self-stimulation. The early work of Olds indicated that reserpine reduces the rate of self-stimulation. This might suggest that your findings may be due to a simple physiological antagonism.

The other question is on your radioactive counts. If you look at just the effect of loud noise or other types of peripheral stimulation, what is the effect?

My comment concerns the importance of the basal level of performance. Dr. Latz in our laboratory did an experiment with discrete avoidance in which he compared the effects of *d*-amphetamine in rats who were at different basal levels of avoidance. The very poor rats were improved by amphetamine, those in the middle range were impaired, and those at the highest level of avoidance showed a slight increase in avoidance behavior.

DR. STEIN: We have many experiments in which we fail to get release. We have no experiments in which we get release unless the electrode is rewarding. Electrodes which fall outside the median forebrain bundle and do not produce self-stimulation do not cause release of norepinephrine. Your explanation of the interaction between reserpine and amphetamine as a physiological (rather than pharmacological) antagonism is logically possible, but the explanation based on norepinephrine depletion seems more appealing when one considers the various lines of evidence that implicate norepinephrine in self-stimulation and in the action of amphetamine, as discussed in detail in our paper in this meeting. There is a very interesting experiment by Dr. Ronald Hill on the effects of various stimulant drugs on extinguished behavior. Hill found that the rate-increasing effects of the drugs depended on the presence of secondary reinforcing cues in the extinction test. Specifically, he presented a tone when food was being delivered in the initial or training phase of his experiment. In the extinction test, the animals were divided into two groups. One group continued to be exposed to the tone when the lever was pressed, although of course no food was delivered. The second group got neither tone nor food. And, as I have indicated, increases in response rate were observed after administration of the stimulants only in the group that received the secondary reinforcing tone.

Hill's experiment thus supports the idea that amphetamine does not simply displace norepinephrine from storage sites in some physiologically passive manner, but that its effects may require the physiological activity of nervous tissue. This may explain the selectivity and smooth physiological action of the drug. This may be the way nature loads the dice in order for us to obtain orderly behavioral effects with amphetamine.

DR. KORNETSKY: How about reserpine by itself? I didn't get the answer to that.

DR. STEIN: Reserpine alone depresses self-stimulation. However, other inhibitors of norepinephrine synthesis or of noradrenergic transmission also block the action of amphetamine. It is true that any one effect can be interpreted a number of ways. But when many drugs and many different types of experiments all point to the same conclusion—that self-stimulation and amphetamine effects depend on transmission at noradrenergic synapses—it seems reasonable to explain the effects of reserpine in terms of its action on norepinephrine.

THE COMBINATION OF GAS CHROMATOGRAPHY AND MASS SPECTROMETRY IN THE IDENTIFICATION OF DRUGS AND HALLUCINOGENS

Bo Holmstedt, M.D.

Department of Toxicology, Karolinska Institute, Stockholm 60, Sweden

The past quarter-century has seen a great change in the approach towards the study of drugs. Important steps include the introduction of the determination of plasma levels as a guideline for dosage, the discovery of the liver microsomal enzymes which metabolize drugs, the emerging significance of genetic variability in metabolism and pharmacologic response, and the introduction of new and more sensitive techniques such as fluorescence spectrophotometry. One would therefore be justified in calling the time from about 1945 to date the era of biochemical pharmacology. It is likely that we are now entering a period wherein physico-chemical techniques will greatly influence progress in drug research. This refers particularly to the combination of gas chromatography and mass spectrometry (GC-MS). The instrument used has been the LKB 9000.

The smallest amounts needed for the scanning of a mass spectrum are in the range of 10–100 ng, and the time required for the practical procedure is relatively short. It must be pointed out that this combined technique gives so much information that it is possible to achieve a *positive identification* of a compound by comparing it to a reference substance. This is not the case when ordinary GC alone is used.

Although the sensitivity of the combined technique may seem to be high, there are situations when it is insufficient. In some drug metabolic studies the amounts available are too small for the scanning of complete mass spectra. It may still be possible, however, to identify by a technique which we have called mass fragmentography. In this technique, advantage is taken of some of the physico-chemical characteristics of a compound or a group of compounds by simultaneous recording of up to three mass numbers representing either the molecular ion or fragments of the molecule. By recording additional characteristic fragments it is possible to obtain information allowing the construction of a "partial mass spectrum," in spite of the fact that the amounts present are insufficient for the scanning of a complete spectrum. This method gives a gain in sensitivity of about 1,000–10,000 times as compared to ordinary GC-MS. The selectivity can be altered by changing the mass numbers monitored which distinguishes mass fragmentography from detectors used in the ordinary GC-system.

The combined gas chromatography–mass spectrometry method and mass fragmentography allow the analysis of drugs in body liquids in very small concentrations. These techniques will no doubt open new fields in clinical pharmacology and toxicology by permitting the measurement of therapeutic or toxic plasma levels of many compounds. Further developments may lead to human pharmacological studies of drugs such as morphine and digitalis which have been used for centuries with only a limited knowledge of the relationship between their pharmacokinetics and their clinical effects. In the future the sensitivity of the techniques mentioned, coupled with the possibility of determining stable isotopes, will permit early experiments in man. "Tracer doses" of drugs labelled with stable isotopes could safely be given even in cases where unstable (*i.e.,* radioactive) isotopes are generally avoided, *e.g.*, in pregnant women and newborns. The appropriate species for further animal experimentations could then be selected on the basis of the knowledge of metabolic patterns in man, eliminating needless and costly experimentation with several species of animals. Correlating the pattern of metabolism with the pharmacologic effects of drugs may also lead to the discovery in man of new active drug metabolites which again do not need extensive testing in animals before clinical trials. It is not unlikely that in the future the pattern of circulating metabolites of any given drug may prove to be as important as the plasma levels of a single compound when correlated with therapeutic effects and side effects. The techniques described together with computer analysis will very likely be the best means to elucidate these problems.[1]

---

[1] This is a summary of the paper given by Dr. Holmstedt. A complete description of the technique and outline of its use will appear in: Hammar, C.—G., Holmstedt, B., Lindgren, J.—E. and Tham, R.: The combination of gas chromatography and mass spectrometry in the identification of drugs and metabolites. *Advances in Pharmacology*, in press.

DISCUSSION

DR. KOPIN: I just wanted to compliment you on a very beautiful technique. I think that this has great potential. Can you tell us how much the instrument costs?

DR. HOLMSTEDT: The cost is high; the instrument costs $60,000, approximately, and then it is preferable to attach a computer to it. You don't have to have one, but it takes a skilled research worker from one to three hours to sit with the UV paper and calculate the mass spectrum, whereas a computer can do it in no time at all. This is an expensive instrument, but as I see it, there is no limit to what you could do with it in pharmacology.

DR. MANDELL: I don't mean to make you the victim of some of the hostility generated in me by our inability to duplicate Dr. Horning's reports of successful derivatization and chromatography of endogenous amines from animal tissue. But since we have been struggling without success with this for almost two years now, do you have some hints about doing regional neurochemical studies on endogenous brain amines using any kind of derivative? Have you had as much trouble as we have had, or is it easy to do?

DR. HOLMSTEDT: I have been in this field since 1963, and it is fairly easy to do the derivatization on the compounds. But before you do this, of course, you need a group separation; that is an essential part of our technique, and this, I feel, is much neglected, including such things as extraction and absorption.

DR. MANDELL: We have had little trouble with the catechol or indole acids. It is the amines which give us difficulty. It is hard to get them to derivatize singly and to work at the low levels at which they are found in brain.

DR. HOLMSTEDT: I think you will find my forthcoming review article in *Advances in Pharmacology* helpful in this regard.

DR. LEHRER: I think that in terms of output per man hour invested, if you were to try to make the derivatives and characterize them at this sensitivity, the cost would rapidly exceed that of the equipment. Besides, you couldn't get this sensitivity out of any other method.

DR. HOLMSTEDT: You are right.

DR. LEHRER: Thus, I think it's rather a reasonable cost for this instrument.

DR. HOLMSTEDT: Yes. Judged by that standard, of course.

DR. EFRON: You mentioned *prominent peak* and *base peak*. If they are two different things, how do you differentiate them?

DR. HOLMSTEDT: Base peak is a general term in mass spectrometry; it is the highest deflection, the highest intensity of any ion in the spectrum, and you calculate the rest from that. This is your one hundred percent point.

DR. USDIN: All of these were free products; none of these you showed were derivatives, or were they?

DR. HOLMSTEDT: Oh yes. There were many derivatives. For example, the nortriptylines. Sometimes you have to make a derivative only for the purpose of getting a peak.

DR. DOMINO: Have you ever applied this to the problem of marihuana?

DR. HOLMSTEDT: No, but a co-worker of mine, Dr. Agurell, has. He is a biochemist, and he has made some good progress in the field.

The thing is that once you get a good gas chromatographic condition you can also turn to mass fragmantography, use the combined instrument and step up your sensitivity 10,000 times. It should be possible to chromatograph the cannabinols in this way.

DR. GESSNER: You have told us your findings relative to the metabolism of 5-methoxy-N, N-dimethyltryptamine. Were these obtained by use of this instrument, or by use of radioactive 5-methoxy-N, N-dimethyltryptamine, or by a combination of these two methods?

DR. HOLMSTEDT: We did both. We used both the labeled compounds and the non-labeled compounds, establishing the structures with this instrument. Actually, there is another thing you can do here. You can use a stream splitter system on the gas chromatograph, get the peaks that are radioactive, and then take their mass spectra.

DR. GESSNER: This is the way you did it?

DR. HOLMSTEDT: We have done it that way, too. All metabolites here have been controlled by their mass spectra, so you know what you have. You don't know, for example, if you have DMPEA in urine unless you have a mass spectrum of it. Everything else is indirect evidence.

DR. GESSNER: Do you know about DMPEA now?

DR. HOLMSTEDT: We have done that. If you take the pink spot positive urine and run it through an ion exchange column, collect the various fractions, establish which fractions have a pink spot, pool them, and run a gas chromatogram, you find three peaks. We have the mass spectra of those. And we will do the peak matching and find out what it is. It's not dimethoxyphenylethylamine. That's for sure.

TURNOVER OF MONOAMINES IN BRAIN UNDER THE INFLUENCE OF MUSCIMOL AND IBOTENIC ACID, TWO PSYCHOACTIVE PRINCIPLES OF *AMANITA MUSCARIA*

Peter G. Waser, M.D., Ph.D. and Petra Bersin, M.D.

Department of Pharmacology, University of Zürich, Zürich, Switzerland

INTRODUCTION

Two years ago, we reported for the first time on some pharmacological and psychotomimetic effects of muscimol and ibotenic acid (Waser, 1967). These compounds had earlier been isolated by separate groups of chemists (Eugster, 1967).

Since then, some new results have been published, and a careful psychiatric study with a small group of volunteers has substantiated some of these findings (Theobald *et al.*, 1968). The symptoms, following injection of the amino acid or of the corresponding amine (Fig. 1), indicate strong central action on the sympathetic system of the brain stem. These symptoms are: a hyperthermic effect in reserpinized mice after muscimol (4 mg/kg i.p.; no change after 10 mg/kg ibotenic acid); central pupillary dilatation after muscimol (4 mg/kg i.p. or 6-8 mg/kg p.o.) or ibotenic acid (16 mg/kg i.p. or p.o.). Another symptom, often caused by hallucinogens, is anorexia after small doses in rats (4.0 mg/kg i.p.) and mice (2.5-3 mg/kg). The central motor system is probably involved with some symptoms in mice, such as ataxia, catalepsy, convulsions and muscle twitches. Sedation of all treated animals is a paramount symptom with higher doses.

In personal experiences after orally taking 15 mg of muscimol, dizziness and ataxia were felt, with stimulation and an elevation of mood, but with no vivid hallucinations and only slight changes in taste and color vision (Waser,

1967). Concentration was difficult, and vision was altered by an endless repetition of "echo pictures" of situations seen a few minutes before (palinopia). Sleep occurred after two hours. With small doses of muscimol (5 mg), mental

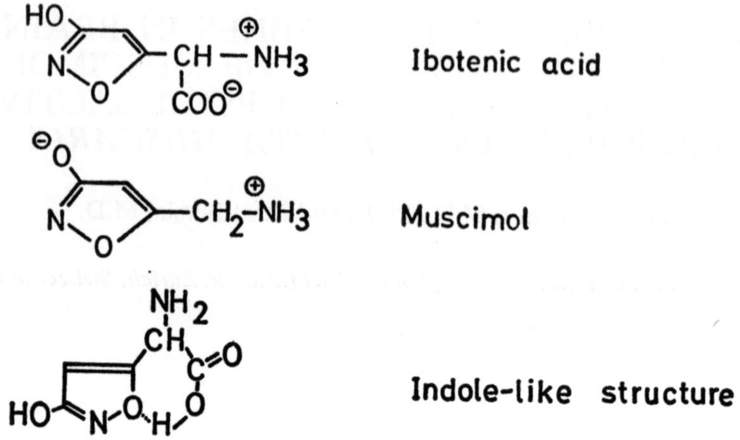

FIG. 1. Molecular structure of muscimol and ibotenic acid.

concentration in psychological tests was improved. Ibotenic acid in doses up to 75 mg had similar, though weaker, effects.

In our present investigation we are trying to correlate these psychotonic effects with neurochemical changes in the brain. Little is known about the distribution of neurotransmitters under the influence of hallucinogenic drugs. Therefore, after preliminary experiments with mice, we limited our studies to investigations of different brain regions of rats injected with muscimol, ibotenic acid or LSD.

METHODS

We used well known methods of fluorescence analysis of norepinephrine (NA), dopamine (DA) and serotonin (5-HT) (Carlsson, 1958; Udenfriend, 1958). Unfortunately, these methods are not very satisfactory, as the recovery of added amines is usually about 90% with a high standard deviation due to the technical procedures.

RESULTS

There is a remarkable similarity between the effects of muscimol and LSD on the overall monoamine concentration in mice and rat brains. Ibotenic acid increased the serotonin concentration in the rat brain, but not in the mouse brain. It increased the catecholamine content in both rat and mouse brain (Fig. 2).

| | Ibotenic acid | | Muscimol | | LSD |
	mouse	rat	mouse	rat	mouse
NA	↑	↑	↓	↓	↓
DA	↑↑	↑	↑↑	↓	↓
5-HT	—	↑↑	↑	↑	↑↑

↑↑ significant change in amine concentration

↑ insignificant change in amine concentration

FIG. 2. Changes in monoamine concentration after drug injection.
↑↑ Significant change in amine concentration
↑ Insignificant change in amine concentration

Our special interest then turned to changes in amine concentration in defined brain areas of the rat. Muscimol (3 mg/kg i.p.) diminished norepinephrine and dopamine concentrations in the 4 sectioned regions: (1) forebrain, hypothalamus, median thalamus and hippocampus, (2) midbrain, (3) pons and (4) medulla oblongata. The same dose of muscimol increased the serotonin concentration in the same parts, most markedly in hypothalamus and midbrain (Fig. 3).

We then investigated the reason for this muscimol-induced increase in serotonin. Forty-eight hours after blocking the serotonin-synthesizing enzyme (tryptophan hydroxylase) with p-chlorophenylalanine (300 mg/kg), the serotonin concentration was markedly reduced to 20% of normal in all

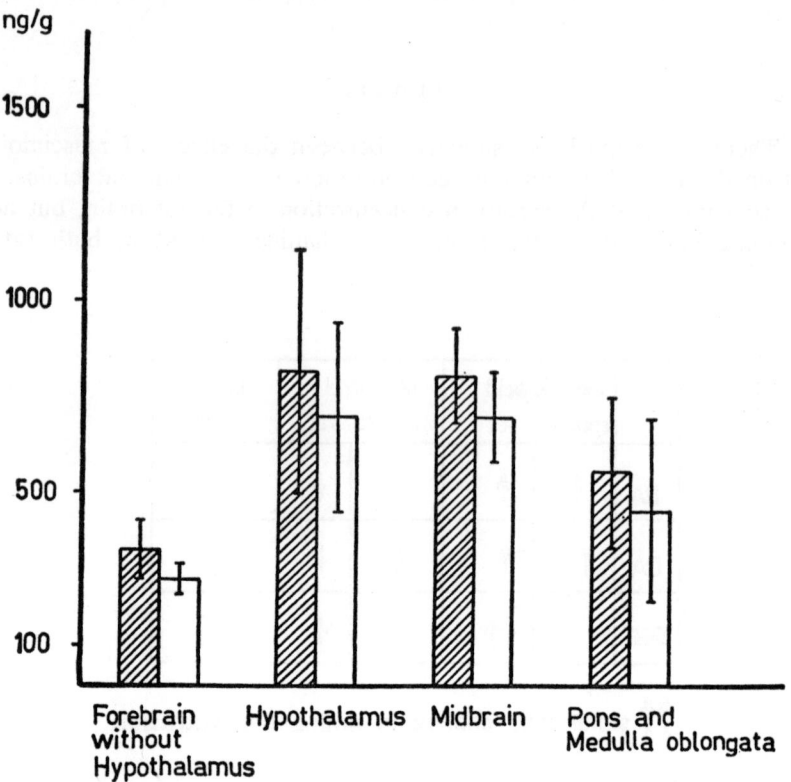

FIG. 3. Serotonin concentration in rat brain after muscimol injection (3 mg/kg i.p.), 2 hours before decapitation. Open bars: controls. Shaded bars: muscimol treatment.

brain regions. Even in this reduced state, muscimol still increased the amine concentration in hypothalamus and midbrain (Fig. 4). Because most serotonergic neurons are located in the hypothalamus and more of their endings in the midbrain, as has been demonstrated by fluorescent histochemical methods, we may conclude that the time-dependent influence of muscimol on serotonin levels is not brought about through an increased rate of synthesis but probably through inhibition of its liberation or degradation.

Finally, the passage of 5-hydroxyindoleacetic acid (5-HIAA) through the neuron membrane was blocked by probenecid (Benemid®) in order to increase the concentration of this metabolite of serotonin. Using this pretreatment, the effect of muscimol on 5-HIAA levels could be observed. The results clearly showed (Fig. 5) that two hours after administration of probenecid (300 mg/kg p.o.), muscimol (3 mg/kg i.p.) tended to mitigate the increase in the concentration of metabolite caused by probenecid block.

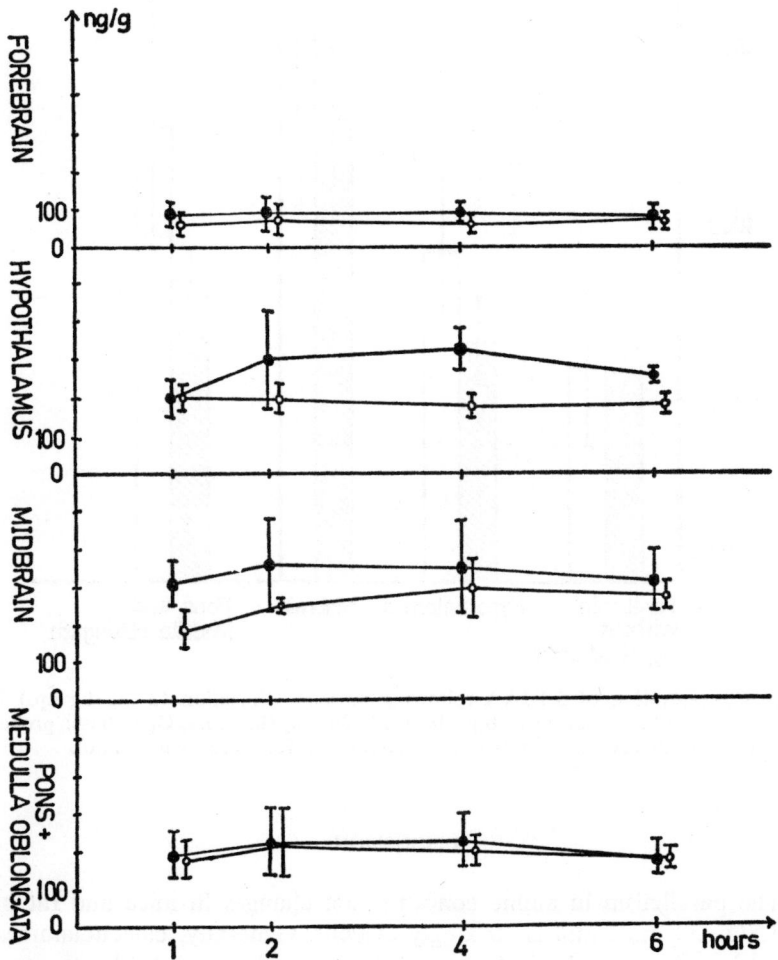

FIG. 4. Serotonin concentration following muscimol injection (3 mg/kg i.p.) in rat brain pretreated 48 hours before with p-chlorophenylalanine (300 mg/kg i.p.). ○ p-CPA alone. ● p-CPA + muscimol.

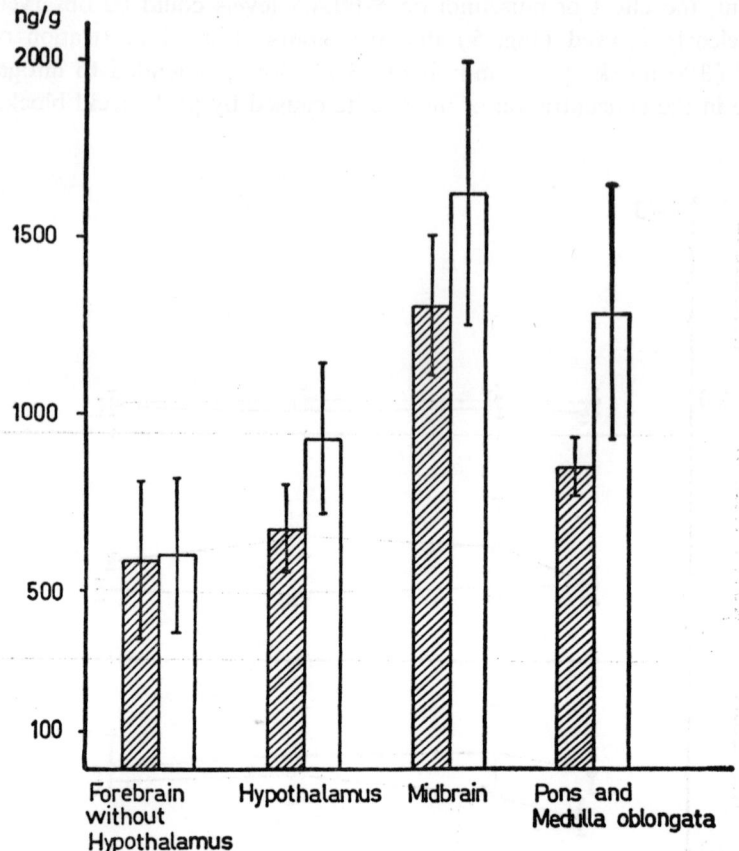

Fig. 5. Concentration of 5-HIAA following muscimol injection (3 mg/kg i.p.) in rat brain pretreated 2 hours before with probenecid (300 mg/kg p.o.). Open bars: probenecid treatment alone. Shaded bars: probenecid pretreatment followed by muscimol.

DISCUSSION

The parallelism in amine concentration changes in mice and rat brains after LSD and muscimol is strikingly evident. Generally, catecholamines are decreased and serotonin is increased by these hallucinogenic compounds. The only exception observed is an increased dopamine content in mice caused by muscimol, instead of a decrease caused by LSD. In contrast to this, ibotenic acid increases the catecholamine concentration, although this compound has a more sedative action.

The increase in dopamine concentration induced by ibotenic acid and muscimol may be related to the observed extrapyramidal symptoms.

All three psychotropic drugs increased serotonin concentration mainly in the hypothalamus and midbrain regions. Although the synthesizing enzyme was blocked by *p*-chlorophenylalanine, muscimol increased the serotonin content. On the other hand, it decreased the formation of 5-HIAA. These effects must be caused by a diminished turnover or liberation of serotonin from neurons, perhaps resulting from a diminshed pulse flow in the neurons.

Substances with LSD-like behavioral effects, *e.g.*, mescaline, *l*-acetyl-LSD, psilocybin or DMT, also tend to produce an increase in brain serotonin concentration (Aghajanian and Freedman, 1967). The isoxazol ring of muscimol and ibotenic acid resembles ring B of the indole system of some hallucinogenic compounds. By hydrogen bonding, another heterocyclic ring (A or C of LSD) might be formed (Snyder and Richelson, 1967).

SUMMARY

Muscimol and ibotenic acid, two psychotomimetic principles of *Amanita muscaria*, have effects similar to those of LSD on norepinephrine, dopamine and serotonin concentrations in the brains of mice and rats. The increased serotonin concentration in the hypothalamus and midbrain is probably caused by a diminished turnover or liberation of serotonin, perhaps resulting from a diminished pulse flow in the serotonergic neurons.

REFERENCES

Aghajanian, G. K. and Freedman, M. D.: Biochemical and morphological aspects of LSD pharmacology. In: *Psychopharmacology, A Review of Progress, 1957–1967*, edited by Daniel H. Efron, pp. 1185–1193. U.S. Public Health Service publication no. 1836 (1968).

Carlsson, A. and Waldeck, B.: A fluorimetric method for the determination of dopamine. *Acta Physiol. Scand. 44:* 293–298 (1958).

Eugster, C. H.: Isolation, structure and synthesis of central-active compounds from *Amanita muscaria* (L. ex Fr.) Hooker. In: *Ethnopharmacologic Search for Psychoactive Drugs*, edited by D. H. Efron, B. Holmstedt and N. S. Kline, pp. 416–418. U.S. Public Health Service publication no. 1645 (1967).

Snyder, S. H. and Richelson, E.: Relationship between the conformation of psychedelic drugs and their psychotropic potency. In: *Psychopharmacology, A Review of Progress, 1957–1967*. Edited by D. H. Efron, pp. 1199–1210. U.S. Government Printing Office, Washington, D.C. P.H.S. Publication No. 1836 (1968).

Theobald, W., Kunz, H. A., Steiger, E. G., Bück, O., Krupp, P. and Heimann, H.: Pharmakologische und experimentalpsychologische Untersuchungen mit zwei Inhaltsstoffen des Fliegenpilzes. *Arzneim.-Forsch. 18:* 311–315 (1968).

Udenfriend, S., Weissbach, H. and Brodie, B. B.: Assay of 5-HT and related metabolite enzymes and drugs. *Meth. Biochem. Anal. 6:* 95–130 (1958).

Waser, P. G.: The pharmacology of *Amanita muscaria*. In: *Ethnopharmacologic Search for Psychoactive Drugs,* edited by D. H. Efron, B. Holmstedt and N. S. Kline, pp. 419–438. U.S. Government Printing Office, Washington, D.C. P.H.S. Publication No. 1645 (1967).

DISCUSSION

DR. EFRON: Thank you very much.

DR. SHULGIN: You mentioned that muscimol had some side-effects at a dose of about 30 mg.

DR. WASER: At the level of 5, 10, and 15 mg as a dose.

DR. SHULGIN: How much mushroom?

DR. WASER: About five mushrooms would satisfactorily intoxicate as well as 15 mg muscimol or 40 mg ibotenic acid. The same amount is contained in 300 to 400 g of mushrooms.

And there is something else I have not told you. You will find muscimol as an excretion product. A very interesting negative experiment was done by a colleague and me. He ate mushrooms and claimed he had hallucinations. I didn't believe him; I then ate a double amount of mushrooms and had no hallucinations or anything, and both of us had no muscimol in the urine.

DR. SHULGIN: And after the mushroom?

DR. WASER: He had some provoked hallucinations which are not explained by muscimol.

SESSION III

PHYSIOLOGY, NEUROPATHOLOGY AND NEUROCHEMISTRY

Morris A. Lipton, M.D., Ph.D. and Wallace D. Winters, M.D., Ph.D., Co-Chairmen

SESSION III

BIOLOGY, NEUROPATHOLOGY AND NEUROCHEMISTRY

LSD AND MESCALINE: COMPARISON OF EFFECTS ON SINGLE UNITS IN THE MIDBRAIN RAPHÉ

George K. Aghajanian, M.D., Michael H. Sheard, M.D., and
Warren E. Foote, Ph.D.

*Department of Psychiatry, Yale University School of Medicine, and
The Connecticut Mental Health Center, New Haven, Connecticut 06519*

Although LSD (*d*-lysergic acid diethylamide) and mescaline (3,4,5-trimethoxyphenylethylamine) are disparate in chemical structure, their effects on autonomic function and behavior are remarkably similar. However, a common mechanism of action cannot be assumed on the basis of like effects, since the same phenomenologic endpoints in behavior may be reached via different pathways. Perhaps more pertinent to the issue of sites of action has been the demonstration that cross tolerance occurs between LSD and mescaline. This relationship has been shown in various species, including man (Balestrieri, 1959) and rat (Appel and Freedman, 1968). Cross tolerance can indicate a sharing of some chemical or cellular site intimately related to mode of action. However, there are a number of other mechanisms that could account for the phenomena of tolerance and cross tolerance, *e.g.*, increased degradation or decreased uptake. Thus, demonstration of cross tolerance does not necessarily indicate an interaction at sites immediately relevant to autonomic or behavioral effects. Nevertheless, it remains a question of considerable theoretical interest as to whether LSD and mescaline produce their similar effects by acting at a common site.

Recently, we have found a specific set of neurons in the brain which are exquisitely sensitive to LSD, and this provides an opportunity to compare the actions of LSD and mescaline on a cellular system. In particular, we have found that LSD in minute parenteral doses (10-20 μg/kg) causes an inhibition of the spontaneous firing of single neuronal units in the midbrain raphé nuclei of the rat (Aghajanian *et al.*, 1968). The entire population of raphé units, which have a characteristic slow rate (~ 30-60 spikes/min) and regular rhythm, are uniformly inhibited by LSD. The results of a typical experiment are illustrated in Fig. 1. The LSD inhibitory effect is specific for raphé units; in other areas of the midbrain (*e.g.*, reticular formation, pontine nuclei) units are mostly unaffected by small doses of LSD. Occasionally, non-raphé units show an increased rate of firing after LSD, but usually at doses higher than are required to just inhibit the raphé units. The dose of LSD needed for threshold inhibition of raphé neurons (~ 10 μg/kg i.v.) is at or below that required for demonstrable behavioral changes.

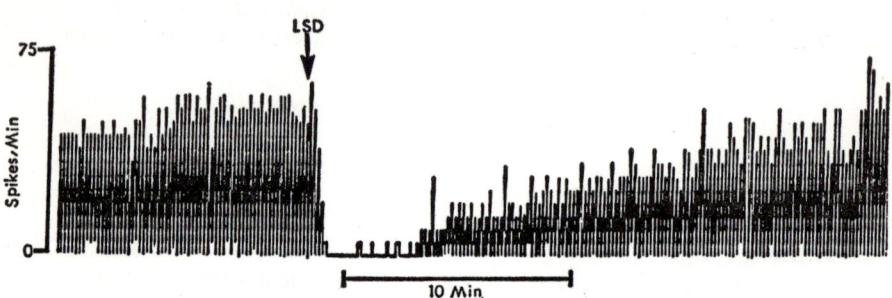

FIG. 1. Inhibition by LSD of a single neuronal unit in the dorsal raphé nucleus.

The spontaneous rate of the unit in this experiment was about 60 spikes/min. An intravenous injection of LSD (10 μg/kg) induces a rapid slowing and temporary cessation of activity. The original rate is gradually restored over a period of about 20 minutes. Rate is calibrated in terms of "spikes/min;" each pen deflection represents a ten second sampling of unit activity.

Although the extreme degree of sensitivity to LSD was unexpected, there is some prior basis for considering that LSD might have an influence on the activity of raphé neurons. The neuronal perikarya which comprise the midbrain raphé nuclei have been shown to contain serotonin (5-HT) by the fluorescence histochemical method (Dahlström and Fuxe, 1965). Although the discovery that the 5-HT in the brain is contained within a specific neuronal system is recent, hypotheses about a possible relationship between LSD and 5-HT are quite long standing. Gaddum (1953) and Woolley (1954) independently suggested, partly on the basis of interactions in peripheral systems, that LSD might produce its behavioral effects by interfering with the normal action of 5-HT in the brain. The biochemical studies of Freedman (1961) showed that LSD induces an increase in 5-HT concentration in the brain. It was later seen that this increase was accompanied by a fall in the concentration of 5-hydroxyindoleacetic acid (5-HIAA), the principle metabolite of 5-HT (Rosecrans *et al.*, 1967). Thus it was evident that LSD had an influence on the metabolism of 5-HT in the brain, although the mechanism for this effect was unknown. One way LSD could decrease 5-HT metabolism would be by inhibiting enzymes involved in its degradation. However, LSD was shown not to inhibit monoamine oxidase, the initial enzyme involved in the metabolism of 5-HT (Freedman and Giarman, 1962).

With the advent of detailed knowledge of the anatomy of the 5-HT-containing neuronal system, the opportunity arose for an experimental analysis of the effect of LSD on these neurons. The fact that the perikarya of these cells are clustered together in the raphé nuclei made it feasible to undertake stimulation and recording studies. Electrical stimulation of the raphé nuclei was found to induce an increased turnover of brain 5-HT as evidenced by a fall in the amine and an increase in the metabolite, 5-HIAA (Aghajanian *et al.*, 1967; Sheard and Aghajanian, 1968). Since the converse was seen after LSD, it was suggested that the inhibition of raphé units by LSD may account for the reduced metabolism of 5-HT caused by the drug (Aghajanian *et al.*, 1968). This possibility is consistent with the notion that, after inhibition of synthesis in the spinal cord and brain, LSD may retard 5-HT depletion by decreasing impulse flow (Andén *et al.*, 1968). Of course, another way LSD could reduce turnover could be by directly inhibiting 5-HT release (Chase *et al.*, 1967). In any case, the mechanism by which LSD induces an inhibition of 5-HT neurons is not known. There has been speculation that if LSD had a postsynaptic 5-HT-like effect, this would signal "excess 5-HT," leading to a neuronal feedback inhibition of the 5-HT neurons (Aghajanian and Freedman, 1968; Andén *et al.*, 1968). Alternative mechanisms are a direct inhibitory action of LSD on raphé neurons, or an indirect effect at sites other than those related to the 5-HT postsynaptic cells.

A large variety of substances were found not to inhibit raphé units. Such diverse compounds as amphetamine and chlorpromazine are not inhibitory. In fact, amphetamine induces an increase in the rate of firing of some raphé units (Foote *et al.*, 1969). Peripheral adrenergic activation does not seem to play a modulating role, since large doses of *l*-norepinephrine given parenterally do not alter raphé activity. 5-Hydroxytryptophan at high doses (100 mg/kg) may cause a slight slowing of raphé units, but it never inhibits completely. Apart from LSD, the only agents of those tested which inhibited raphé neurons were 2-brom-LSD (BOL) and N,N-dimethyltryptamine (DMT) (Aghajanian, Sheard and Foote, in preparation). For these compounds, as with LSD, inhibition of raphé units was uniformly observed. BOL has about 1/20 and DMT 1/25 the inhibitory potency of LSD; this is in the approximate ratio of their behavioral potencies in the rat (Appel and Freedman, 1965; Smithies *et al.*, 1967). However, BOL, unlike LSD and DMT, does not inhibit all raphé units completely.

We had a strong expectation that mescaline, like LSD, BOL and DMT, would inhibit the raphé units. The first few cells tested did in fact become inhibited after intravenous injections of mescaline. The threshold dose for a complete cessation of firing was between 2 and 4 mg/kg of mescaline sulfate (Fig. 2). Thus, mescaline seemed an effective inhibitor of raphé neurons,

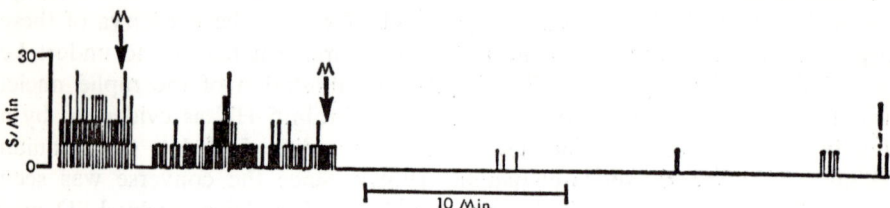

FIG. 2. Inhibition by mescaline of a dorsal raphé unit. An intravenous injection of 2 mg/kg of mescaline (M) induces a brief inhibition. A second injection of mescaline (4 mg/kg) causes a prolonged inhibition with recovery beginning about 20 minutes after injection.

although it had less than 1/100 the potency of LSD; this ratio corresponds to the relative potency in behavioral tests in the rat (Appel and Freedman, 1965). However, when the effects of mescaline were observed in a larger series of raphé cells, it became apparent that not all the raphé cells were responsive to mescaline. Figure 3 illustrates a raphé unit which is typically inhibited by LSD but which is unaffected by mescaline. We have now observed the effects of mescaline on 24 raphé cells (mostly in the dorsal raphé nucleus), and 14 of them have been unresponsive even to large doses of this agent. This result was quite surprising because responses to all the other inhibitory drugs (*i.e.*, LSD, BOL and DMT) were invariably observed in raphé cells.

Moreover, it is now becoming evident that there is a non-random pattern of response to mescaline. The only units that have been inhibited by mescaline are located in the ventral portion of the dorsal raphé nucleus. It is unclear at this time whether or not this selectivity of response indicates a functional differentiation of various portions of the raphé nucleus. The dorsal raphé neurons do receive a catecholamine fiber input (Fuxe, 1965), and variations in this innervation could account for differential responses to mescaline. However, a closer analysis of the pattern of distribution of the catecholamine fibers in this nucleus would be necessary to establish such a correlation. Of

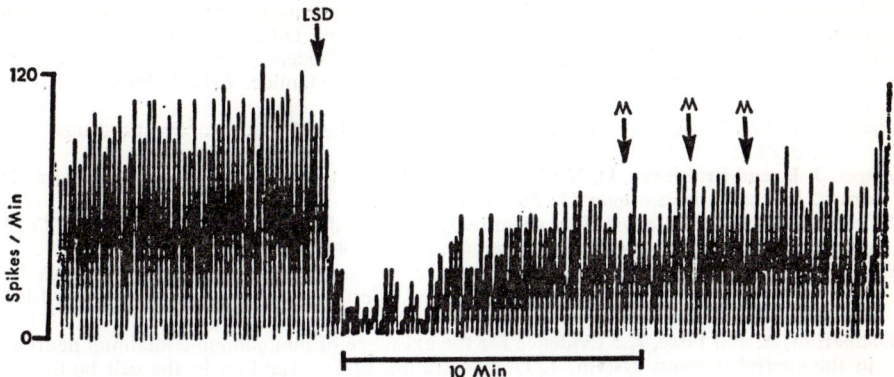

FIG. 3. Failure of mescaline to inhibit a dorsal raphé unit. This unit was first shown to be sensitive to LSD; a dose of 10 µg/kg produced a brief slowing of activity. Repeated doses of mescaline (M) reaching a total of 12 mg/kg failed to give any inhibition. Such a failure of mescaline to inhibit was also demonstrated in cells where there had not been a prior injection of LSD.

course, the major portions of the inputs to raphé neurons are unknown, and it is difficult to evaluate their contribution in determining the response to mescaline.

We began this study with the need to explain the similarities between the behavioral effects of LSD and mescaline. A close relationship between the two drugs was indicated by the existence of cross-tolerance. Such lines of evidence, although suggestive, cannot provide definitive proof that two drugs share a common site of action. Studies on the raphé neurons have provided a means of testing for a common site of action on a cellular level. The results of our experiments are unexpectedly complicated in that the effects of mescaline on raphé units overlap, but are not identical to, those of LSD. Thus a second need emerges, that of explaining the basis for differences as well as similarities, at least in the rat, between the actions of mescaline and LSD on single neurons. The finding of differences on a cellular level in turn leads to questions concerning the autonomic and behavioral effects of the two drugs. For example, do the subtle differences between the effects of mescaline and LSD on autonomic function and behavior (Wolbach *et al.*, 1962) correspond to a difference in the pattern of action on raphé units?

REFERENCES

Aghajanian, G. K., Rosecrans, J. A. and Sheard, M. H.: Serotonin: release in the forebrain by stimulation of midbrain raphé. *Science* 156: 402–403 (1967).

Aghajanian, G. K., Foote, W. E. and Sheard, M. H.: Lysergic acid diethylamide: sensitive neuronal units in the midbrain raphé. *Science* 161: 706–708 (1968).

Aghajanian, G. K. and Freedman, D. X.: In: *Psychopharmacology; A Review of Progress,* edited by D. H. Efron. U.S. Government Printing Office, Washington (1968).

Andén, N.-E., Corrodi, H., Fuxe, K. and Hokfelt, T.: Evidence for a central 5-hydroxytryptamine receptor stimulation by lysergic acid diethylamide. *Brit. J. Pharmacol. 34:* 1-7 (1968).

Appel, J. B. and Freedman, D. X.: The relative potencies of psychotomimetic drugs. *Life Sci. 4:* 2181-2186 (1965).

Appel, J. B. and Freedman, D. X.: Tolerance and cross-tolerance among psychotomimetic drugs. *Psychopharmacologia 13:* 267-274 (1968).

Balestrieri, A. and Fontanari, D.: Acquired and crossed tolerance to mescaline, LSD-25 and BOL-148. *A.M.A. Arch. Gen. Psychiat. 1:* 279-282 (1959).

Chase, T. N., Breese, G. R. and Kopin, I. J.: Serotonin release from brain slices by electrical stimulation: regional differences and effect of LSD. *Science 157:* 1461-1463 (1967).

Dahlström, A. and Fuxe, K.: Evidence for the existence of monoamine-containing neurons in the central nervous system. 1. Demonstration of monoamines in the cell bodies of brain stem neurons. *Acta Physiol. Scand. 62:* Suppl. 232, 1-55 (1965).

Foote, W. E., Sheard, M. H. and Aghajanian, G. K.: Differential effects of LSD and amphetamine on midbrain raphé units. *Nature, 222:* 567-569 (1969).

Freedman, D. X.: Effects of LSD-25 on brain serotonin. *J. Pharmacol. Exp. Therap. 134:* 160-166 (1961).

Freedman, D. X. and Giarman, N. J.: LSD-25 and the status and level of brain serotonin. *Ann. N.Y. Acad. Sci. 96:* 98-106 (1962).

Fuxe, K.: Evidence for the existence of monoamine neurons in the central nervous system. IV. Distribution of monoamine nerve terminals in the central nervous system. *Acta Physiol. Scand. 64:* Suppl. 247, 41-85 (1965).

Gaddum, J. H.: Antagonism between lysergic acid diethylamide and 5-hydroxytryptamine. *J. Physiol. 121:* 15P (1953).

Rosecrans, J. A., Lovell, R. A. and Freedman, D. X.: Effects of lysergic acid diethylamide on the metabolism of brain 5-hydroxytryptamine. *Biochem. Pharmacol. 16:* 2011-2021 (1967).

Sheard, M. H. and Aghajanian, G. K.: Stimulation of the midbrain raphé: effect on serotonin metabolism. *J. Pharmacol. Exp. Therap. 163:* 425-430 (1968).

Smithies, J. R., Bradley, R. J. and Johnston, V. S.: The behavioral effects of some derivatives of mescaline and N,N-dimethyltryptamine in the rat. *Life Sci. 127:* 1887-1893 (1967).

Wolbach Jr., A. B., Isbell, H. and Miner, E. J.: Cross tolerance between mescaline and LSD-25. With a comparison of the mescaline and LSD reactions. *Psychopharmacologia 3:* 1-14 (1962).

Woolley, D. W. and Shaw, E.: A biochemical and pharmacological suggestion about certain mental disorders. *Proc. Natl. Acad. Sci. 40:* 228-231 (1954).

DISCUSSION

DR. DOMINO: Could you define the parameters of stimulation? Usually neurons speed up their rate of turnover of a transmitter, which would of course explain the increase in 5-HIAA levels. I am a little surprised that you find a significant, although small, decrease in 5-HT levels. It would appear that the raphé nuclei cannot keep up with the synthesis of 5-HT. Therefore your stimulation procedures must be rather demanding.

DR. AGHAJANIAN: Yes, they are demanding, but only in a relative sense. We stimulated at 10 pulses per second, which ordinarily would not seem like a high rate of stimulation, but it is important to note that raphé units have very low spontaneous rates. With lower rates of stimulation we fail to see the fall in 5-HT levels, but still see some increase in 5-HIAA levels.

DR. DOMINO: What is your pulse wave form?

DR. AGHAJANIAN: It is a biphasic square wave pulse, one millisecond in duration.

DR. DOMINO: Is this measured as current or as voltage?

DR. AGHAJANIAN: This is by voltage.

DR. DOMINO: You don't know what the current wave form is?

DR. AGHAJANIAN: That is correct. The stimulation happens to be 6 volts, but that voltage was not critical. The effect on 5-HIAA (but not on 5-HT) levels was obtained over an enormous range of voltages and frequencies of stimulation. The only thing we found to be critical was the site of the electrode. The electrode had to be either in or very close to the raphé nucleus.

DR. DEMENT: It is nearly a cliché that a state of behavioral suppression may involve so-called sleep processes, which in this case may relate to the raphé system. My question is simply, do you feel that behavioral state did change the turnover rate of 5-HT? Not that it makes any difference to the results.

DR. AGHAJANIAN: I think that almost any stimulus will change the turnover of 5-HT in a transitory way. It is a very responsive system.

DR. DEMENT: In the anesthetized animal did you find an increase in turnover of 5-HT in terms of percentage of controls? In other words, I am asking whether the anesthetic state requires the activity of the raphé system?

DR. AGHAJANIAN: The turnover of 5-HT was lower in anesthetized as compared to unanesthetized rats, but not a great deal lower.

A VOICE: Do you know what behavioral signs occurred during raphé stimulation in the unanesthetized rats?

DR. AGHAJANIAN: There were behavioral signs in the unanesthetized animals, and, in brief, they consisted of enhanced reactivity to sensory stimuli. This was not the case when regions lateral to the raphé were stimulated.

A VOICE: Were any behavioral tests done to see whether it was positive or negative reinforcement?

DR. AGHAJANIAN: No.

DR. STEIN: Were your controls unstimulated or unimplanted?

DR. AGHAJANIAN: The controls were implanted with electrodes, but no current was passed.

DR. STEIN: I ask that because the electrode itself might cause some destruction and account for the drop in 5-HT.

DR. AGHAJANIAN: There is a drop in 5-HT but only on a chronic basis. When an electrode is placed in the raphé nucleus there is destruction of some neurons and eventually axonal degeneration.

A VOICE: What happens to the cells in the central gray after LSD?

DR. AGHAJANIAN: The breakdown of the data would be something like this: We have tested cells in various parts of the central gray, in the third and fourth nerve nuclei and in other midbrain areas. Many cells show a slight increase in rate of discharge after LSD. We found an occasional cell outside the raphé that has slowed in firing rate after LSD. But these cells never stop completely, even at very high doses.

Incidentally, the threshold for getting responses in cells outside the raphé is higher, so that is a distinguishing feature. It takes about 40 or 50 μg/kg to get the increased response rate of some cells outside the raphé. Perhaps half to two-thirds of the non-raphé cells actually were not affected at all.

DR. STEIN: How do you know which are the 5-HT-containing cells and which are not?

DR. AGHAJANIAN: From the fluorescence microscopy it appears that the only type of neurons present in the raphé are those showing fluorescence for 5-HT.

DR. FREEDMAN: Do you see any tolerance in the raphé cells to LSD or mescaline?

DR. AGHAJANIAN: No. But we haven't studied this on a meaningful tolerance schedule. We have given repeated threshold doses of LSD to get several inhibition and recovery cycles in a row, but what we haven't done—and this is one of the things we expect to do shortly—is to prepare rats that have been on a tolerance schedule (*i.e.,* receiving daily doses of LSD) to see if their threshold would be different.

DR. STEIN: I was very impressed by those findings. They are quite interesting. And I am curious as to how you conceive these actions, which apparently are on cell bodies, to influence transmission at serotonergic synapses which presumably would be located outside the raphé nucleus.

DR. AGHAJANIAN: Let us consider an axon, a raphé unit terminating in the hypothalamus or elsewhere in the forebrain. There would be a post-synaptic cell although it would be unidentified from a chemical standpoint. This post-synaptic cell might be involved in a feedback loop to the original cell, either directly, or via intermediate cell. Now, one can postulate that LSD could act at a post-synaptic receptor site by either blocking or mimicking the action of 5-HT released onto it by the serotonergic cell. If LSD blocked the action of 5-HT, a positive feedback should result. The message carried by the feedback loop would be that the 5-HT output of the cell is insufficient or blocked and the raphé units would be accelerated in rate. On the other hand, if LSD were mimicking 5-HT at the post-synaptic site, the message conveyed over the feedback loop would be that an excessive 5-HT output was occurring, and the effect would be to shut off the raphé unit. This would be a negative feedback effect. Our data fits best with the latter possibility, since LSD produces an inhibition of raphé unit activity.

DR. STEIN: We do know that electrical stimulation of the raphé and LSD action have opposite effects.

DR. AGHAJANIAN: How do we know that?

DR. STEIN: From your earlier studies.

DR. AGHAJANIAN: I am not sure just how to compare the effects of electrical stimulation of the raphé nuclei and LSD action. They do not have opposite effects. They certainly share one effect: LSD in various animals, including rat and man, produces an enhanced responsivity to sensory stimuli. One particular aspect of this is a failure of habituation[1] to repeated stimuli, an effect we also get with raphé stimulation.

DR. STEIN: I was referring to your data showing levels of 5-HT and levels of 5-HIAA going in the opposite direction depending on the procedures used: Electrical stimulation of the raphé, or LSD injection.

DR. AGHAJANIAN: Yes, but I think those data precisely fit the interpretation that raphé stimulation has an LSD-like action.

DR. LEHRER: One of the obvious experiments that suggests itself would be to supply the drug iontophoretically through a double-barrelled electrode. Have you considered doing this, or have you done it?

DR. AGHAJANIAN: We are collaborating on such a study with Dr. Floyd Bloom, and it is just getting under way. Only a few cells have thus far been tested, but let me say this: I wouldn't reject the idea that LSD has a direct action on the cells.

DR. SNYDER: Have any results been forthcoming yet?

DR. AGHAJANIAN: We have studied a few raphé cells according to the following experimental design: LSD was giving intravenously to establish its inhibitory effect on raphé unit after systemic administration. LSD (100 μg/ml) was then applied iontophoretically in an extremely dilute concentration, much more dilute that has been used in previous iontophoretic studies. At higher concentrations LSD may have a local anesthetic or non-specific toxic effect. In our cases in which extremely dilute solutions of LSD were employed, the drug inhibited the cells. This was followed by a recovery of the raphé unit. It remains to be shown that LSD at the same concentration does not inhibit other, non-raphé cells.

---

[1] The term "habituation" is used here to describe a decrement in the alerting response to repeated sensory stimili. (Ed.)

DR. SNYDER: Could you comment about the candidate for the inhibitory interneuron?

DR. AGHAJANIAN: A few cells that we have studied have increased enormously in rate in response to very low doses of LSD. Those cells happen to have been in the ventral tegmental nucleus which is lateral to the median raphé. An increased firing rate would be one of the characteristics one would expect of an inhibitory interneuron. However, there may be many other nuclei that have similar properties.

DR. KOPIN: I should like to make a comment, and then pose a question. Using stimulation-evoked release of amines from brain slices, Dr. Richard Katz and I have studied the effects of LSD at doses about ten times those you are using. We found an inhibition by LSD of release of norepinephrine, 5-HT, and some amino acids. The dosage range that is needed to inhibit release of 5-HT is about one-fifth to one-tenth of that needed to inhibit release of other transmitters. The active isomer of LSD has this effect; the inactive one does not. Mescaline has this effect, but at a much higher concentration.

So much for the comments. The question: Have you considered using 5-hydroxytryptophan or 5-HT itself to see whether or not you can inhibit raphé cells?

DR. AGHAJANIAN: Yes, in just a few studies we have given 5-hydroxytryptophan. After l-5-hydroxytryptophan is given in fairly large amounts, of the order of 50 mg/kg, there is a moderate slowing of discharge rate by 30 to 50 percent. The difficulty with such an effect is that we will need a lot more cells to be sure that this slowing wouldn't have occurred anyway, although I must say that these cells characteristically maintain rather constant rates.

DR. HOLMSTEDT: There is a recent paper by Andén *et al.* (*Brit. J. Pharmacol.*, 34: 1–7, 1968) in which they report on a study of the effects of LSD by biochemical and histochemical techniques.

DR. AGHAJANIAN: I mentioned that study yesterday. That was a study in spinal cord and brain, and LSD had several effects. It slowed the depletion of 5-HT after inhibition of synthesis, which I think corresponds nicely to the experiments of Dr. Freedman. I think the histochemical data here is really not quantitative.

DR. HOLMSTEDT: No, it never is.

DR. AGHAJANIAN: In any case, their results are quite in agreement with Dr. Freedman's results. They have also looked at tremor in spinal animals after injections of LSD and 5-hydroxytryptophan. They found that the effects of LSD and 5-hydroxytryptophan when injected intra-arterially were similar. Others have had similar results in the past.

DR. FREEDMAN: I think one of the elegant things about your study from my own standpoint is that the findings obtained from our tedious biochemistry so faithfully predicts what is probably its cause, namely, the altered activity of these neurons.

As I recall, your threshold dose of 10 μg/kg of LSD produces only a very brief inhibition of raphé unit, but higher doses produce a longer lasting inhibition that has about the same duration as both the behavioral and biochemical changes that one can observe.

DR. AGHAJANIAN: I think you were finding changes in 5-HT and 5-HIAA concentrations with doses of around 130 μg/kg intraperitoneally.

DR. FREEDMAN: Right.

DR. KORNETSKY: This doesn't necessitate a direct effect, does it?

DR. FREEDMAN: I think there are biochemical sequences that are unaccounted for by the parameters that have been studied so far, such as the binding of 5-HT that Dr. Szara found with DMT and that we found with LSD. One wonders if turning off a nerve somehow changes the avidity of particles in the nerve ending for 5-HT. If so, why? Those are rather subquestions as to what nerve activity has to do with vesicles and the traffic of 5-HT in the nerve endings. We have been going through as many of the psychotomimetics as possible to see if the original paradigm-increased binding, decreased 5-HIAA-holds for the various classes.

Dr. Aghajanian asked me yesterday—I see why today—what I remembered about the effect of mescaline on 5-HT metabolism. It seems different from the indoles. Psilocybin has the same pattern with respect to 5-HIAA. The time course is different. There are many differences to account for: 5-HIAA levels drop before 5-HT levels rise, for example. So there may be peculiar biophysical and biochemical sequences which may or may not be relevant to the effects, but the overall pattern for indoles is startling. All this shows biochemists that perhaps it's sometimes easier to get to measures of neural activity rather than bother with complex biochemical changes.

The other thing that is important to do (and to remember when you are doing it) is that in tolerance studies, which are tedious studies to do, dose and time are critical for the tolerance effects of LSD. There are always effects that do not show tolerance to LSD, just as with morphine. So what I am saying is that I am becoming more and more interested in the neurobehavioral significance of the raphé pathway, for which we have little insight. And there is the fact that habituation seems to be influenced in some of the experiments, both with drugs and with neural stimulation. Thus the neurobehavioral significance of these systems in perception, constancies and regularities in behavior is at issue. It hasn't been approached. I think this is what we are going to have to know about if we want to tie these studies in with behavior.

DR. TEUBER: Have you tried BOL (brom-LSD) on this system?

DR. AGHAJANIAN: Yes. It is about one-tenth to one-twentieth as potent as LSD in producing partial inhibition. Its effect differs from that of LSD in that complete inhibition of raphé units is usually not obtained even with very high doses of BOL.

DR. DOMINO: I am reminded that LSD-25 is a rather effective cholinesterase inhibitor, although the enzyme's relationship to hallucinations is controversial. Have you tried agents which would increase brain acetycholine, such as physostigmine?

Since the Betzold-Jarisch reflex is stimulated by these compounds, I wonder if you have tried various deafferentations to rule out an indirect, peripheral action?

DR. AGHAJANIAN: Just to get to the last point, I don't think we have ruled out anything so far as the site of action is concerned. In terms of cholinergics, we haven't tried cholinesterase inhibitors. We did try atropine, and found that it doesn't affect the firing of raphé units.

DR. DIAMOND: Was there any modification of the effect on forebrain when you used LSD? Did the drug effects involve cells in the third nerve nucleus?

DR. AGHAJANIAN: That is a very interesting point about the third nerve nucleus. We had one atypical cell in the dorsal raphé region which was phasic instead of regular in rhythm but it responded to LSD; the drug inhibited the cell at the usual threshold dose. Histological examination showed the cell to be further forward than with any of our other raphé placements. It was in the caudal portion of the Edinger-Westphal nucleus. I went back to Dahlström and Fuxe's work and reread the paragraph on the distribution of 5-HT cells. They said that the cells in the caudal portion of the Edinger-Westphal nucleus are 5-HT-containing. This nucleus thus seems to be a forward extension of the dorsal raphé nucleus.

DR. DIAMOND: Did you observe the pupils while the animals were experiencing LSD effects?

DR. AGHAJANIAN: This has been studied, and there is dilation.

DR. DIAMOND: Was this accompanied by increased activity in the cells of the third nerve nucleus?

DR. AGHAJANIAN: I don't think I can answer that.

DR. DIAMOND: Did you stimulate the animals after they had been dosed with LSD?

DR. AGHAJANIAN: Yes. Pretreatment with LSD markedly reduced the increase in 5-HIAA levels after electrical stimulation of raphé nuclei. Actually, Sheard and I reported this at the VIth International Congress of Neuropsychopharmacology last year (1968) (Excerpta Medica Foundation, Amsterdam, in press).

Dr. Leon Harmon's paper entitled "Visual Information Processes" is not being published for reasons beyond the control of the Editor. The discussion following the presentation of this paper is, however, included.

DISCUSSION

DR. DIAMOND: There is clearly a need on the basis of your presentation to understand what the phenomena really are before we attempt to study their physiological basis. For example, in the matter of stabilized images, there is great controversy which is only gradually resolving. Evans has shown by clever use of afterimages that the phasic appearance and disappearance of the image does not result from a subject's inability to maintain stabilization. When phenomena are well understood on a descriptive level, then the approach you suggest will of course be very profitable. This has been proved by the achievements of neuropsychologists like Professor Teuber, who have systematically investigated patients with brain lesions. Many normal sensory mechanisms have been suggested by investigating the perceptual exaggerations and distortions that occur in the course of brain disease. I think the same approach can be profitably applied to psychotrophic drug studies. It is also clear that additional important information can be obtained by investigating drug effects on patients with reduced nervous systems, that is, on patients who have central nervous system lesions and already show some degree of dysfunction.

DR. OSMOND: I was very interested in your remarks about the use of hypnotic techniques. My friend and colleague, Dr. Bernard Aaronson, has worked on these matters for many years. He can produce extraordinary behavioral changes by inducing very simple alterations in perception using hypnosis. He finds that alterations in the experience of time and space are especially effective and produce a widespread disintegration of the experiential world of his subjects. While different people are more or less susceptible to such changes in perception, it seems that no one is completely unsusceptible.

DR. WEST: I would like to add one comment regarding the way hypnosis may relate to certain other things.

One of the bright young men at Oklahoma, Dr. G. H. Deckert, has been able recently to differentiate (in terms of a bioelectrical record) among a given visual experience as it actually takes place, as it is imagined to take place, as it is pretended to take place, as it is hallucinated through the use of hypnosis, and as it is dreamed. The differences are not great, but they are distinctive enough so that you can tell them apart objectively from the record. Dr. Deckert used a swinging pendulum of a known frequency. The image of this beating pendulum was then conceived under one circumstance or another. The recording involves an EEG, EMG, electro-oculogram, and so forth.

One of the interesting things Deckert found, incidentally, was that contrary to what we have always thought, it's possible for people to move their eyes in smooth pursuit movements rather than in sacchadic[1] movements while following an imagined target. We had thought that only truly watching a pendulum would produce this smooth type of tracing. Actually, in a clear-cut conscious pretense, you would have expected always to find sacchadic movements. However, some people are able to "pretend" a pursuit movement that looks much like the real thing. It's smooth, in other words, but the timing is a little bit off. It is not exactly the frequency it is supposed to be.

DR. DEMENT: I would like to add to Dr. West's remarks. In addition an hallucination is not real in the sense that you could not distinguish what the nervous system does inside. And in ocular motor performance it is possibly a little bit better to have the pursuit movement. There is also optokinetic nystagmus—for example, the subject could imagine looking out the window of a moving train at the telephone poles. There has been some work showing that under hypnosis this specific ocular motor performance can be duplicated in the absense of stimuli. I have always been skeptical about it, but recently we finally succeeded in inducing beautiful opticokinetic nystagmus with hypnotic suggestion in our own laboratory. Thus, we considered the hallucinatory experience giving rise to the nystagmus to be "real". We then attempted to substitute "real" hallucinations during the day for dreams during the night. The results have not been conclusive, but it is not impossible that if the hallucination is "real", it will offset a REM deprivation rebound. We have obtained in collaboration with Leo Hollister a similar effect, or REM rebound, with marijuana extract, in cases when there were vivid hallucinations.

My main point is that whether or not any particular hallucination is real, and how to judge this, is terribly important. Not every mental image or thought is hallucinatory.

DR. GRIFFITH: From a theoretical standpoint, could one predict that illusions that depend upon binocular vision would be sensitive to drugs as opposed to these color illustrations that have just been demonstrated?

CHAIRMAN: I think you will get some very interesting answers to that question in Dr. Julesz's presentation which follows next.

DR. LEHRER: Dr Dement raised an important point which has been bothering me. I don't know if it is the proper time to bring this up, but on the question of drug-induced "hallucinations" versus the classic definition of hallucination, can one really fit the drug-induced abnormal sensory state into the classical definition of hallucination, or is there a difference between the two kinds of phenomena?

DR. DEMENT: What is the classical definition, actually?

---

[1] Irregular, abrupt

DR. LEHRER: Well, the classical definition I was taught in my medical school psychiatry course was that hallucination involves experience or response which has no relation to the external input, whereas most of the things that we see after drugs, in my experience or in what I have read about it, involves a response to a subliminal stimulus or a distorted perception of the stimulus in the environment. And I am not familiar with any evidence of seeing things that are truly not there; in other words, that there is no cue in the environment which triggers the response.

DR. DEMENT: These considerations should be emphasized because the issues are very confused. For example, Horowitz has raised the possibility that schizophrenics "see" their own retinal processes which they elaborated into hallucinations; they could see their own arterial pulsations. Again, what is a real hallucination? Can it ever be demonstrated? I am convinced that dreams are "real" hallucinations, and may be the only ones.

DR. BERGER: I think the next two papers will clear this up somewhat, and I think if we can save these problems for the general discussion we will get better continuity.

A VOICE: If I could make one final point. I think the hypnotically induced hallucination is, in my experience (and I used to play with hypnosis quite a bit), a true hallucination because obviously your subject is seeing something suggested which is completely independent of the environment.

DR. DEMENT: The question is, is he really seeing it or not. In many cases he obviously isn't.

A VOICE: He is responding to it.

A VOICE: I have one question on your hypothetical IBM 7094 computer, on the desert island, having some acquaintance with computers and using the computer model in terms of mental functions for the human. We have an apparently infinite set of programs with no known human meaning which can be created in an IBM 7094. Does one call these distortions, hallucinations, delusions, or psychotic states?

VOICE I: With respect to the computers in mind, or harassing?

VOICE II: This is what I am asking.

VOICE I: Well, you are getting here at the question of language and metalanguage and program and subprogram and super-program.

VOICE III: And meta-program.

VOICE II: And I think perhaps the best way for us to come to some agreement on what is significant here would be to observe that it is entirely conceivable to me that the language that we use in this course as I am talking to you and you to me is of a different kind from the language that the neural signals operate in. It is also conceivable to me that the output interface, that is our conscious mind, whatever that is, that enables us to examine this and put this into some articulated form, that this is a vastly reduced kind of information process with respect to the mechanism that is giving rise to it. And it may very well be, I am afraid, that the intellectual searchlight that we can consciously bring to bear on any of these languages with respect to underlying mechanism may not be potent enough ever to come to a complete and satisfactory analysis in the sense it would be—as the mathematicians have it—an incompleteness there in which it says no system is ever capable of explaining or modeling itself fully. I think this is a very real possibility.

A VOICE: Well, you slipped the question back into machine language out of soft ware at a high level. My question was totally within soft ware and at a pretty high level.

A VOICE: Well, if you look at the Fortran program, for example, which is used to implement some algorithms for pattern recognition of printed letters —and we have been working on these things—it's impossible, literally impossible for anyone not knowing the intent of that algorithm or the grand plan at the highest level of language, to look at that program and to say what is going on and why.

A VOICE: Right. But if I were to introduce a noise source anywhere in that program it woul dgenerate an infinite set that you couldn't possibly understand.

A VOICE: My point is you don't have to introduce that noise and I am still in trouble.

DR. OSMOND: I doubt if one can discuss hallucinations usefully without going back to Galton's great work on imagery done during the 1880's. One of the great difficulties regarding scientific discussion of imagery is that a number of scientists who are themselves really good imagers is smaller, perhaps much smaller than the good imagers in the general population. Many of us here, for instance, might be unwilling to believe that someone in good health could produce and enjoy a three dimensional image of a small black chihuahua which would run to and fro in front of us. As a small girl, one of my daughters used to do this easily. Her mother, who is also a good imager, would do the same thing and they were both greatly amused by it. I, on the other hand, was profoundly puzzled and even disturbed. There are people who can produce three dimensional audiovisual images of this kind, such a one would hear the chihuahua bark as well as see it gambol around. As a non-imager, I find this strange and sometimes feel that I have been cheated of a great source of fun. As far as I can make out imagery at the complex level that I have sometimes called maxi-hallucinations, is very rare in either health or illness. I mean by this three dimensional "solid" images which are perceived as solid objects by at least one person and behave that way. These are the viridical hallucinations described by the Society for Psychic Research in the 1880's. Yet in the Maudsley archives, I am told, Guttman and MacClay give an account of an artist to whom they had administered a large quantity of mescaline. He hallucinated a three dimensional, apparently solid, sweet-smelling and sweet-behaving dancing girl. The question was whether the girl was "real" or not. The artist saw her and was convinced that she existed. MacClay and Guttman did not see her and did not believe that she existed. In normal circumstances, the consensus being that the girl was not there, this might have persuaded the artist that he was mistaken, but he was so sure that the investigators became very anxious.

I believe that as we become able to use these substances, and techniques derived from them, more skillfully, we shall be able to inquire better into difficult questions of this kind. Such questions are not only difficult, but they are very important, because at certain times it appears that all of us become susceptible to changes in what we consider to be our real world. I think John Lilly would say we change our program and it is then that we can be in real trouble. It is not only the ill who run into these changes of perception. The same kind of things happens to whole societies; just how and why we do not know. It appears that we resist such changes desperately and perhaps on the whole we are well advised to do so. But today with the logarithmic rise of technology, unless we understand the meaning of these changes and their psychosocial consequences, we may be in very grave trouble. For at least a century we have been led to suppose that the technological revolution will make life easier and easier. Perhaps we must accept the harsh fact that it won't necessarily be any easier, but simply different and much less familiar. What you gentlemen are doing, I believe, is to allow us to change our programming a bit more quickly and, I hope, a lot less brutally than in the past. The evidence is accumulating here; it seems to me, to be cause for both sober thought and some exhilaration.

DR. DEMENT: It is important to know whether your daughter can image well, and also whether she is really seeing—I mean whether she is producing the exact same brain processes that would in fact be produced by the chihuahua.

Obviously, we couldn't have survived if distinguishing between images and perceptions were a universal problem. We must see the real world without internal contamination.

THE SEPARATION OF RETINAL AND CENTRAL PROCESSES IN VISION

Bela Julesz, Ph.D.

Bell Telephone Laboratories, Inc., Murray Hill, New Jersey 07974

Human visual perception can be important for many disciplines, but for psychotomimetics it is crucial. In a way, the definition of this entire field is based on some subtle perceptual changes induced by certain chemicals. Undoubtedly, some of these perceptual changes might be inferred from behavioral studies on animals, but the most sensitive methods are based on introspective reports by human subjects.

The importance of perceptual experiments has been well appreciated by contributors to this meeting, as attested by the several reports that involve psychophysical methods. However, as a worker in visual perception, I observed that the psychological methods mentioned here were gathered from rather old-fashioned textbook psychology. The only reason why, as an outsider, I accepted Dr. Efron's kind invitation is my belief that I would be able to draw your attention to a new perceptual technique that I developed a decade ago. The findings might be more relevant to your research than the classical ones.

I must begin with the great neurophysiological breakthroughs that took place in the last 15 years. With the technique of microelectrode recordings of the visual cortex of the cat and monkey, Hubel and Wiesel (1960; 1962; 1968) in particular have found early feature extractors for edges, slits, corners, movements, parallel lines, etc. of a given locale and orientation. Some of these features are already extracted at the stage at which the left and right visual pathways combine. There are at least four synaptic levels, such as bipolars, ganglion cells, lateral geniculate cells and simple cortical cells in area 17 which, in the monkey, belong to the monocular pathways prior to binocular combination. At each synaptic level, thousands of neurons are connected, and the complexities at the neural stage where binocular combination occurs are enormous.

Obviously, if these first synaptic levels could somehow be skipped, and the information portrayed on the "mind's retina" at some cortical level, one could simplify perception. It would be possible to "repeat" almost every experiment of classical psychology by such *postretinal* stimulation and determine whether a given phenomenon is *peripheral* or *central*. From now on I will call this postretinal stimulation *cyclopean* stimulation, the word referring to the mythological giants with one center eye, or, in our case, with one "central" eye. Let me assure you that I will not stimulate this "cyclopean retina" by surgical intervention, although Brindley and Lewin (1968) implanted a few dozen electrodes in a blind woman's cortex and produced an array of visual phosphenes. Neither do I want to skip the peripheral processes by painting images on the cyclopean retina by hypnotic suggestions, induced hallucinations or by observing dreams. Instead, I use classical psychological techniques of retinal stimulation by light, except for an innovation.

In the fall of 1959 I was able to produce binocular shapes from monocularly shapeless and contourless random textures. I called these displays *random-dot stereograms* (Julesz, 1960). Figure 1 shows such a random-dot stereogram. When monocularly viewed, it gives an entirely random impression, but when binocularly fused, a certain center area jumps out in vivid depth in front of a random surrounding. Figure 2 explains how such a stereogram was

FIG. 1. Random-dot stereogram of 100 × 100 black and white dots of equal probability. When monocularly viewed the left and right images appear uniformly random. When stereoscopically fused a center square jumps out in vivid depth. Of course, instead of a square, any figure or text can be similarly portrayed.

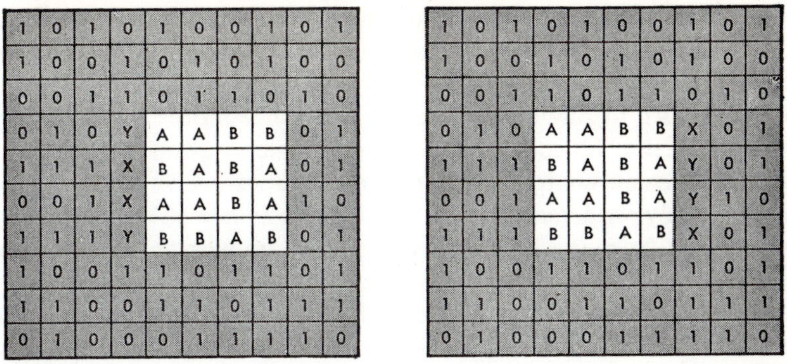

FIG. 2. Schematic illustration on a small array of how Fig. 1 has been generated. (1, 0), (A, B) and (X, Y) correspond to black and white picture elements.

produced by a computer. Except for a 100 × 100 array size, this schematic illustration uses a small array. As you can see, both the left and right fields are composed of black and white, randomly-selected cells of equal probability. Certain areas are point-by-point identical in the two fields; certain other areas are also identical, but are shifted horizontally relative to each other as if they were a solid sheet. Of course, instead of a center square, any other surface or pictorial information can be portrayed by this method. The important difference between classical stimuli and random-dot stereograms is that the former portray the information by brightness changes, while the latter uses depth changes.

As I point out in my book to be published on *Foundations of Cyclopean Perception,* this technique is the visual generalization of the "musical counterpoint." In counterpoint, the constituent independent musical textures produce a new melody in the listener's mind. In my technique, the constituent melodies are random textures, while the counterpoint can be a visual form of any shape desired. Of course, only with the advent of fast computers and accurate visual displaying devices could this research paradigm become a reality. Nor does this method need to be restricted to binocular depth perception. At any stage, and for any modality which combines in the central nervous system, one can produce a counterpoint pattern that has not existed before. One can then portray any stimulus shape that produced some classical perceptual phenomenon by cyclopean techniques, and ask whether the cyclopean phenomenon is identical to the classical one or not. In the case of identity, one can infer that the phenomenon in question, *e.g.,* the Müller-Lyer optical illusion, is of central origin. If only the classical phenomenon can be obtained, and no cyclopean counterpart exists, one can postulate the peripheral origin of this phenomenon. Finally, if only a cyclopean phenomenon exists without its classical counterpart, one can assume that the phenomenon is central but overshadowed by the powerful peripheral processes.

Let us return to random-dot stereograms once more. If you look around you will notice that objects are the same whether viewed with both eyes or only one. The same contours, textures and shapes are seen monocularly as binocularly. Only with random-dot stereograms is it possible to separate the monocular cues from the binocular ones. Since in everyday life the monocular cues are inseparable from the binocular ones, Nature performs many of the preprocessings in the monocular pathways. It is not surprising that these powerful monocular processes overshadow the workings of the more central processes. Only after an "eclipse" of these strong monocular cues can one expect to study a new, hitherto unobserved psychology.

It would take too long to summarize the many new perceptual phenomena that have been obtained by colleagues, my coworkers and myself using random-dot stereograms (Julesz, 1960; 1967; Fender and Julesz, 1967; Julesz and Payne, 1968). It would take even longer to review those classical problems that have been clarified by this technique (Julesz, 1964; 1965). The interested reader is referred to the reference list of this paper. I would like to mention briefly a recent development by Steve Johnson and myself which we call *mental holography*. We were able to generate random-dot stereograms that can portray any two surfaces, but only one of them can be perceived at a time (Julesz and Johnson, 1968 a,b). The other organization can be perceived at will. Figure 3 shows such a reversible ambiguous presentation in which one can perceive either a plane in front of the printed page or a wedge behind it. A distinct margin at the top and bottom help the viewer to obtain perceptual reversals. This technique might provide a sensitive tool in studying drug-induced mental changes. The two surfaces and the hidden surfaces of objects can be seen. Whereas in the case of holograms the viewer has to move around the object in order to see it from different angles, in the case of ambiguous stereograms the viewer can sit still. It is his mind that wanders around. Because organization changes in mental holography are not a result of physical movements but rather of mental attention changes, these ambiguous stereograms might be very sensitive indicators of subtle mental changes.

It is impossible to go into detail in a short presentation and I can only hope to convey the flavor of this research. The essence of my talk was twofold. First, I tried to shift your interest to techniques which enable the researcher to separate peripheral processes from central ones. I think it is of the utmost interest to your research to locate the probable activation sites of your chemicals. Second, I gave an example of a new phenomenon from a repertoire of many new phenomena that was obtained by the random-dot stereo-

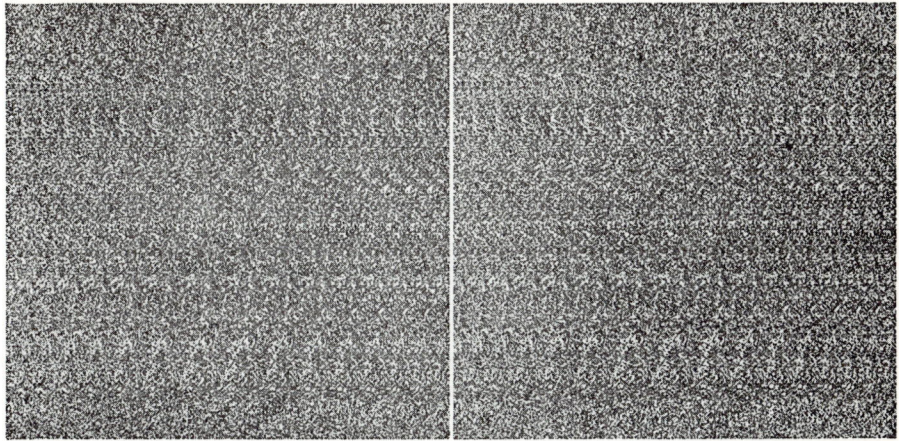

Fig. 3. Ambiguous random-dot stereogram with distinct margins in the upper and lower areas. Surface A is a horizontal plane in front of the printed plane, while surface B is a wedge behind the printed plane.

gram technique and that provides possibly a more sensitive indicator of mental changes than the ones you have been using.

REFERENCES

Brindley, G. S. and Lewin, W. S.: The sensations produced by electrical stimulation of the visual cortex. *J. Physiol.* 196: 479–493 (1968).
Fender, D. and Julesz, B.: Extension of Panum's fusional area in binocularly stabilized vision. *J. Opt. Soc. Am.* 57: 819–830 (1967).
Hubel, D. H. and Wiesel, T. N.: Receptive fields of single neurons in the cat's striate cortex. *J. Physiol.* 148: 574–591 (1959).
Hubel, D. H. and Wiesel, T. N.: Receptive fields, binocular interaction and functional architecture in the cat's visual cortex. *J. Physiol.* 160: 106–154 (1962).
Hubel, D. H. and Wiesel, T. N.: Receptive fields and functional architecture of monkey striate cortex. *J. Physiol.* 195: 215–243 (1968).
Julesz, B.: Binocular depth perception of computer-generated patterns. *Bell Syst. Tech. J.* 39: 1125–1162 (1960).
Julesz, B.: Binocular depth perception without familiarity cues. *Science* 145: 356–362 (1964).
Julesz, B.: Texture and visual perception. *Scientific American* 212: 38–48 (1965).
Julesz, B.: Suppression of monocular symmetry during binocular fusion without rivalry. *Bell Syst. Tech. J.* 46: 1203–1221 (1967).
Julesz, B. and Johnson, S. C.: "Mental holography": stereograms portraying ambiguously perceivable surfaces. *Bell Syst. Tech. J.* 47: 2075–2093 (1968).
Julesz, B. and Johnson, S. C.: Stereograms portraying ambiguously perceivable surfaces. *Proc. Natl. Acad. Sci.* 61: (2) 437–441 (1968).
Julesz, B. and Payne, R. A.: Differences between monocular and binocular stroboscopic movement perception. *Vision Res.* 8: 433–444 (1968).

DISCUSSION

DR. EFRON: If you have a subject that received one of the psychotomimetic compounds, would you be able, using your technique, to distinguish if a change in his perception occurred on the retina or on the central level?

DR. JULESZ: If I were to produce phenomena which exist only retinally or phenomena which exist only centrally by my technique, and if the psychedelic behavior were to change only for one case and not for the other, I could pinpoint the site of the phenomenon in question.

DR. EFRON: Would you be willing to do this?

DR. JULESZ: Well, if I don't have to take the drug, but provide only stimulus material, of course. If I would have to, I would never undertake such experiments.

Let me give you concrete illustrations of my technique. For instance, you look at a waterfall, or in another case, you are in your car driving for hours and you see the road moving; then you close your eyes, and suddenly everything flows in the opposite direction.

Now, the question comes up, is this illusion retinal? We know in the rabbit from Barlow and Hill that motion perception is retinal; however, in the cat and the monkey it is cortical (Hubel and Wiesel).

If I make a movie with random-dot stereograms and have a column (which doesn't exist monocularly) appear to move from right to left in depth, and then I stop movement, the stimuli appear to move in the opposite direction, so I know that the illusion is partly central.

Now, if a drug were given which would affect the cyclopean stimuli but wouldn't affect the classically produced movement aftereffects, then we would know that the active site of the drug after stereopsis has been central. This means it is located after area 18.[1]

DR. DIAMOND: There are several perceptual anomalies experienced by patients with lesions of the central nervous system, especially those producing bilateral dysfunction, which are possibly relevant to this discussion. The one Dr. Lehrer referred to is the inability of some patients to identify written symbols, like ciphers or line drawings of common objects, when the contours are discontinuous. This is true even if the discontinuous contours are not formed in the usual way by dots, but by a small alphanumeric charac-

---

[1] According to the cytoarchitectural map of the human cortex by K. Brodman (*Vergleichende Lokalisationlehre der Grosshirnrinde in ihren Prinzipien dargestellt auf Grund des Zellenbaues.* J. A. Barth, Leipzig, 1909).

ter replacing each dot. In such cases many patients will be able to identify these small figures even though they are unable to see the larger one whose contour they form. Thus, for example, the number 4 or the outline of a pear can be traced by closely spaced 3s. In each case the patient will say that he sees a 3 or a number of 3s, but even when the 4 or the pear is suggested to him, he cannot make it out. Dr. Peter Schilder has tried a variant of this with macaques who have been trained to go to either triangles or circles. When they are presented with a number of circles arranged in the shape of a triangle or, conversely, with small triangles forming the boundary of a circle, the monkeys respond only to the smaller figures. It would be interesting to hear your comments on this sort of behavior.

DR. JULESZ: This illustrates nicely how visual perception is carried out on both local and global levels. The small figures that serve as elements of a larger shape are representing the local level. Patients with cerebral lesions tend to have difficulties with global features, while the local stimulus features might be processed at a more peripheral level which has been less affected by the trauma. Animals with less developed global processes might process only the smaller, more local features. The advantages of my technique are that we can study the relations between local and global processes in normal humans. With random-dot stereograms it is possible to separate or juxtapose local and global processes. It is possible to present the local features monocularly and the global features binocularly or *vice versa*.

DR. DIAMOND: Yes, but the implication is that you will lose some of the global.

DR. JULESZ: This loss of global information processing can be easily studied with random-dot stereograms. The monocular perception of the random-dot textures is the local processing, while the binocularly perceived shapes correspond to the global processing. It is interesting that recently Edward Bough at Harvard Medical School could train macaques to see the center figure of random-dot stereograms in depth. Whether lower level animals with good local stereopsis could still see the global shapes in a random-dot stereogram remains to be tried. But even more importantly, Carmon and Bechtoldt (*Neuropsychologia, 7:* 29–39, 1969) were able to show recently that patients with right hemispheric lesions required considerably more time and made more errors than normal controls or patients with left hemispheric lesions to perceive the global shape in random-dot stereograms. Thus, the non-dominant (speechless) hemisphere is concerned with the processing of global features. On the other hand, with classical stereoscopic targets (such as a few lines or dots) that stimulate only a few edge detectors, no such deficiency could be revealed in similar patients.

DR. SNYDER: A test that has been very predictive of psychedelic drug potency in man has been its effect on the discrimination of sizes of circles by squirrel monkeys. I recall that Dr. Efron wondered whether a stereoscopic perceptual test might be even more sensitive to disruption by psychedelic drugs.

DR. JULESZ: In the previously quoted work by Carmon and Bechtoldt, and in other reports, right hemispheric-injured patients had no measurable deficiencies in simple perceptual tasks, particularly when familiar shapes were presented. Whether the perception of a simple stereogram or even a random-dot stereogram of the simpler kind (such as my Fig. 1) is more affected by drugs than a circle discrimination task is easy to determine. However, I am fairly confident that some of the random-dot stereograms portraying complex or ambiguous surfaces might yield percepts that are much more vulnerable to drugs than the percept of the size of a circle. But of course, this is only my guess.

DR. FREEDMAN: I tried some very poorly designed stereoscopic studies some years ago with LSD. Stereopsis was not different under LSD than with normal subjects. But we noticed another phenomenon: during LSD experience there is a failure to suppress a prior image. If one looks at an object and then shifts his vision to another, the two objects appear superimposed.

DR. JULESZ: As I said before, stereopsis of simple targets (that have monocular brightness contours) is a much simpler process than the binocular fusion of complex textures without monocular cues. I am not surprised that stereopsis of classical targets is such a relatively simple task that it is not disrupted by drugs. It would be interesting to try stereoscopic fusion of complex stereograms in your experiments. Your second observation, the failure of one image to erase another after intake of LSD, could lead to a most sensitive test using random-dot cinematograms. Here the global information is portrayed by successive textures in which certain areas are correlated. Failure of suppression of the prior image could be exploited. Two random-dot patterns could be generated whose superposition portrayed a global figure. Normals could not see this figure, since only the last presentation is always seen, which is a random texture. However, in drug-influenced states, the two patterns could be shown with increased time intervals between them, and the global form would still be seen. The longest time interval between the two presentations might serve as an indicator of drug potency. If the left image and the *negative* of the right image of Fig. 1 is presented to one eye in temporal succession, such a test pattern is obtained. The aligned surround will form a gray average, while the center area which is not aligned will appear textured.

Your perceptual persistence phenomenon raises an interesting question. Is it a retinal afterimage of unusually long duration, or is it a central aftereffect that can be gradually built up during scanning through the image. If the latter were the case there might be some relation between **LSD**-induced states and the rare instances of eidetic memory.

DRUG INDUCED STATES OF CNS EXCITATION: A THEORY OF HALLUCINOSIS

Wallace D. Winters, M.D., Ph.D. and Marshall B. Wallach, Ph.D.[1]

*Department of Pharmacology and the Brain Research Institute,
U.C.L.A. School of Medicine, Los Angeles, California 90024*

I. INTRODUCTION

It is obvious from the discussions during this meeting that evaluation of drug efficacy is difficult. The simplest technique involves administering various doses of a drug and observing the resultant gross behavior. Inherent in this approach is an inbred bias which most observers seem to maintain, namely, that when a subject is less active or lies down and is quiet, he is depressed. Further, if one adds to this the finding that the subject is unresponsive, then one is even more convinced that the subject is depressed. For many years, pharmacologists have utilized this incorrect type of observation and added the loss of the righting reflex as a further indication of depression. We have recently observed that drugs which induce CNS excitation, *i.e.*, cataleptoid and epileptoid states, can likewise induce an appearance of depression with a loss of the righting reflex (Winters and Spooner, 1965a,b; Marcus *et al.*, 1967; Winters, 1967) (Fig. 1).

It was obvious that better techniques were required in order for us to assess the state of the CNS following drugs. The technique which we now utilize involves an assessment of brain activity by examining the gross behavior, cortical and subcortical EEG, auditory and visual averaged evoked responses and multiple unit activity in the midbrain reticular formation. Utilizing these techniques, characteristic changes were noted for each control state, *e.g.*, wakefulness, slow wave sleep and rhombencephalic sleep (RPS or paradoxical sleep) (Figs. 2, 3, and 4), and following drug induced states

---

[1] Present address: Department of Psychiatry, New York University Medical Center, 560 First Avenue, New York, New York 10016.

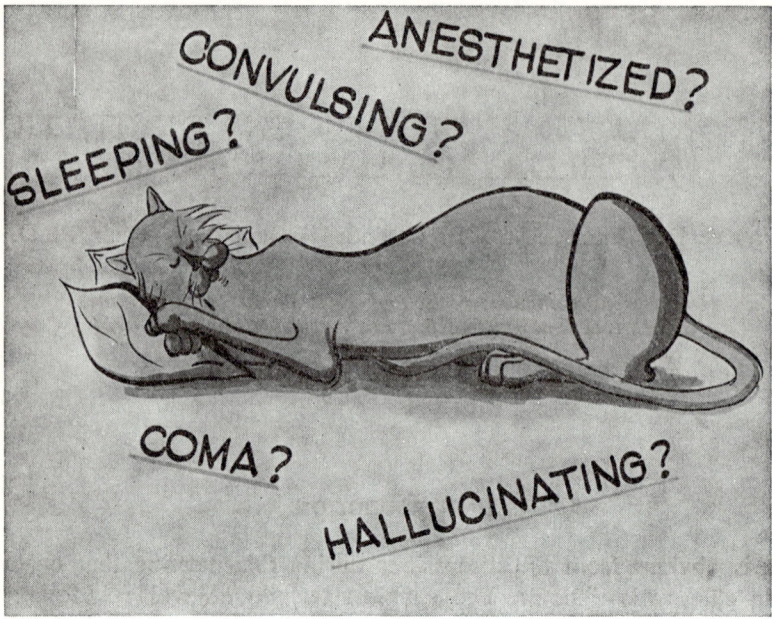

FIG. 1. Cartoon characterization of possible misinterpretations of CNS activity when behavioral manifestations are the only criteria assessed.

of CNS depression and excitation in the chronic cat with brain and muscle electrodes implanted (Winters, 1964; Winters, *et al.*, 1967b; Mori *et al.*, 1967).

II. CONTINUUM OF STATES

On the basis of studies with various CNS excitatory agents, a progression of CNS excitation has been proposed (Winters *et al.*, 1967a; Winters, 1968). All the agents examined have the same general initial EEG and behavioral patterns, and differ only in the degree of progression. The least active CNS excitant agents induce only the initial phases of the progression (Fig. 5); for example, 2 to 8 mg/kg of *d*-amphetamine induces only the initial desynchronization and motor excitability; 50 to 100 µg/kg of LSD-25 induces desynchronization followed by intermittent hypersynchrony; 25 mg/kg of mescaline and 80 to 90% nitrous oxide induce desynchronization, intermittent and then continuous hypersychrony associated with bizarre postures and inappropriate behavior; 10 to 15% diethyl ether similarly induces

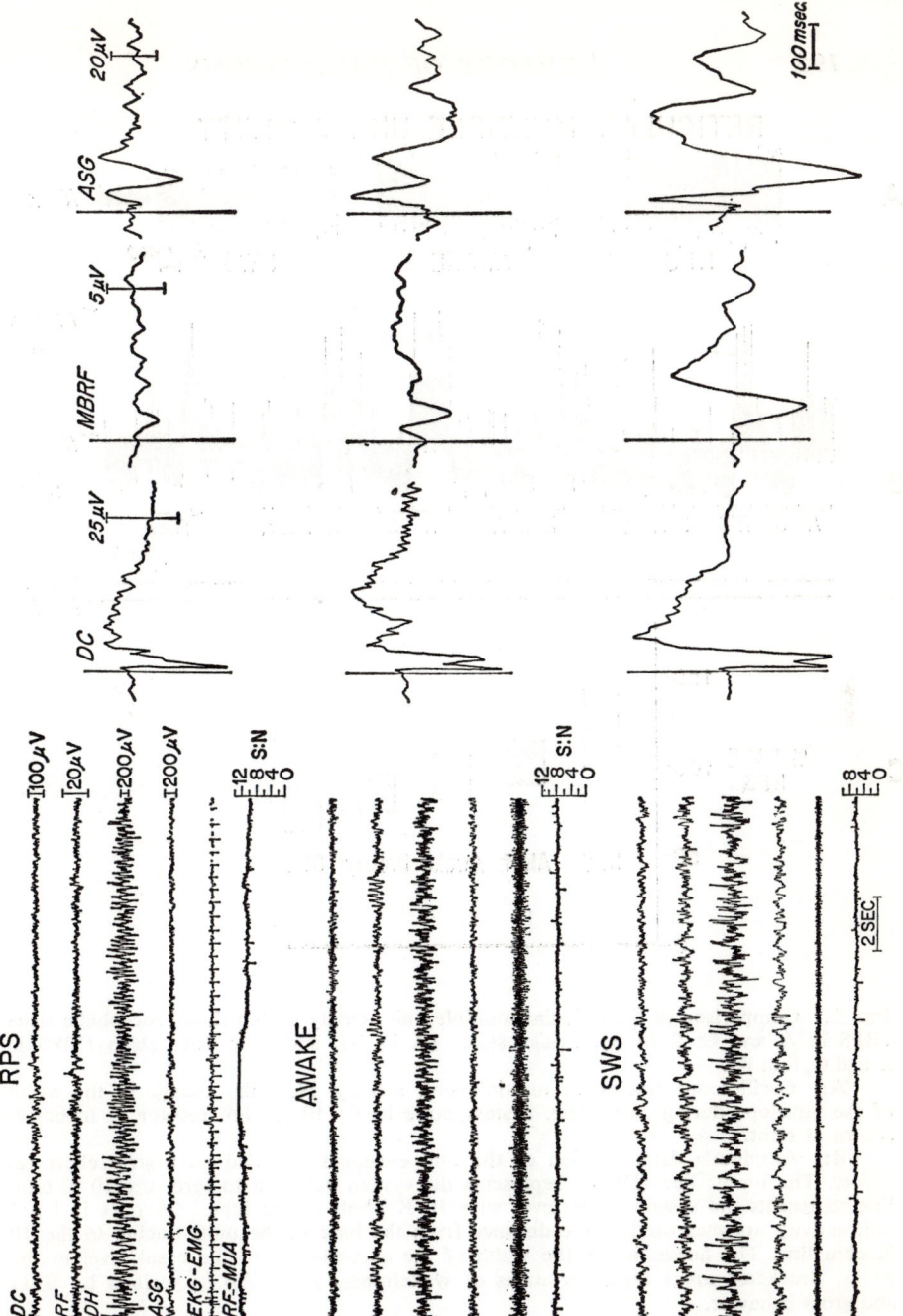

FIG. 2. Comparison of EEG (*A*) and auditory evoked response (*B*) during rhombencephalic sleep (RPS), awake, and slow wave sleep (SWS). The leads are as follows: dorsal cochlear nucleus (*DC*), midbrain reticular formation (*RF*), dorsal hippocampus (*DH*), anterior suprasylvian gyrus (*ASG*), electrocardiogram—electromyogram (*EKG-EMG*), and reticular multiple unit activity (*RF-MUA*). The signal-to-noise level scale (*S:N*) is given in units equal to the level obtained with a 10 K ohm resistor at the input. (From Winters *et al.*, 1967*b*).

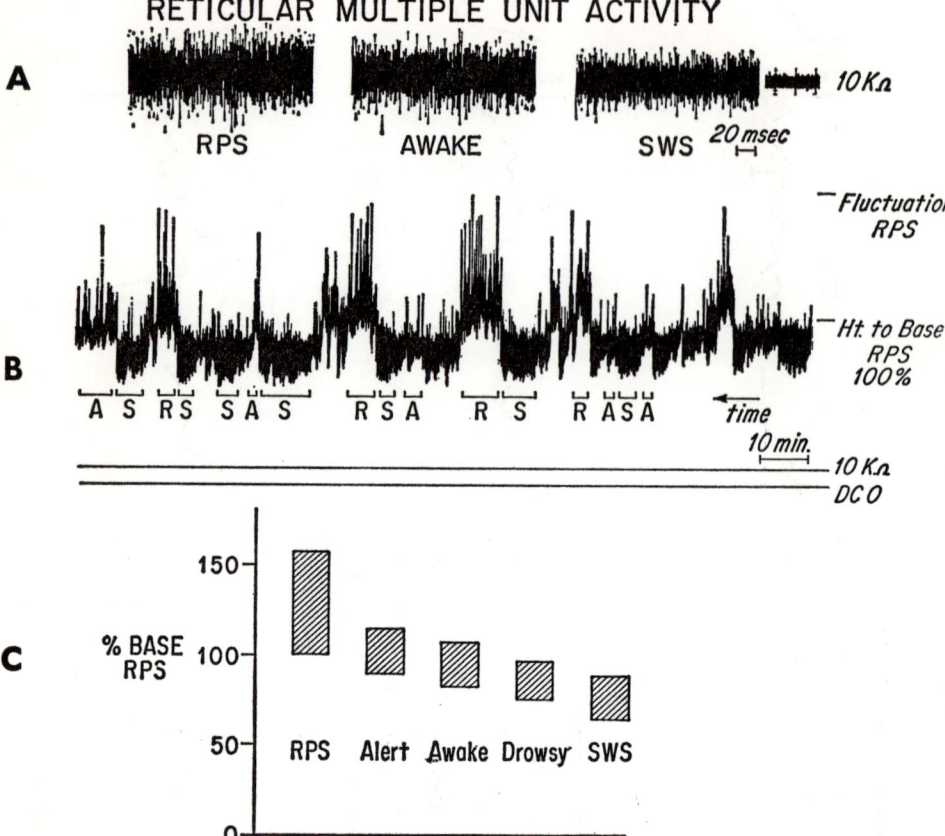

Fig. 3. Comparison of the reticular multiple unit activity during rhombencephalic sleep (RPS in **A** and **C**; R in **B**), awake states (A in **B**), and slow wave sleep (SWS in **A** and **C**; S in **B**).

A: Oscilloscope tracing of multiple unit activity. Note the change in the width of the envelope during each state. System noise level (10 K ohm resistor at input) is shown at right.

B: Amplitude demodulation of the unit envelope recorded on a strip chart recorder. The lowest line (DC 0) represents the system balanced to zero, the 10 K ohm line represents the system noise level with 10 K ohms at the input. Changes in basal unit activity are measured as the distance from the base of the units tracing to the 10 K ohm line. The fluctuation is the width of the excursion from the basal level to the peaks. Bracketed areas represent states of wakefulness and sleep as verified by EEG and gross behavior.

C: Represents the basal height and fluctuation of unit activity as measured from the amplitude demodulated data and expressed as percent of the basal rhombencephalic sleep. (From Winters et al., 1967b).

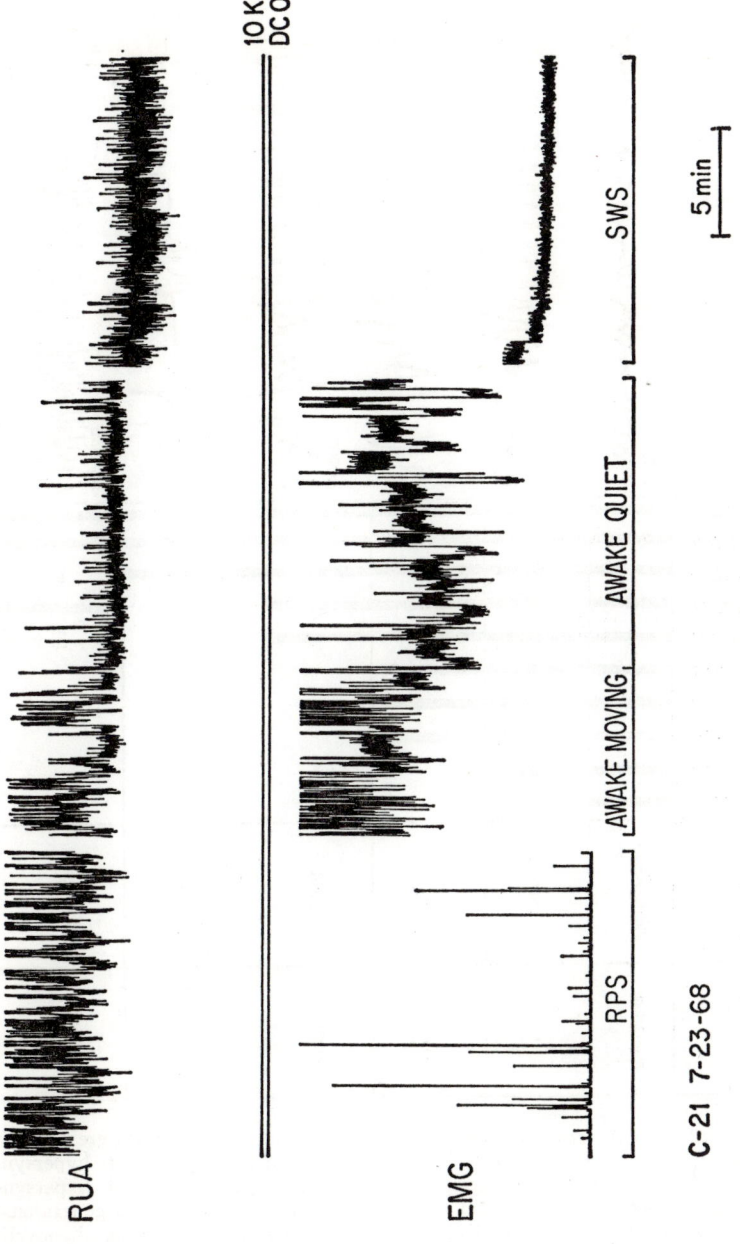

Fig. 4. Recordings of the amplitude demodulated signals of the midbrain reticular formation unit activity (RUA) and EMG. The RUA and EMG are recorded during the control states of RPS, wakefulness, and SWS. See also Figs. 2 and 3.

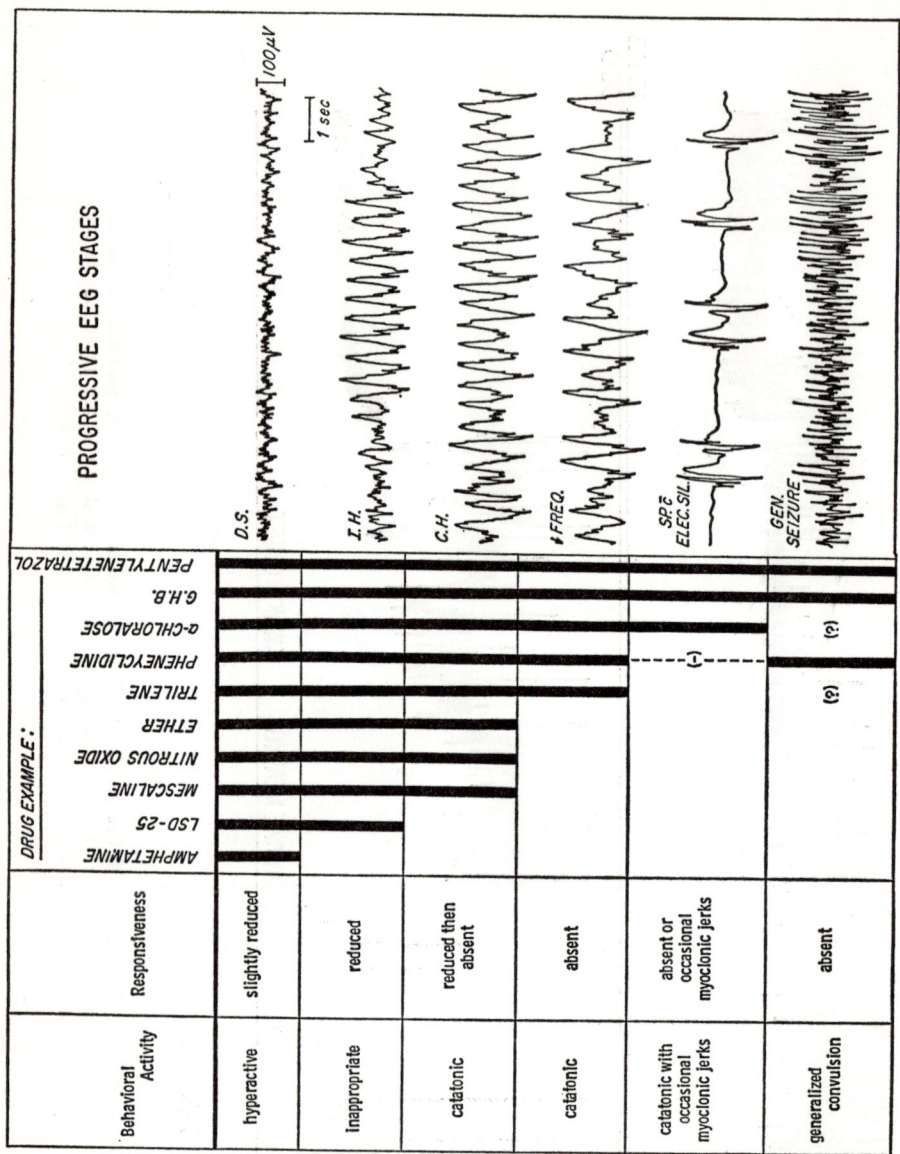

Fig. 5. Behavioral activity, responsiveness, EEG stages following the progression of effects induced by various drugs. Desynchronization (*D.S.*), intermittent hypersynchrony (*I.H.*), continuous hypersynchrony (*C.H.*), reduced frequency of hypersynchrony (↓ *FREQ.*), spikes with electrical silence (*SP. c̄ ELEC. SIL.*), and generalized seizure (*GEN. SEIZURE*). Spikes with electrical silence rarely noted following phencycliene were not observed in our studies. (From Winters *et al.*, Wisc. Med. J., 66: 299–303, 1969).

the initial progression up to continuous hypersynchrony and then induces the characteristic EEG and behavioral patterns of anesthesia; 2 to 8 mg/kg of phencyclidine, 500 to 800 mg/kg of gamma-hydroxybutyrate and 20 mg/kg of pentylenetetrazol transcend the initial phases and induce the total progression to generalized seizure.

While the initial state (Fig. 6) is clearly a behavioral and electrical psychomotor stimulation, the next three induced states are less clearly defined. These states are characterized by inappropriate behavior coupled with abnormal postures indicative of "hallucinatory" behavior. Obviously one cannot be certain that this induced state in cats is an hallucinatory phenomenon similar to that which occurs in man; however, this behavior is pronounced in the cat following agents such as LSD, mescaline and psilocybin which induce profound hallucinatory actions in man. In addition to the induction of hallucinatory behavior in man, these agents induce 2.5 to 3 cps hypersynchronous EEG wave patterns during the hallucinatory state in man (Heath and Mickle, 1960). Further, Adey *et al.* (1962) demonstrated that LSD induced an apparent intermittent loss of contact with the environment at the same time that the hypersynchronous 3 cps EEG waves appeared in the EEG of cats performing in a T-maze. Thus, there is strong presumptive evidence that the induced state of intermittent and continuous hypersynchrony, coupled with inappropriate behavior and inappropriate postures, represent an *hallucinoid* state in the cat. For convenience, I would like to refer to these states as hallucinoid with the clear realization that this is entirely speculative in the cat.

LSD usually induced hallucinations in man in which the subject is aware of the experience. Since the EEG (Fig. 7) is characterized by intermittent bursts of hypersynchronous activity during the LSD induced state, the periodic episodes of desynchronization between hypersynchrony may indicate that the subject returns intermittently to an excited, non-hallucinating, alert state. This pattern of alternating hypersynchrony and desynchrony we will refer to as *hallucinatory A* (Fig. 7). The intermittent appearance of the alert EEG may indicate that during LSD, as in the studies reported above by Adey *et al.* (1962), the hallucinating experience is intermittent, thus the subject is unaware of the experience. The EEG pattern during the state induced by mescaline, nitrous oxide, ether and phencyclidine is one of continuous hypersynchrony (Fig. 8) (Winters *et al.*, 1968). The subjects hallucinate following these agents but are apparently not aware that they are in an abnormal state and usually have some later recall; we shall call this state *hallucinatory B* (Fig. 7). We postulate that the unawareness of subjects during this induced state may be a manifestation of the induced continuous hypersynchrony, with no return to the desynchronized EEG patterns as was characteristic following

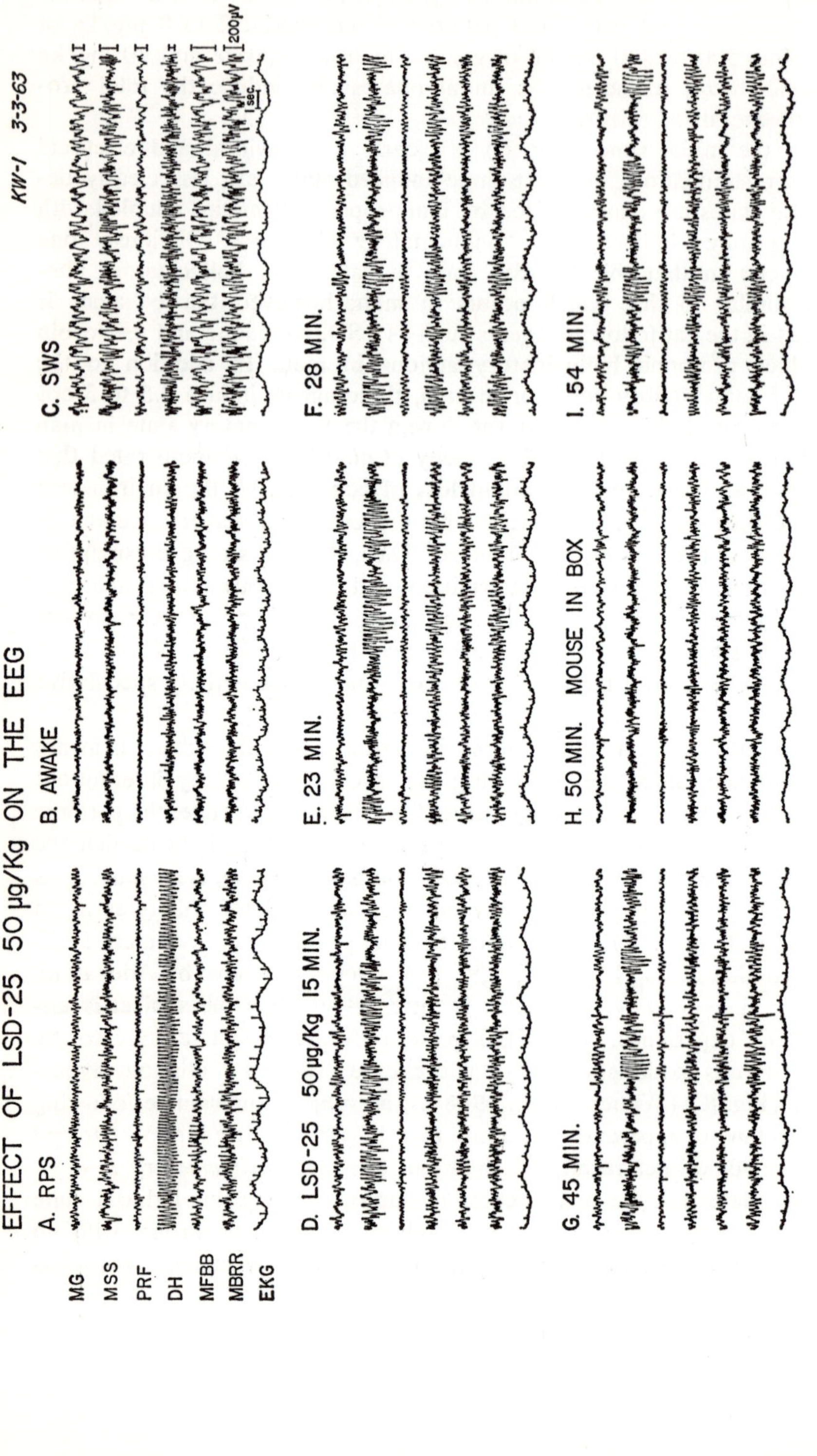

FIG. 6. EEG records from a cat during rhombencephalic sleep (RPS), wakefulness (AWAKE), slow wave sleep (SWS) and following 50 µg/kg i.p. LSD-25. Medial geniculate (MG), median suprasylvian gyrus (MSS), pontile reticular formation (PRF), dorsal hippocampus (DH), median forebrain bundle (MFBB) and electrocardiogram/respiration (EKG). (From Winters et al., 1967a).

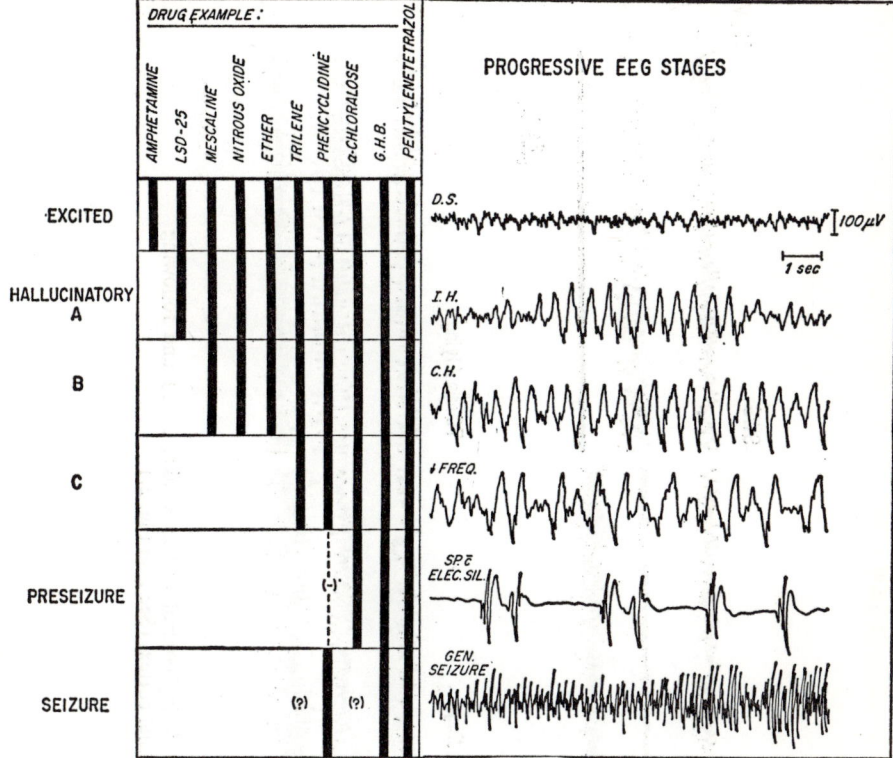

FIG. 7. Representation of the division of the continuum of CNS excitation. (See Fig. 5 for explanations of abbreviations.)

LSD. During the transition to reduced frequency hypersynchrony induced by phencyclidine, gamma-hydroxybutyrate and pentylenetetrazol, which we refer to as *hallucinatory C* (Fig. 7), the patients apparently are completely unaware that they are hallucinatory, are not rousable and have no recall. Of interest is the finding that the hallucinatory C phase is utilized in anesthesiology as a "pseudo" state of general anesthesia. For example, both phencyclidine and gamma-hydroxybutyrate have been reported to be anesthetic agents (Winters *et al.*, 1967a). Our interpretation of this would be that these agents apparently meet the major requirements of an anesthetic agent, *i.e.*, loss of responsiveness and amnesia. It is of interest that both gamma-hydroxybutyrate and phencyclidine traverse the continuum and induce generalized seizures (Winters and Spooner, 1965a,b; Winters *et al.*, 1967a) in a manner similar to the progression induced by pentylenetetrazol (Fig. 9). The hal-

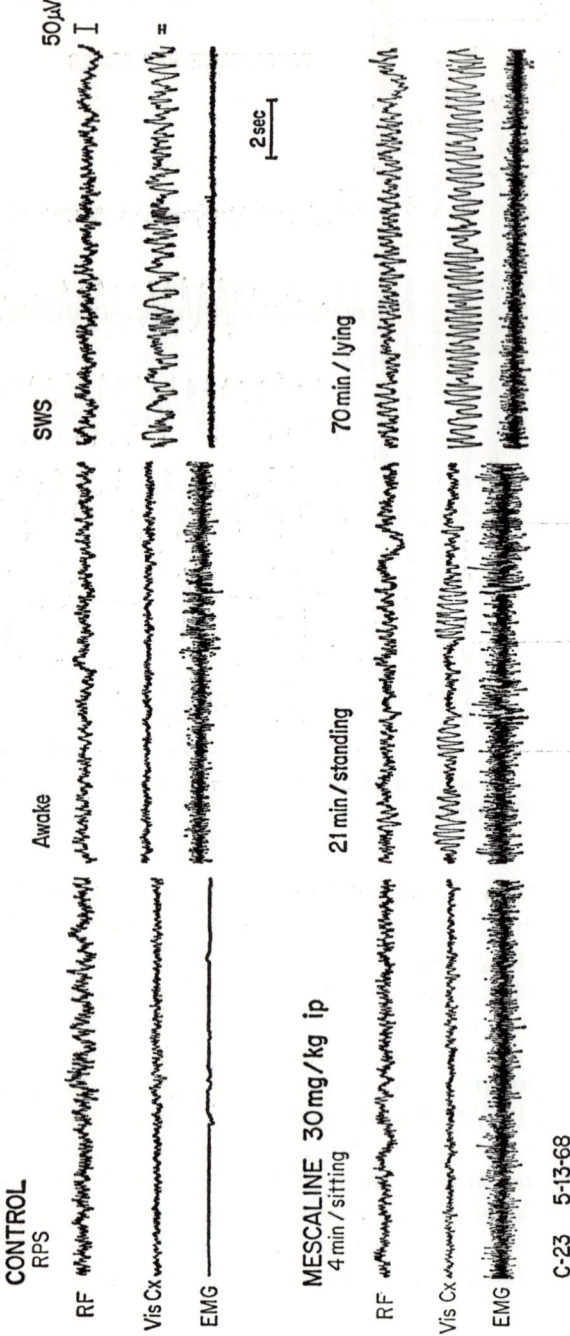

Fig. 8. EEG comparison recorded during control (RPS, Awake, SWS) and following mescaline, 30 mg/kg i.p. *Vis Cx* = visual cortex. (See also Fig. 2.)

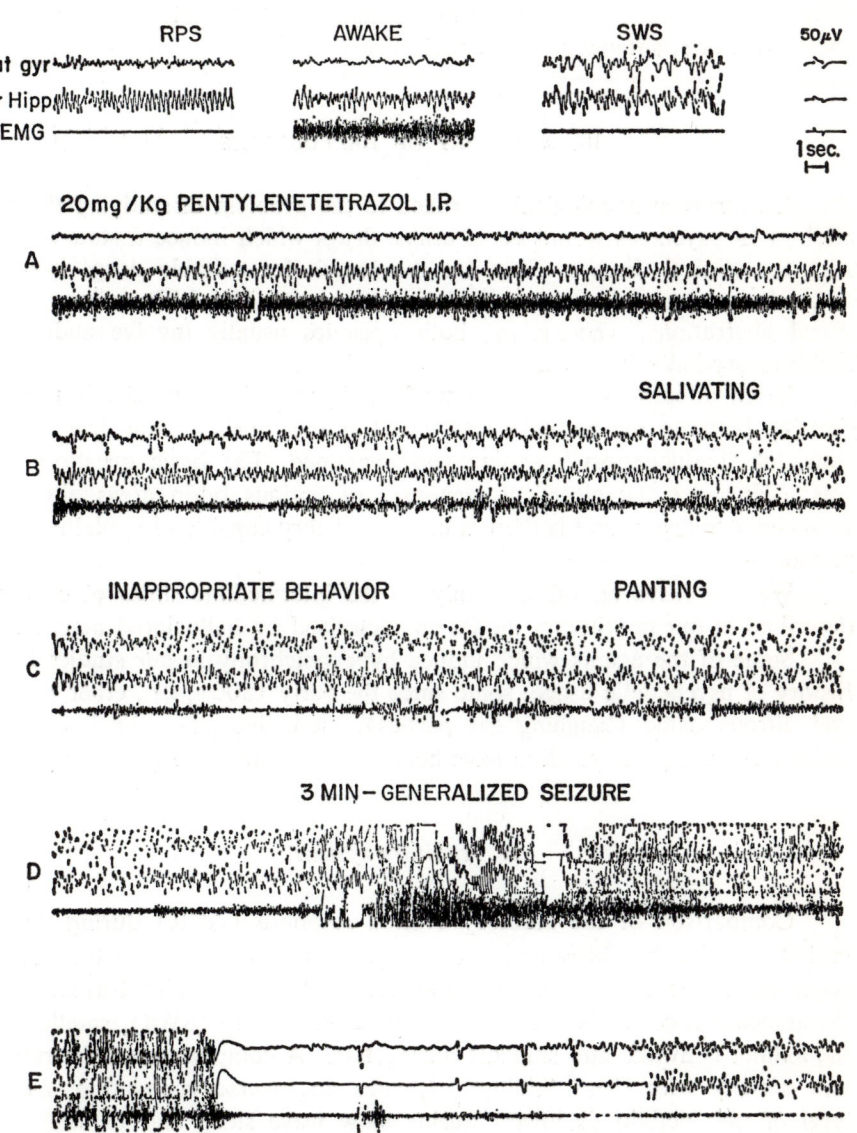

FIG. 9. EEG comparison recorded during control (RPS, AWAKE, SWS) and following pentylenetetrazol, 20 mg/kg i.p. *Lat. gyr* = lateral gyrus, *Dor Hipp* = dorsal hippocampus. (See also Fig. 2.)

lucinoid activity preceding the generalized seizure activity induced by these convulsant agents may be similar to the aura noted clinically prior to pentylenetetrazol or spontaneous grand mal seizures.

III. A THEORY OF HALLUCINOSIS

A neuropharmacological approach to the problem of studying the basic etiology of psychosis would be to utilize drugs which induce a state identical with the clinical disease. Thus far the search for suitable drugs has been deemed unsuccessful since hallucinogenic agents like LSD induce mainly visual aberrations, whereas psychotic episodes usually involve auditory or multisensory hallucinations.

In an attempt to develop a working hypothesis of psychosis the relationship between the auditory and visual system during acute drug induced states of "hallucinatory" activity was examined. The basic question asked was: "How are the electrical responses of various brain areas altered by hallucinatory drugs, and is there a unifying theory capable of explaining these phenomena?"

We will focus attention mainly on the intermediate states of excitation described in our continuum model characterized by hallucinoid activity.

Some of the agents which induce hypersynchrony in our studies have a history of psychedelic usage; some since the early 1800's, *i.e.,* ether (frolics) and nitrous oxide (laughing gas parties), mescaline since the late 1800's, while LSD and phencyclidine have been utilized within the past few years.

A. Auditory system

Comparison of the auditory evoked response (AER) during the natural states of wakefulness and sleep (Fig. 2) demonstrates that the potential recorded at the dorsal cochlear nucleus, midbrain reticular formation and the association cortex is largest during slow wave sleep (SWS), smaller when the animal is awake and smallest during RPS. A comparison of the reticular unit activity with these findings indicates an inverse correlation, *i.e.,* the level of unit activity is lowest during slow wave sleep and highest during RPS. Since the level of reticular neuronal activity is directly correlated with the level of arousability, *i.e.,* wakefulness and sleep, it appears likely that this level of neuronal activity is likewise related to the degree of modulation which the reticular system exerts on the auditory sensory input system

(Winters et al., 1967b). The model states that when reticular unit activity is reduced there is less modulation exerted at the peripheral input system; therefore, the transmitted sensory signal is larger; thus the evoked response is larger. Conversely, when the animal is highly alert, reticular unit activity is elevated, modulating activity is elevated, the transmitted sensory input signal is reduced and the evoked response is smaller.

Those drugs which induce desynchronization, intermittent hypersynchrony and early continuous hypersynchrony (*i.e.*, amphetamine, LSD, nitrous oxide, mescaline and moderate doses of gamma-hydroxybutyrate, phencyclidine or pentylenetetrazol) all induce a slight fall in the amplitude of the evoked responses as compared with the awake control. During this activity the reticular unit activity is high, the animals are markedly aroused and sensory modulation is increased; thus, there is an apparent reduction in the amplitude of the sensory input, and evoked responses are reduced.

During the later phase of the hypersynchronous activity, the animal does not arouse either electrically or behaviorally, the evoked potentials are slightly larger than controls and the basal level of unit activity begins to fall, but the units appear to fire in synchronous bursts. Since the arousal response disappears at the same time that this intermittent bursting of units occurs, it appears that the reticular unit activity has undergone a partial functional disorganization (Schlag and Balvin, 1963; Winters and Spooner, 1966), and while highly excitable, it exerts a reduced control over the level of arousal and sensory modulation (Figs. 10 and 11). As this functional disorganization becomes more profound, the EEG pattern changes to the spiking phase, and the bursting pattern of unit activity becomes more pronounced. At this time there is a more profound loss of reticular modulation, the sensory input becomes markedly elevated and the evoked response in all brain areas is enlarged (Fig. 12).

Reviewing the action of agents on the auditory system during the hallucinatory phase of action, it appears that those drugs which induce only intermittent hypersynchrony, *i.e.*, LSD, result in a reduction in the auditory evoked response, whereas the agents which induce a progression of action to continuous 2.5-1.5 cps hypersynchrony, *i.e.*, mescaline, nitrous oxide, ether, phencyclidine and gamma-hydroxybutyrate, can induce an augmentation of the auditory evoked response. This augmentation appears when the modulation of auditory input is reduced due to the functional disorganization of the reticular system (Fig. 10). Thus it appears that agents inducing 2.5-1.5 cps hypersynchronous activity may be useful tools for investigating states of auditory aberration more closely associated with the clinical symptoms of the psychotic hallucination.

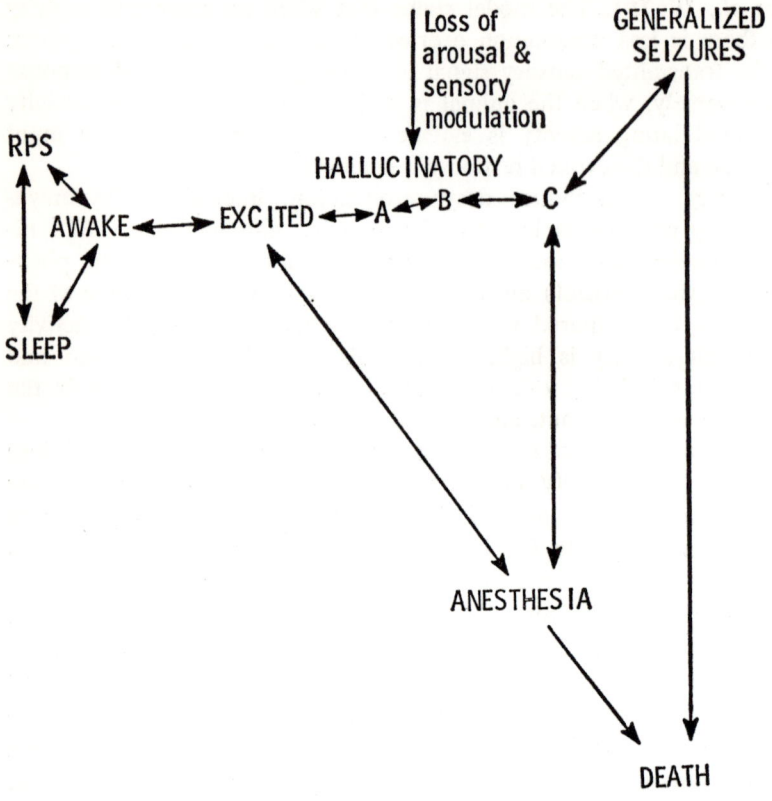

FIG. 10. A simplified representation of the continuum of states of CNS excitation and depression demonstrating the approximate position at which the loss of reticular control occurs.

B. *Modulation of sensory systems*

In order to clarify the dichotomy between drug induced hallucinatory states and those found in psychotic patients, the modulation control of various sensory inputs was examined during spontaneous and drug induced states, and a model was postulated (Winters and Spooner, 1965a,b; Winters, 1967; Winters, 1968). The model is based on the assumption that sensory inputs are directly controlled by a subcortical modulating system located in the midbrain reticular formation, and that the reticular system varies the level of modulation in accordance with the regulation of the state of arousal. The

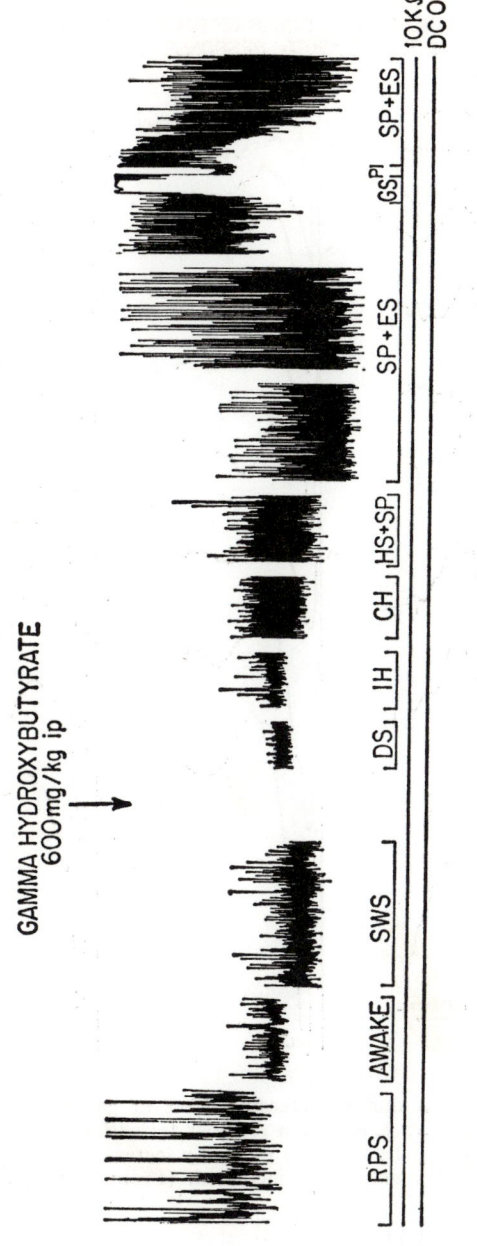

FIG. 11. Multiple unit activity of midbrain reticular formation recorded during the control states of RPS, AWAKE, and SWS, and following gamma-hydroxybutyrate, 600 mg/kg i.p. Desynchronized (DS); intermittent hypersynchrony (IH), continuous hypersynchrony (CH), hypersynchrony with spikes (HS + SP), spikes with electrical silence (SP + ES), generalized seizure (GS), postictal depression (PI). (See also Fig. 3.) Hallucinatory A, B and C occur during IH, CH, and HS + SP, respectively.

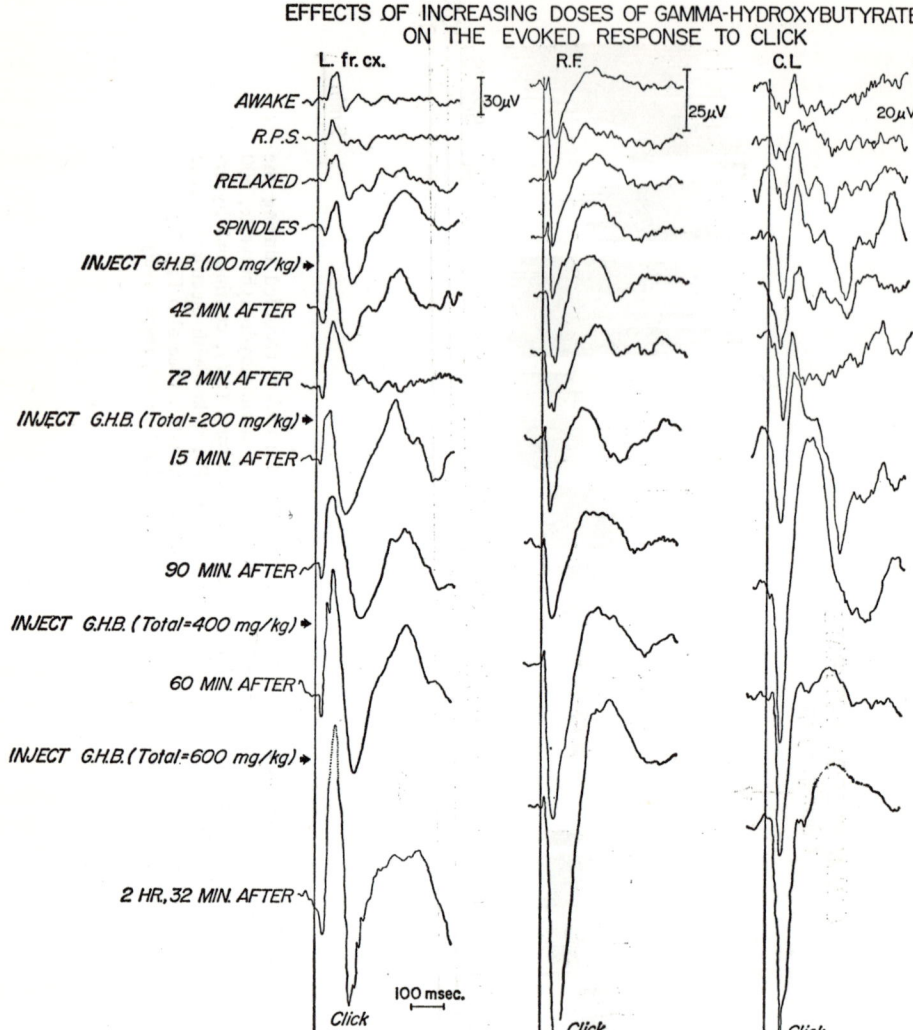

Fig. 12. Computed average of 40 clicks during increasing doses of gamma-hydroxybutyrate (G.H.B.). Frontal cortex (*L. fr. cx.*), midbrain reticular formation (*R.F.*), and centralis lateralis (*CL.*). The amplitude of the response markedly increases in all of the above leads as the dose of gamma-hydroxybutyrate is increased. (From Winters et al., 1965a).

existence of an inhibitory system in the reticular formation which acts on the first synaptic relays within each of the classical afferent systems has been postulated previously. Killam and Killam (1958) suggest that this inhibitory system filters incoming information in order to control the priority level of incoming information. Scheibel and Scheibel (1962) have demonstrated that reticular neurons bifurcate and send ascending branches into the diencephalon and cortex and descending branches caudal as far as the receptors and spinal cord. Therefore, there appears to be anatomical evidence for the proposed modulatory system.

C. Visual system

To understand better the role of LSD action on the visual system, studies paralleling those described for the auditory system were performed. Apter and Pfeiffer (1957) reported that the visual system activity induced by LSD starts in the retina and travels through visual pathways up to the visual cortex. They also describe clinical studies indicating that LSD does not induce hallucinations when administered to patients whose optic nerves were severed.

Visual hallucinations can be postulated to result from an abnormally large number of visual stimuli entering the CNS which overload the visual system, thus resulting in bizarre sensory manifestations. Evidence in favor of this premise is noted by the studies of Purpura (1956a, 1965b) which demonstrated an increase in the visual evoked response (VER) in both the lateral geniculate and cortex following LSD at the same time that the AER was reduced. Preliminary studies in our laboratory demonstrate that the VER is largest during wakefulness, smaller during SWS and smallest during RPS (Figs. 13 and 14). These findings are in agreement with Granit (1955) who demonstrated that reticular activation induces facilitated responsiveness of retinal cells. Thus the cat appears to demonstrate an *inverse* relationship between the level of reticular neuron activity and that of the auditory system activity, but a *direct* relationship between the visual system and the reticular system level of activity. The exception to this is noted during RPS since both auditory and visual responses are reduced during this state. It appears that during sleep the cat is an "auditory animal," while when awake he is a "visual animal," and during RPS both auditory and visual inputs are markedly reduced.

Following amphetamine, and during the initial desychronous activity induced by the more potent CNS excitant agents (*i.e.*, LSD, mescaline, nitrous oxide, ether, phencyclidine, gamma-hydroxybutyrate and pentylene-

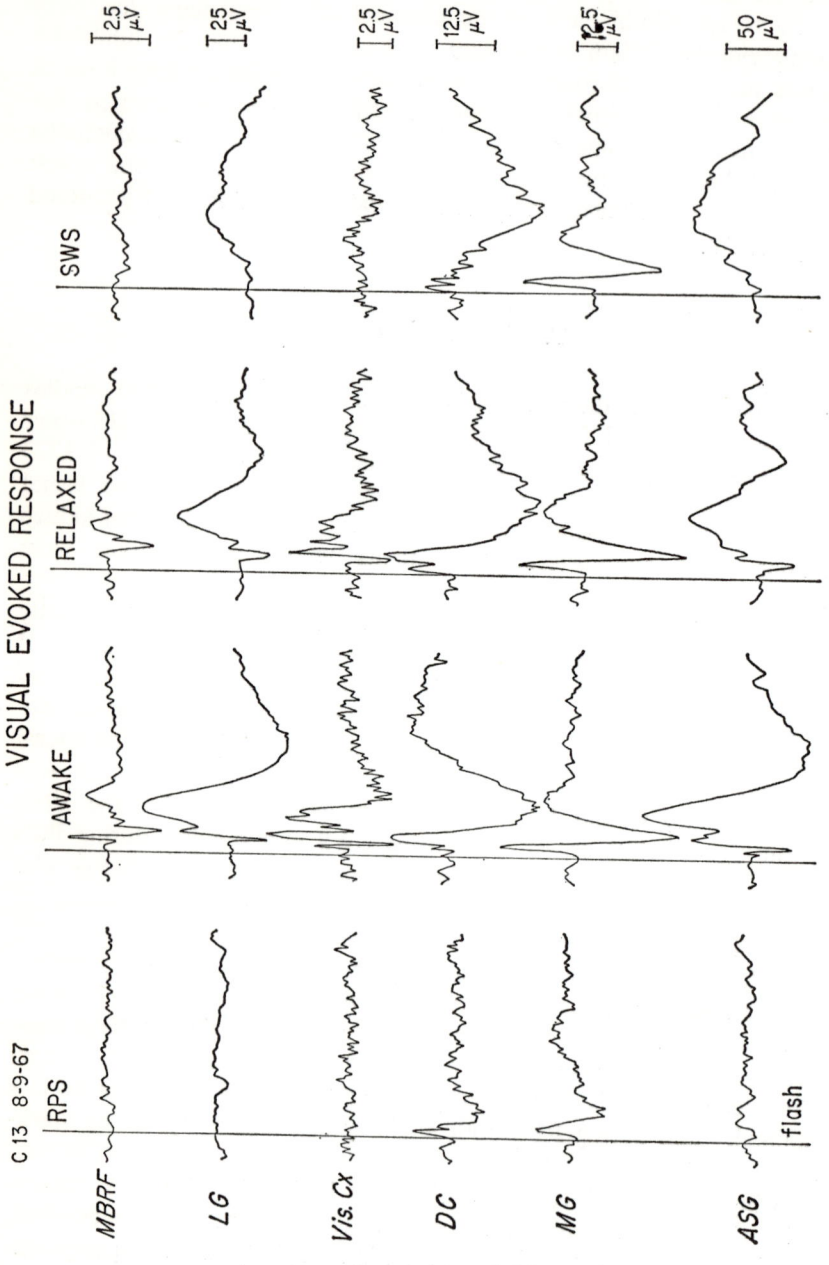

Fig. 13. Averaged visual evoked response recorded during the control states of RPS, AWAKE, RELAXED and SWS. Midbrain reticular formation (*MBRF*), lateral geniculate nucleus (*LG*), visual cortex (*Vis. Cx.*), dorsal cochlear nucleus (*DC*) medial geniculate nucleus (*MG*), and anterior suprasylvian gyrus (*ASG*). (See also Fig. 2.) (From Winters, 1968).

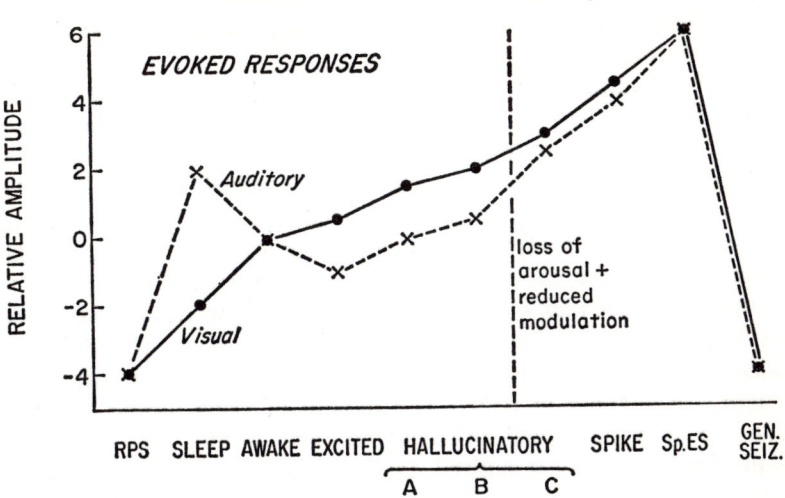

FIG. 14. Representation of the relative amplitude of the auditory and visual evoked response utilizing the effect of gamma-hydroxybutyrate as an example. The amplitude of the responses were normalized such that both auditory and visual responses are zero during the awake state. There is a loss of the arousal response and a reduction in modulation during the hallucinatory B-C stage. The modulation action is progressively reduced as the functional disorganization of the reticular formation progresses during spikes, spikes with electrical silence (SP. ES) and generalized seizure (GEN. SEIZ.).

tetrazol), the visual evoked response increases in size over the awake control. During the intermittent hypersynchronous activity (hallucinatory A), the visual evoked response is further enhanced, apparently to the point that abnormal amounts of visual information are transmitted within the CNS, resulting in the visual hallucinations. This state is characterized by an enlarged evoked response, elevated reticular unit activity and intermittent 2.5 cps hypersynchronous EEG bursts.

Following mescaline, nitrous oxide, ether, phencyclidine and gamma-hydroxybutyrate, and during the progression of increasing reticular functional disorganization (*i.e.*, 2.5-1.5 cps hypersynchrony, hallucinatory C) to spikes with electrical silence, there is a progressive increase in the VER reaching markedly enlarged response amplitudes during the latter phases.

It appears that the visual system, which has a high priority of action during the awake state, can be excessively activated to the point of disruption by overloading the input system during states of increased excitation induced by LSD. As the CNS excitation continues to the point of inducing a functional disorganization of the reticular formation modulation system, other sensory systems, such as the auditory system, begin to become functionally disrupted due to a reduction in the modulation of these sensory systems; thus multisensory aberrations are induced.

Three points are relevant regarding the relationship of visual and auditory systems to reticular formation modulation of input signals (Fig. 14): (1) As evidenced by the amplitude of the evoked response, the asleep cat is an auditory animal and the awake cat is a visual animal. (2) As one progresses through the continuum as outlined, the AER is reduced and the VER is progressively increased through hallucinatory A and B. (3) During hallucinatory C the animal is no longer arousable, the AER begins to enlarge, and both AER and VER are markedly enlarged during the pattern of spiking with electrical silence. The increase in size of the AER during hallucinatory B and C and the loss of the arousal response correlates with the progressive increase in RUA. The pattern of firing during hallucinatory B begins to lose functional organization, and during hallucinatory C is essentially functionally disorganized, thus sensory inputs are no longer modulated and the AER increases.

Since the psychotic hallucination involves more than one modality, *i.e.*, auditory, visual, somatosensory, etc., perhaps an abnormality in the general modulation system in the reticular formation exists during this disease. The psychotic hallucination may be triggered by abnormally large numbers of sensory stimuli entering the CNS which would normally be inhibited at the peripheral sense organ. In psychosis or after LSD these stimuli can enter the CNS and overload one or more sensory systems, resulting in bizarre sensory experiences.

IV. SUMMARY

To recount, we have postulated:

1. That there is a continuum of CNS excitatory states.
2. That hallucinatory activity is a part of this continuum, falling between motor excitation on one side and either general anesthesia or convulsions on the other.
3. That visual hallucinations occur prior to multisensory aberrations, presumably due to the higher priority of the visual system during states of increased excitation.
4. That hallucinations are manifestations of abnormally increased amounts of sensory input.
5. That multisensory aberrations probably occur as a result of a loss of reticular modulation of these sensory systems.
6. That psychosis may be a disorder of modulation control.

The psychotic state appears to fall in the general range of hallucinatory B. As the modulatory control of the prepsychotic becomes increasingly more disrupted, the total environment of the patient becomes more and more bizarre. Thus the lack of a clean symptomatology in schizophrenic states may be a function of the patient's individuality, past experiences and rate of change in sensory control.

It should be noted that the theories proposed above represent only a working hypothesis which serves as an aid in the design and performance of studies of these phenomena. Our strategy has been to test various aspects of the model in the cat, relate the conclusion to man and alter the model as necessary. This process will continue until a final model arises that can pass all of the critical tests and improve our understanding of the basic processes involved in disease states and the therapeutic rationale of effective controlling agents.

ACKNOWLEDGMENTS

The authors wish to acknowledge the most valuable collaborative assistance of Doctors C. E. Spooner and A. J. Mandell and the technical assistance of Mrs. Susan Miller and Mrs. Merrilyn Kvan, without whose help these studies would not have been feasible.

This work was supported in part by grants 1-R01-MH-12121 (U.S.P.H.S.), 5-TI-MH-6415 (U.S.P.H.S.), NB02501 (N.I.N.D.B.). Bibliographic assistance was received from the U.C.L.A. Brain Information Service which is part of the Neurological Information Network of N.I.N.D.B. and is supported under contract # DHEW PH-43-66-59.

REFERENCES

Adey, W. R., Bell, F. R., and Dennis, B. J.: Effects of LSD-25, psilocybin, and psilocin on temporal lobe EEG patterns and learned behavior in the cat. *Neurology, 12:* 591–602 (1962).

Apter, J. T. and Pfeiffer, C. C.: The effect of the hallucinogenic drugs LSD-25 and mescaline on the electroretinogram. *Ann. N.Y. Acad. Sci., 66:* 508–514 (1957).

Granit, R.: Centrifugal and antidromic effects on ganglion cells of retina. *J. Neurophysiol., 18:* 388–411 (1955).

Heath, R. G. and Mickle, A. W.: Evaluation of seven years' experience with depth electrode studies in human patients. In: *Electrical Studies on the Unanesthetized Brain,* edited by E. R. Ramey and D. S. O'Doherty, pp. 214–247. Hoeber, New York (1960).

Killam, K. F. and Killam, E. K.: Drug action on pathways involving the reticular formation. In: *Reticular Formation of the Brain,* edited by H. H. Jasper, L. D. Procter,

R. S. Knighton, W. C. Noshay and R. T. Costello, pp. 111–122. Little, Brown, Boston (1958).

Marcus, R. J., Winters, W. D., Mori, K. and Spooner, C. E.: A comparison of gamma-hydoxybutyrate, gamma-butyrolactone and short chain fatty acids on the EEG and behavior of the rat. *Int. J. Neuropharmacol.*, 6: 175–185 (1967).

Mori, K., Winters, W. D. and Spooner, C. E.: Comparison of reticular and cochlear multiple unit activity with auditory evoked response during various stages induced by anesthetic agents. II. *EEG Clin. Neurophysiol.*, 24: 242–248 (1968).

Purpura, D. P.: Electrophysiological analysis of psychotogenic drug action. I. Effect of LSD on specific afferent systems in the cat. *Arch. Neurol. Psychiat.*, 75: 122–131 (1956a).

Purpura, D. P.: Electrophysiological analyses of psychotogenic drug action. II. General nature of lysergic acid diethylamide (LSD) action of central synapses. *Arch. Neurol. Psychiat.*, 75: 132–141 (1956b).

Scheibel, M. E. and Scheibel, A. B.: Hallucinations and the brain stem reticular core. In: *Hallucinations*, edited by L. J. West, pp. 15–35. Grune and Stratton, New York (1962).

Schlag, J. and Balvin, R.: Background activity in the cerebral cortex and reticular formation in relation with the electroencephalogram. *Exp. Neurol.*, 8: 203–219 (1963).

Winters, W. D.: Comparison of the average cortical and subcortical evoked response to clicks during various stages of wakefulness, slow wave sleep and rhombencephalic sleep. *EEG Clin. Neurophysiol.*, 17: 234–245 (1964).

Winters, W. D.: Neuropharmacological studies and postulates on excitation and depression in the central nervous system. In: *Recent Advances in Biological Psychiatry*, edited by J. Wortis, pp. 313–345. Plenum Press, New York (1967).

Winters, W. D.: Neuropharmacological studies utilizing evoked response techniques in animals. In: *Psychopharmacology: A Review of Progress, 1957–1967*, edited by D. H. Efron, pp. 453–477. U.S. Government Printing Office, Washington, D.C. (1968).

Winters, W. D., Mori, K., Bauer, R. O. and Spooner, C. E.: The neurophysiology of anesthesia. *Anesthesiology*, 28: 65–80 (1967a).

Winters, W. D., Mori, K., Spooner, C. E. and Kado, R. T.: Correlation of reticular and cochlear multiple unit activity with evoked responses during wakefulness and sleep. I. *EEG Clin. Neurophysiol.*, 23: 539–545 (1967b).

Winters, W. D., Mori, K., Wallach, M. B., Marcus, R. J. and Spooner, C. E.: Reticular multiple unit activity during a progression of states induced by CNS excitants. III. *EEG Clin. Neurophysiol.* (in press).

Winters, W. D. and Spooner, C. E.: A neurophysiological comparison of gamma-hydroxybutyrate with pentobarbital in cats. *EEG Clin. Neurophysiol.*, 18: 287–296 (1965a).

Winters, W. D. and Spooner, C. E.: Various seizure activities following gamma-hydroxybutyrate. *Int. J. Neuropharmacol.*, 4: 197–200 (1965b).

Winters, W. D. and Spooner, C. E.: A neurophysiological comparison of alpha-chloralose with gamma-hydroxybutyrate in cats. *EEG Clin. Neurophysiol.*, 20: 83–90 (1966).

DISCUSSION

DR. DEMENT: Is the multiple unit absolutely foolproof? How do you know that you really are dealing with anatomical units?

DR. WINTERS: We can't say we are recording only unit firing. What we say is that the biological activity which we are assessing has a band pass between 500 cycles and 2.5 KC.

DR. DEMENT: And so, it might just be some curious condition that is *not* necessarily related to many units firing.

DR. WINTERS: We don't know any more than the electrophysiologist who puts a microelectrode into a cell. We probably know a little less, but all we can say is that the spikes have a one msec duration. They look very much like a spike which one sees with microelectrode techniques. It's related to biological activity because it disappears when we poison the animal with anesthetic agents, and it has a relation to behavioral states.

DR. GESSNER: In terms of your working model here, as I understand it, pentylenetetrazol does not cause hallucinations in man.

DR. WINTERS: Yes it does. Pentylenetetrazol induces a profound hallucinatory phase with intermittent and continuous EEG hypersynchrony followed by hypersynchrony of reduced frequency prior to the generalized seizure.

DR. GESSNER: If you administer it to man there is no record of it being hallucinatory?

DR. WINTERS: My understanding is that pentylenetetrazol seizures are preceded by a hallucinatory aura.

DR. DIAMOND: I would support that. Metrazol produces significant psychic changes in subconvulsive doses. These auras of terror, confusion and sense of doom are frequently so intense that psychiatrists appear to have grown much more hesitant to use the drug.

A VOICE: Operationally what you are calling the hallucinatory phase is EEG hypersynchrony. Was it intermittent to continuous hypersynchrony picked up in different brain areas?

DR. WINTERS: Yes.

A VOICE: That's all you really know about hypersynchrony?

DR. WINTERS: We see intermittent hypersynchrony associated with the behavioral syndrome which is associated with inappropriate posture and behavior in the animal, and we call it hallucinatory behavior.

We fully realize the fact that one cannot prove that a cat is hallucinating, but behaviorally he certainly looks as if he is. This behavior always appears when we see the electrical phenomena described. On the basis of the behavioral and associated electrophysiological records, we postulate the existence of three states, hallucinatory A, B, and C.

A VOICE: Would the changes in amplitude noted for the visual evoked response occur at the receptor level?

DR. WINTERS: The modulation is probably mainly at the receptor level.

DR. TEUBER: You mean there is no control over the pupil in these experiments?

DR. WINTERS: That's right. The eyes are closed when the animal is asleep. We are just reporting the phenomenon as it occurs.

DR. TEUBER: It might reflect changes in the pupils, eyes, or in general muscle tension.

DR. WINTERS: Right.

DR. DOMINO: Would you agree that the change is peripheral?

DR. WINTERS: Yes. I think it is mainly peripheral, but induced via a central control mechanism.

DR. DIAMOND: What is the magnitude of the visual stimulus as compared to the auditory?

DR. WINTERS: The auditory stimulus is 10 db above noise; we have not quantitated it.

DR. DIAMOND: A global stimulus?

DR. WINTERS: Yes. The visual and auditory stimuli were set arbitrarily at levels which enabled us to obtain responses which were above threshold and which changed significantly with changes in state.

DR. UNGER: You don't think these stimulus parameters affect the magnitude of the auditory or visual response? Do you think that you can just make a flat statement that this is an auditory animal, not a visual one, independent of parameters of the input?

DR. WINTERS: I'm not sure that it is possible to equalize two different input systems in a meaningful way. However, the data in Fig. 14 were normalized such that the amplitudes of the evoked response were the same when the animal was awake. I don't see why it is so difficult to assume that when an animal goes to sleep his auditory system is a more protective sensory input system for him than is his visual system, and that when he is awake his visual system is a more protective sensory system than is his auditory system.

DR. UNGER: On what basis do you infer that LSD induces mainly visual hallucinations? Which cat experiment showed this? We can get auditory hallucinations with LSD.

DR. WINTERS: I was referring to clinical studies and trying to explain the clinical data on the basis of our model and data obtained in the cat. My impression is that LSD induces mainly visual hallucinations in man.

DR. UNGER: On occasion, auditory hallucinations under LSD do occur, if you want to call them hallucinations. However, man appears to be a visual animal.

DR. DOMINO: Dr. Winters, you have stuck your neck out, but frankly I am glad you did. You have taken a great deal of very complex electrophysiological data and tried to make some sense out of it. I might disagree here and there with your scheme; still, you have been very courageous and I personally would like to say thank you for doing it, because you are making me do a lot of thinking about what is going on.

For example, a subject on LSD who has a hallucinogenic episode develops theta waves. That seems to fit with your cat story.

DR. WINTERS: I might mention that fifteen years ago Heath recorded similar types of EEG patterning with electrodes implanted in brains of men, *i.e.,* hypersynchronous activity following psilocybin, LSD, and mescaline. This was associated with hallucinatory behavior. He reported further that schizophrenics during acute exacerbations have hypersynchronous activity and septal spiking, whereas, during regression, this activity subsides. These studies were looked upon with distrust for a long time. However, studies of two schizophrenic patients with implanted electrodes at U.C.L.A. have confirmed Heath's findings.

DR. DOMINO: I was a little surprised that you would take the position that the decreased response in the visual system during slow wave sleep was a strictly peripheral phenomenon. Do you have data to support that?

DR. WINTERS: I didn't say it was strictly peripheral. I didn't want to get into an argument about the cat's eyes being closed, thus there is less illumination on the retina, and so on. More important is the finding that going from the point of wakefulness up the continuum of CNS excitation, reticular activation facilitates unit firing of the retina, and would indicate a central control of the input system such that arousal induces facilitation (Granit, 1955).

DR. STEIN: Could we return to someone's previous question about where dreaming fits into your scheme?

DR. WINTERS: We obviously don't have any evidence as to whether cats dream during RPS[1] or not. They certainly look like they are sleeping and dreaming, but I suppose I am not to be permitted the same clinical observation that one is permitted in the case of man.

DR. WEST: If they can hallucinate, they can dream.

DR. WINTERS: Cats hallucinate begrudgingly, though. My concept is that there are two general types of hallucinations. The type that was seen with these drug-induced states of increased excitability represents a reduction in modulation of sensory input, so that more information from a given stimulus impinges upon the nervous system. As a result, the learned relationships are lost and bizarre representation of the stimulus occurs. The second type is represented by dreaming, and perhaps also sensory deprivation represents an endogenous dream state characterized by a reduction in exogenous sensory

---

[1] RPS = rhomboencephalic phasic sleep, the phasic component of REM; however, in this case, the term is used interchangeably with REM. (Ed.)

input. For example, during RPS, the auditory and visual responses are markedly reduced. It would appear that peripheral sensory inputs are reduced, and it is like a state of sensory deprivation. Now, what the mechanism for the hallucination in this state is, I don't know.

DR. STEIN: So on your chart it goes before sleep, rather than in hallucination through excitation?

DR. WINTERS: Yes, I regard RPS as an entirely different phenomenon, and it is not in the CNS continuum. I don't know where to put RPS, but it is off to the side somewhere. On the basis of unit activity and PGO spikes, RPS represents CNS excitation, not deep sleep. On the basis of evoked responses, responsiveness to stimuli, and EEG, it is like a deep sleep.

DR. UNGER: What about hypersynchrony?

DR. WINTERS: I have never seen 2.5 to 3 cps hypersynchrony in RPS sleep. I have seen theta activity in the frequency range of 5 to 7 cps which is localized only in the hippocampus but does not appear in other areas, except in something like the rat which has a very thin cortex. You can often get theta activity reflected on the surface of the posterior cortex in the rat.

DR. UNGER: As I understood you before, the sort of hypersynchrony observed was the operational index for what you called hallucinations. Now, if you don't see hypersynchrony in REM (RPS) sleep, then, in your use of terms, I think one would conclude there are no hallucinations during REM sleep.

DR. WINTERS: As I just stated, there appears to be a difference between the hallucination of the excitatory state which appears to be characterized by hypersynchrony as opposed to dreaming and the hallucination of sensory deprivation. I have not studied the electrophysiology of sensory deprivation.

DR. MANDELL: If you move to man, you can't see the hippocampal theta activity in depth electrode studies of sleep, not even with the aid of a computer.

DR. UNGER: Regarding this hypersynchronous period which you call hallucinatory A, B, and C, if you left out "hallucinatory," I think we could communicate more effectively in an objective data-level language and then discuss the interpretation of these phenomena separately.

DR. WINTERS: You can call it anything you wish.

DR. UNGER: Well, why not first stick to describing the phenomena which you are actually observing?

DR. WINTERS: I call it on the basis of the phenomenon which I have observed. I am using hallucinatory drugs. These are drugs which produce hallucinations in man.

DR. UNGER: Well, but that is perhaps an arguable point.

DR. WINTERS: The point being what?

DR. UNGER: The point being that many investigators have found that *true* hallucinations (with loss of insight) are rare occurrences after the administration of this class of drugs. Hence, it's been a somewhat confusing and prejudicial kind of presumption to have labeled these drugs hallucinogenic.

DR. WINTERS: I am unaware of this group of people and their argument. Whatever the effect is in man and whatever you want to call it in man, something similar to this seems to occur in our animals.

DR. KOPIN: Another question relates to the effect of cutting off the efferent impulses to the sensory organs. Would you expect to have a continual state of hallucination, or would you expect that LSD and other hallucinogens would not work?

DR. WINTERS: I have not studied this. You are pulling me into sensory deprivation experimentation.

DR. KOPIN: I did not mean cutting off incoming signals, but outgoing ones to the sensory organs. If you had cut off these sensory efferents by destruction of the pathways, would you then expect that LSD would no longer have an effect, or that there would then be a continual state of hallucination?

DR. WINTERS: I would guess that there would be a continual state of hallucinations.

DR. KOPIN: Would this be a continual state? If the reason hallucinations are caused is that there is a diminished amount of efferent control of the receptor, then if this were cut off completely there would be a continual state of hallucination.

DR. MANDELL: I don't want to talk for Dr. Winters, but I don't think he implied purely efferent receptor modulation, but rather a more complex, integrative type involving sensory collaterals, the reticular formation, and perhaps more anterior structures, such as the midline thalamic nuclei.

DR. KOPIN: Originally I had asked about the receptor, and his answer was that yes, he did think it was at the receptor.

DR. WINTERS: I think there is a modulation at the receptor, and the geniculate is very important in terms of the visual system. The main responsibility for modulation of sensory input systems probably lies within the control of the reticular formation. We have the idea that psychosis is a state in which modulatory control of input is disrupted, and this is why multisensory aberrations are observed in this disease.

DR. KOPIN: Modulation can occur at any level. The question is, where is it occurring? I think Roy John has demonstrated that you can shift the site of modulating control from one area to another. This is part of the feedback mechanism of the brain. The primary modulating control of sensory input may be from the reticular formation down to the peripheral sense organ, but there are also ways of modulating impulses at many levels.

DR. TEUBER: How many of these effects might be in a strict sense peripheral, so that they are due to those well-known mechanisms for modulating input, even mere changes in the directions of the head and eyes relative to a visual stimulus, etc. These are questions that have plagued this field for quite a number of years now. But to assure Dr. Domino, I did not mean to say that if we admit these peripheral components we have thereby excluded the central ones; of course not. Unfortunately, all these analyses are still in a rather primitive state. As we begin to investigate these regulations with more refined tools, going from massive stimulation of midbrain (and watching what happens in the retinal pathway) to actual microelectrode recordings, say during certain phases of sleep and REM sleep, for instance, you find that in the cat you do have a presynaptic inhibition at the lateral geniculate nucleus. This effect during rapid eye movements in the dark was discovered by Emilio Bizzi (*J. Neurophysiol. 29:* 1087–1095, 1966). But when Bizzi tried the same thing in the monkey he could not find this particular geniculate interaction during REM sleep, and I do think we are closer to the monkey than to the cat. So this, you see, is one of the many reasons why it is easy to get discouraged at times in looking at these phenomena.[2]

DR. WINTERS: I can't say anything about the monkey in terms of sensory input-output systems. I could add, though, that the pharmacological effects that we observed were also observed in the chimpanzee, which is really a young primate, in the rat, and for some of them, in the chick.

DR. KORNETSKY: I do not think the question whether or not cats or dogs hallucinate or dream is really the relevant question. That is, can you observe and measure physiological and behavioral changes after certain drugs in infrahuman species that are similar to those seen in man when he is dreaming? The question of dreaming in animals is an interesting one. Since animals do not have language, dreaming may be functionally quite disrupting for them. We can use language to test to distinguish reality from non-reality of a dream against the reality of others. How does an animal do this? If an animal dreams as we do and it dreamed that he had eaten, he would be put in immediate conflict when he awakened. He would feel hungry, but would have a memory of eating. I think this would be functionally quite difficult for the animal.

DR. KOPIN: I would think he would have just as much trouble remembering how long ago he ate. If he were hungry he could be hungry again.

DR. DEMENT: That is an interesting point, whether the confusion that

---

[2] References for all parts of Dr. Teuber's comments of Session III appear at the end of this discussion.

arises is based upon memory or not. Part of the judgment is made by comparing the dream to reality in terms of spatial configuration and so forth. If you don't remember doing something, is the need still satisfied? How much is remembering part of the really essential aspect of fulfillment?

A VOICE: He would believe in his stomach rather than his memory.

DR. DEMENT: Yes, but for subjects that were not related to his stomach, there could be a traumatic experience.

I would like to pose a question: If someone had a traumatic experience and was amnesiac for this experience; and the memory of the experience came back first in a dream, would it then be experienced as if it had been experienced for the first time, and would the emotional consequences be what they were the first time?

DR. FREEDMAN: What they could have been the first time?

DR. DEMENT: If you have repressed the experience, will eventual recall be as if it were the first time it had happened?

A VOICE: Generally speaking, no. The closest experimental approach to this is in hypnosis and hypnotic amnesias, but a number of experiments show that while a person may claim that he is experiencing the repressed materials, and that he does not remember at all the information that has been blotted out by hypnotic association which is presumably related at least to the mechanism of the traumatic amnesia—I assume emotionally traumatic amnesia is what you are describing—the kind that would come back first in a dream and then little by little as a person could tolerate.

Anyhow, these hypnotic experiments I think may go back in time, and in subtle ways the person reveals that he is aware of the information and behaves in some fashion accordingly.

DR. FREEDMAN: That is not the condition he described—not the subtle way with which he would monitor the behavior and so the amnesia. But with war casualties—we have seen this clinically, I don't know about experimentally—traumatic dreams or sudden confrontations, sudden breaks in the amnesia occur. I think you see this sometimes in LSD. A break of the barrier can be very traumatic.

DR. WEST: From a theoretical view point, wouldn't it be proper to say that the material that began to come back, first in dreams and then in bits and fragments of recollection, was something the person was now psychologically more capable of recalling, more prepared to integrate at a conscious level?

DR. FREEDMAN: You are speaking of adaptive processes in dreams, and they are there.

QUESTION: What if you have a break?

DR. WEST: With sodium amytal you do break into it.

DR. FREEDMAN: Or with LSD.

DR. WEST: I have never known a case where the dream of a normal person, recalled by him, posed a problem that he was so unable to face that he disorganized on account of it.

DR. LEHRER: You talk about a break after a period of amnesia. I wonder if the recall is the equivalent of the original experience or if it may have been amplified, added to or modified in the meantime?

DR. FREEDMAN: Obviously this is possible. That may be the definition of the condition under which a person disorganizes. He doesn't have the option, the alternatives, the feedback from reality—all the things that you might need to have a sort of gyroscope that keeps you going. I think that's probably what we are defining.

DR. STEIN: Isn't the question of whether or not a break occurs separate from the discussion of what processes are involved in retrieving traumatically repressed memories? The retrieval may or may not cause a break. I would like to second Dr. Freedman's idea that the retrieval in narcoanalysis may be similar to the kind of retrieval that occurs in sleep. In both states, the drug state and the dream state, and perhaps in fatigue states as well, one is in a condition of lowered inhibition (lessened activity of the periventricular mechanism). Under these conditions of low inhibition, the forbidden retrieval is more likely to occur.

DR. WEST: I would like to say one more thing about this, if I might, in response to a point Dr. Dement brought out.

I think there are two different kinds of circumstances in which material reappears in a dream that might be pertinent; one augurs well, and the other augurs ill.

If a person is in a state of psychological improvement and is now able to deal with information he couldn't manage before, it might start to appear in dreams as manifest dream content even before he recalled it during wakefulness. This is what you may see in a person who is routinely reporting his dreams during psychotherapy, perhaps following recovery from a psychotic break, and is now being followed along.

However, the opposite significance would hold in the case of a person who is beginning to disintegrate psychologically, and is not able any longer successfully to repress previously unconscious material or process ideation. This previously repressed material may start appearing in dreams as a harbinger of what is soon going to appear even in the waking state. In that respect it would be a sign that things were getting worse.

DR. DEMENT: Well, the trouble is that we remember so few of our dreams. If you could have the experience of being awakened every time a dream occurs night after night, it might get to be confusing just on its own terms; that is, there would be so many dream memories that you might easily have trouble sorting them out from real experiences. We are protected from this by not remembering; but in terms of what a recall experience is and what it should do to the organism, if dreams are real at the time—and they certainly seem to be when you remember them vividly—how do we separate them, really, from our waking experience? How is that memory barrier accomplished?

When you add up two hours a night, night after night, that is a lot of experience. Where does it go?

DR. STEIN: Perhaps there are two mechanisms for separating dreams from real experiences. One of them is simply forgetting the dream, and that may account for some of it. The other is labeling a dream as a dream. When I see a motion picture I don't pool these events into my own set of experiences. I remember that they occurred in a movie. And I see no reason why the events that occur in dreams couldn't somehow be labeled and remembered as dreams.

DR. DEMENT: I am only telling you that if you remember all of your dreams, you don't do that so well. You start saying, "Gosh darn it, did that happen in the dream or didn't it?" You can't tell.

DR. STEIN: That may be why we forget some of them.

DR. DEMENT: We don't want to do this too much on a continuing basis.

DR. FREEDMAN: In response to that problem, we have to interpose another step in experiences of vividness and reality. Anything experienced really can't be denied reality. The question is how do you locate it; which order of reality do you locate the "real" experiences in?

DR. OSMOND: I think that schizophrenic patients often attempt to cope with their peculiar and unfamiliar experiences by looking upon them as a dream, or perhaps, more exactly, as a nightmare. When they begin to recover, some patients are very much afraid that the waking nightmare will recur. It is only as they become more confident of their recovery that some of them become much concerned to know what "really" happened to them; then they need help to categorize strange, even bizarre happenings which they can recall with various degrees of reality. They must be helped to distinguish what "really" happened, as perceived by others, from what they experienced, from what might have happened and what never happened. Some people have great difficulty in doing this; some have very little.

DR. DEMENT: I think that the only animal who could get confused is the human. I could give you a whole list of reasons for saying this. I think humans are the only ones for whom dreams and reality are the same. I don't think cats see the real world in REM sleep, and I don't think, with rare exceptions, that monkeys do either. What I am saying is that the internal stimuli of REM sleep are not capable of replicating the real world in cats, but that they are in humans.

DR. HOLMSTEDT: Why do you say that?

DR. DEMENT: You are asking for a 10 minute discourse. Let me mention just one kind of data relevant to this issue. If you give cats p-chlorophenylalanine (PCPA) and follow them while the brain 5-HT level drops to virtually zero, you will see in the waking state of the cat electrophysiological (PGO spike) phenomena which are usually seen only in REM sleep; you can't tell the difference. You can, however, tell that the cat is not in REM sleep. He is, in a sense, in two states at the same time, REM sleep and wakefulness. In this condition, he doesn't act as if he is seeing formed activity. When REM events occur, he acts only as if expecting to see something, or as if you made a click. The cat never seems to be seeing a mouse and then reacting to that appropriately. Never does he ever do anything that would confirm there is a real honest-to-goodness image out there.

The monkey, when given PCPA, falls somewhere in between on the hallucination scale. Most of his behavior is nondescript, like the cat, but every once in awhile—infrequently—you see him do something that could only occur in response to complex stimuli. For example, when you approach the monkey's cage, he bares his teeth and makes threatening motions. Occasionally, he will do that in the PCPA state when no one is there.

The human, from what I have read in the literature, can have continuing complicated hallucinations when treated with PCPA.

But at any rate, this and some other things make you suspect that the cat simply doesn't see in REM sleep what he sees when he is awake, and likewise with monkeys. Human beings are the only animals that really duplicate the real world in REM sleep in most of its properties.

DR. LUDWIG: I would just like to cover a couple of clinical observations which may resolve some of what has been said—perhaps even make it more complex in a way. We are asking the question what is real in terms of dreaming or the waking state? When a man is dreaming he is doing something more than dreaming, since on some level of consciousness he often is aware that he is dreaming. And in many dreams which are disturbing, for example, he can tell himself that he is dreaming, and can go back to the dream and try to resolve it. Is this reality if something is very vivid for him? Well, it is reality plus the additional knowledge that he is dreaming.

For example, under a drug state, such as LSD, things are real, but by the same token the person is often aware that what he is experiencing is due to the drug; it's real but it isn't real at the same time. The really scary part comes when he's no longer aware that he is dreaming or under the influence of drugs.

DR. DEMENT: There is one other aspect of that. Many people have had the experience of knowing that they are dreaming when they are presumably dreaming; at least so they say. But there is another quality: being impelled along and not having time to stop and really contemplate the events; for example, you look at something, it's a person you know perfectly well is dead, or it's writing you know you shouldn't understand, or you are playing a piano. You know full well you didn't take lessons. You don't seem to be able to stop and reflect on the improbability of that—you are on to the next event. So I think that there is some aspect that is missing in this state that is present in wakefulness.

DR. FREEDMAN: Dr. Dement, the Lord was merciful; in view of some of our dreams perhaps he was making sure we were impaired during that state.

A VOICE: Dr. Teuber, what happens in the split-brain preparation in the course of subjective experiences?

DR. TEUBER: I can't speak much about that, having seen only one case, but certainly they don't seem to be very different with respect to the things we are now discussing. Each hemisphere, apparently, can process and store sensory impressions, but only one hemisphere can talk about them. What may be more relevant is another clinical condition, namely, post-traumatic amnesia, not in the sense of hysterical repression but of apparently genuine forgetting due to a cerebral trauma. Following a concussion, as you all know, there may be this inability to recall events immediately preceding the blow, as if some crucial stage in the processing of material had been disrupted. You see particularly severe retrograde effects of this sort after certain surgical assaults upon the brain, as in bilateral hippocampectomy. We have had the privilege of seeing the famous Scoville-Milner case, patient H. M., in our laboratory on several occasions (Scoville and Milner, *J. Neurol. Neurosurg. Psychiat.* 20: 11–21, 1957; Milner, Corkin and Teuber, *Neuropsychol.* 6: 215–234, 1968), and one is certainly struck by the retrograde effect of the operation in this case (he apparently has a gap of more than a year preceding the hippocampal removal); the anterograde amnesia is very severe. This man lost his father about two years ago. We dare not ask him about that, because he has forgotten the event so completely that if you inadvertently bring it up, you get the complete bereavement reaction all over again, as if he heard the news for the first time. Note that this can happen only because his earlier attachment is still there; he does recall the time he spent with his father up to the operation, except for the last 18 months or so before surgery.

In trying to come to grips with these forms of amnesia, one has to assume that some crucial step in the categorizing of ongoing events is missing after these mesial temporal lobectomies (and, transiently at least, after certain lesions in the upper brainstem; cf. Milner, Corkin and Teuber, *Neuropsychol.*

6: 215–234, 1968). Events are perceived but not put into the form in which they can be stored and retrieved.

The difficulty we experience in recalling dreams may be quite similar, and perhaps so is the trouble in retrieving childhood events as well. It is certainly paradoxical: children learn such a great many things, including language and all sorts of complicated motor skills, but the recall for events of one's early childhood is quite poor; this or that incident resurfaces, often in a manner similar to the notorious "islands of memory" that surface from a sea of forgetting in the post-traumatic amnestic state. Some functional level on which we transform individual experiences into a more permanent store is not reached by the child, even though he is extremely competent in acquiring implicit rules (as in first-language learning). To come back, finally, to the unanswerable question, Dr. Winters, of whether cats are dreaming: I am much more ready to concede them their dreams than to assume they could ever give us their autobiography![2]

DR. WINTERS: The point I was making was that gamma-hydroxybutyrate is one example of an agent which induces an epileptoid progression, yet is used clinically in Europe and Asia and is in clinical trial in this country as an anesthetic agent. If you check the clinical literature, there are many clinical statements of the efficacy of the agent, and on the basis of the neurophysiological effect on the cat—and I hasten to add on the chimp, monkey, rat, and chick—one would assume that this agent induces epileptic activity, and the only criteria which we can come up with to understand how this agent can be used clinically is that this drug induces a state of unresponsiveness and amnesia, so that the surgeon can perform his surgery and the subject will not recall the events.

DR. FREEDMAN: The reason you can't use the term catatonic is that the catatonic with waxy flexibility is monitoring very clearly what goes on and doesn't really have amnesia.

A VOICE: There is a fascinating discussion going on here about dreams and the reality thereof, and I wonder if I might address myself to this concept: that is, that people who have experienced psychedelic drugs appeared later to revise for a time thereafter their concept of what is real. I think this is the meaning in which this should be discussed.

DR. MANDELL: I think it would have been of interest to invite to this conference Kenneth Kesey, who has done in addition to his novel writing some informal clinical research in this area. He was the one, you remember, who wrote *One Flew Over the Cuckoo Nest*. He drove a psychedelic bus with a

---

[2] References for all parts of **Dr. Teuber's** comments of Session III appear at the end of this discussion.

rock band and had a hobby of dropping LSD into the punch at parties without telling anyone. I have talked to two people who were at such parties and what resulted is similar to what Dr. Dement is talking about. The unknowing acid takers began to experience their aberrations within the context of normality without the "drug-taking" set. Is this what the REM-deprived person with a high REM deficit experiences? Is the capacity for reflection against reality necessary to make a dream a dream and not reality without the knowledge of the drug ingestion?

Perhaps Hoffman's original experiment with LSD and his initial subjective "psychosis" (not "drug experience") may be another example of the need a person has to have an actual reality against which to reflect an induced reality. These kinds of drug experiences (sans set) add considerable substance to the issue Dr. Dement introduced.

DR. FREEDMAN: Hoffman noticed the difference. He noticed the difference and took certain behavioral measures, such as going home and not working.

DR. WASER: He felt sick!

DR. MANDELL: The second time he knew better.

DR. WEST: Kenneth Kesey is an author who isn't driving his psychedelic bus around anymore because he was jailed for possession of marihuana, and has subsequently withdrawn to recover on a farm in Washington. His case history appears in a recent book by Tom Wolfe entitled *The Electric Kool-Aid Acid Test*.

DR. JULESZ: I have one book I would like to recommend, *The Mind of a Mnemonist* by Luria (Basic Books) translated a year ago from Russian to English. There is a strange, abnormal man whose problem is that he *cannot* forget. He does not have childhood amnesia, and so on. He doesn't have the next process which we have, namely, he just doesn't have symbolic thinking. Probably in this man the ability for symbolic processing did not develop; for instance, he could not imagine the notion of "nothing." For him "nothing" meant a gray cloud, whereas "something" was a cloud of another color. In his childhood he would sometimes forget to go to school because he so vividly visualized that he was going to school. He was already "at school" when his father said, "Oh, why didn't you wake up?" So maybe the sense of reality is something that operates on a higher level.

DR. TEUBER: May I add one footnote to what Dr. Julesz just said? The book is an amazing account of a "hyperamnestic" rather than amnestic condition. Yet with all these tremendous accomplishments of memory, this man had a remarkable and selective difficulty in recognizing faces. I just want to underscore this. We are utter primitives in dealing with these phenomena. To think that we have a single word, *memory,* for such a tremendous diversity of behavioral achievements! The term *memory* is one of the main barriers that keeps us from coming to grips with the question of basic mechanisms.

References for Dr. Teuber's portions of the discussion

Bizzi, E.: Discharge patterns of single geniculate neurons during rapid eye movements of sleep. *J. Neurophysiol., 29:* 1087–1095 (1966).

Broadbent, D. E. and Gregory, M.: Accuracy of recognition for speech presented to the right and left ears. *Quart. J. Exp. Psychol., 16:* 359–360 (1964).

Kimura, Doreen: Functional asymmetry of the brain in dichotic listening. *Cortex, 3:* 163–178 (1967).

Köhler, W. Zur Theorie des Sukzessivvergleichs und der Zeitfehler. *Psychol. Forschung, 4:* 115–175 (1923).

Kraepelin, E. Der psychologische Versuch in der Psychiatrie. *Psychol. Arbeiten, 1:* 1–91 (1896).

Lange, J. and Specht, W. Neue Untersuchungen über die Beeinflussung der Sinnesfunktionen durch geringe Alkoholmengen. *Z. Pathopsychologie, 3:* 155–256 (1914–1919).

Milner, Brenda, Corkin, Suzanne and Teuber, H.-L. Further analysis of the hippocampal amnesic syndrome: 14-year follow-up study of H.M. *Neuropsychologia, 6:* 215–234 (1968).

Soville, W. B. and Milner, Brenda. Loss of recent memory after bilateral hippocampal lesions. *J. Neurol. Neurosurg. Psychiat., 20:* 11–21 (1957).

Specht, W. *Die Beeinflussung der Sinnesfunktionen durch geringe Alkoholmengen. I. Teil: Das Verhalten von Unterschiedsschwelle und Reizschwelle im Gebiet des Gehörsinnes.* Leipzig: Engelmann, 1907.

SESSION IV

CLINICAL CONSIDERATIONS:
a. Model Psychosis
b. Therapeutic Use and Therapeutic Potential

Daniel X. Freedman, M.D. and Louis J. West, M.D., Co-Chairmen

THE RELEVANCE OF CHEMICALLY-INDUCED PSYCHOSES TO SCHIZOPHRENIA

Morris A. Lipton, M.D., Ph.D.

Department of Psychiatry, University of North Carolina School of Medicine, Chapel Hill, N.C. 27515

Contemporary psychiatry is not without its paradoxes. One of these is in the area of psychotomimetic agents. Of the many defensible reasons for interest in research on these agents, two of the foremost deal with opposing propositions. The first states that psychotomimetic agents may produce psychoses which are useful models of spontaneous or endogenous psychoses like schizophrenia, and may, therefore, offer insight into their biochemical or metabolic etiology. The other proposition is that psychotomimetic agents may be therapeutically useful. I call these opposites because if the first is true, then the second implies that the production of a transient psychosis is therapeutically useful in the treatment of certain types of mental illness. Offhand, this would seem to be absurd, but need not necessarily be so. I shall try to examine both propositions critically.

The concept that schizophrenia is an illness caused by a toxic metabolite is, of course, hardly new and dates back at least to Thudicum (1884), who felt that many forms of insanity were the result of intoxications. The toxic model of mental illness fits the traditional model of many somatic illnesses which can be caused by poisonings of some sort. This model reached its height with the infectious, or germ, theory of disease. The success of this model with repeated demonstrations that so many somatic illnesses are caused by external noxious agents or internally produced aberrant metabolites makes it persistently attractive in the field of mental illness. Fashions have changed somewhat over the years, and what used to be viruses or ptomaines are now products of an autoimmune reaction, an ingested amino acid, or an aberrant transmethylation, yet they ultimately fit into a toxic model. Some chemical enters or is produced somewhere in the body, and this affects the function of the brain to produce a psychosis.

The discovery of a substantial number of psychotomimetic compounds, frequently derivatives of the neurohumors, has led to the most recent resurgence. Within the past decade taraxein, bufotenin, adrenochrome, dimethoxyphenylethylamine, and perhaps other compounds suggested by the transmethylation hypothesis have been candidates (Smythies, 1967).

You will recall, of course, that Koch about 100 years ago established four postulates which had to be met in order to satisfy the requirements for the etiology of an infectious disease. He required that the organism be isolated, that it be cultured in pure medium, that when administered to an organism it produced the illness, and that it could again be isolated from the new organism after it had been made ill. These are very rigorous criteria, but they are the standards which have consistently been met by investigators in the field of infectious disease. Modified but similarly rigorous criteria have been employed by pharmacologists and toxicologists investigating other types of toxic illnesses.

It would seem appropriate, then, to ask to what extent have Koch's postulates or some modification of them been met by those who are proponents of the chemical models of psychoses. Before doing so, however, it is worth emphasizing that this is by no means the only model of illness which the physician and investigator has, and that it is inappropriate to some forms of illness. A strong competitor, for example, is the deficiency model. For reasons which are not at all clear, the toxic model and deficiency model have competed throughout the ages, with the toxic model usually being more popular initially. Thus, toxicity, in the form of demons, miasmas, and germs held sway for hundreds of years before deficiencies were taken seriously. It is, after all, only since the beginnings of the 20th century that illnesses due to vitamin or mineral deficiency were thoroughly established. In the area of psychiatry, too, even Freud initially attributed the origins of mental illness to a traumatic (toxic?) environment and only much later to deprivation. In the field of mental retardation it is hardly a decade since emphasis has been placed upon emotional or cultural deprivation as a cause of illness.

These are not the only two models available. Another, which intrigues the oncologists, deals with carcinogenic agents which trigger a process which goes inexorably on long after the initiating agent has been metabolized. Many chemical carcinogens are metabolized and disappear long before the tumor becomes established. Still other disease models exist, but time does not permit their discussion. It is worth keeping in mind that these models need not be mutually exclusive. In the inborn errors of metabolism, for example, an enzyme deficiency may result in the accumulation of toxic metabolites that may be related to the pathogenesis of the illness and the nature of its symptoms.

Returning to the toxic model of endogenous psychoses and the relevance of the chemical psychoses to these, we may attempt to examine them from the perspective of Koch's postulates. First, are there any agents which seem to be uniquely present in the tissues or excreta of psychotic patients and which, when administered to normals, will render them psychotic? The answer is no, or at most a very weak yes. Of the many potent agents which produce chemical psychoses, none have been isolated from the urine or tissues of schizophrenics. Compounds isolated from such patients have little or no psychotomimetic potency and are not absolutely unique to their illness. For example, dimethoxyphenylethylamine (DMPEA), the compound discovered by Friedhoff (1967), is present in 65% of acutely ill schizophrenics and 8% of normal controls. It seems not to be present in the urine of chronic schizophrenics, and it disappears from the urine of acute schizophrenics when phenothiazines are given, even though some symptoms of the illness remain. Friedhoff's findings have been questioned, but even if they are correct, we are left with a dilemma. Eight percent of the population, or 16 million people, in this country presumably excrete the compound but not more than one percent have schizophrenia. At the very most, then, the DMPEA may be a necessary but not sufficient condition for the illness. Thirty-five percent of acute schizophrenics do not excrete it. This may imply a subtype or subtypes which are different, and we have long suspected that the schizophrenic condition may be a syndrome encompassing several illnesses. Chronic schizophrenics and schizophrenics on phenothiazines do not excrete it. We have no explanation for this, but perhaps the compound is formed only by subjects with a genetic diathesis during the stress of the initial psychotic turmoil and disappears when a relatively peaceful psychotic resolution is achieved. In a somewhat loose sense, the compound may resemble the carcinogen which initiates a process which is continued after the agent is gone. Since Sachar *et al.* (1963) have shown that there is extremely intense anxiety associated with both entering into and coming out of a psychotic equilibrium, it is possible that patients are maintained in a psychotic state by the Damoclean threat of encountering the same metabolic psychotogen when coming out of the psychotic state. Speculation of this sort may be attractive since it might help to explain Friedhoff's data, but it is utterly lacking in evidence.

If the situation regarding the presence of dimethoxyphenylethylamine in the urine of schizophrenics is muddy and Koch's first postulate isn't clearly met, we find ourselves even more disappointed when we examine this compound with respect to the second postulate. DMPEA administered in high doses to normal subjects does not produce a psychotic state (Friedhoff and

Hollister, 1966). Recently, Friedhoff demonstrated that DMPEA could be acetylated to N-acetyl DMPEA, and this compound has five times the hallucinogenic properties of mescaline when administered in rats. However, it too has no psychotomimetic properties when administered to man (Friedhoff, personal communication).

Bufotenin (5-OH dimethyltryptamine) presents us with similar problems. This compound, as well as tryptamine and indole metabolites, has been reported to be present in elevated concentrations in the urine of schizophrenics during an exacerbating phase of schizophrenia (Brune and Himwich, 1963; Tanimukai et al., 1967), but here, too, the results are controversial. Furthermore, there is a consensus that bufotenin administered to human subjects is not psychotomimetic (Turner and Merlis, 1959). Clearly, neither the first nor the second of Koch's postulates have been met with either compound.

Compounds with true psychotomimetic properties have not been isolated from the urine or blood of psychotic patients, and those compounds claimed to be present in schizophrenia have no psychotomimetic properties when administered to normals. One exception to this generalization seems to be found in Heath's work with taraxein. Here, the claim is made that a compound is present in the blood of schizophrenics and that this compound administered to either humans or monkeys will produce a similar clinical or electroencephalographic condition (Heath and Krupp, 1967). This work, while highly controversial and badly in need of replication, at least has a systematic logic, and if correct, does fulfill the first two postulates.

Recently, I have heard of an unusual compound, isolated from schizophrenic sweat by Dr. K. Smith of Washington University. This compound presumably accounts for the unusual odor of schizophrenic patients. The compound is *trans*-3-methyl-2-hexenoic acid. Whether it is psychotomimetic or possesses any unusual biological activity is not known. But its chemical structure seems established beyond a doubt by the techniques of gas chromatography, mass spectrometry and nuclear magnetic resonance spectrometry. In an era of frequent disappointment one can only hope that this compound will not be an artifact and will offer a clue.

The problems in isolating compounds unique to schizophrenia are formidable, and I do not mean to discourage the continuing search. Humane considerations thus far limit us to readily accessible tissues like blood or excreta like sweat or urine. The mere facts that neurohumors are present in micro quantities in the brain, that psychotomimetic agents chemically related to these neurohumors are potent in exceptionally small dosages and that the brain is homeostatically insulated from the remainder of the body all generate technical difficulties that make direct evidence difficult to obtain. Technological advances such as that described by Dr. Holmstedt yesterday may lead to new advances. But we must confess that we are presently at the stage where indirect and suggestive evidence is the best available. Attractive hypotheses, like the transmethylation hypothesis, exist and the pharmacological evidence like that derived from the exacerbation of schizophrenia by the administration of methyl donors are persuasive, but direct evidence is still lacking (Kety, 1967).

Another approach to the problem of the relevance of the chemically induced psychoses to the spontaneous ones is to move directly to the question of whether the syndromes produced by psychotomimetic agents resemble the psychoses, and if so, to what extent. This is again a difficult and controversial area in which opinions are rampant and hard data very difficult to achieve. For example, Rinkel, one of the very early workers with LSD, concluded, "The psychotic phenomena produced were predominantly schizophrenia-like symptoms, manifested in disturbances of thought and speech, changes in affect and mood, changes in perception, production of hallucinations and delusions, depersonalizations and changes in behavior. Rorschach tests and concrete-abstract thinking tests showed responses quite similar to those obtained with schizophrenics" (Rinkel and Denber, 1958). Rinkel encountered a few difficulties with the autonomic effects of LSD not encountered in schizophrenia, but was otherwise apparently satisfied with the model.

Just a few years later Manfred Bleuler stated that "modern neuropharmacology has hitherto contributed nothing to the understanding of the pathogenesis of schizophrenia." He also stated that "both important arguments in support of the assumption that noradrenaline or 5-hydroxytryptamine metabolism might explain the pathogenesis of schizophrenia thus become untenable: agents influencing their metabolism neither induce schizophrenia nor constitute a specific remedy for it" (Bleuler, 1958).

Bleuler's argument that LSD or similar agents do not induce schizophrenic psychoses of short duration is based on his concept of schizophrenia. He argues that "the type of disease designated by us as schizophrenia can never by any means whatever be characterized by the presence of any particular isolated symptoms and not even by the apposition of any particular symptoms." Psychotic thinking disturbances can be seen in organic brain disease and fatigue. Depersonalization occurs in severe anxiety states and endocrinopathies; hallucinations in thirst, encephalitis and temporal lobe epilepsy. It is only the constellation of symptoms lasting many days and certainly much longer than the duration of the drug-induced state that to him is pathognomonic of schizophrenia. To Bleuler the psychotomimetic agents have contributed to our understanding of the organic psychoses, not of schizophrenia.

More recent comparison of the gross clinical states of schizophrenia and the chemically induced psychoses reveals striking differences. Hollister (1968) has pointed out several of these. Withdrawal from interpersonal contacts is characteristic of schizophrenics; it is atypical of the drug-induced psychoses. Schizophrenics and drug subjects communicate poorly, but the former seem not to care; the latter are greatly concerned about it. The nature of the hallucinations is different. In schizophrenia they tend to be auditory and threatening; in the drug-induced states they are visual and pleasant or impersonal. Subjects under drugs tend to be highly suggestible; that is why the drug tends to be cultogenic. Schizophrenics are highly resistant to suggestion. In a blind study of tape-recorded mental status interviews of six schizophrenics and six subjects under drugs, a large group of professional raters had little difficulty in distinguishing between the two groups (Hollister, 1962).

Since the gross comparison of drug-induced state and the endogenous clinical state does not resolve the problem, attention has turned by psychologists toward the comparison of what might be termed the microscopic features of the syndromes. Two approaches have been used. In one Linton and Langs (1964) have employed a questionnaire approach in which a large number of specific questions like "Have you ever felt like this before?" "Are you happy?" "Is the room steady?" are clustered into a variety of constellations that are designed to tap into motives, defenses, thought processes, body senses, memory, cognition, etc. The results of the questionnaire were compared between subacute or perhaps chronic schizophrenics and a group of 50 actors, otherwise normal, in a drug-induced state. The results show interesting similarities and differences. Paranoid schizophrenics resembled LSD subjects in the area of feelings of unreality, lack of control, changes in the meaning of experience and suspiciousness, but differed in their affective changes and in their altered body images. The responses of undifferentiated schizophrenics, on the other hand, differed greatly from those of drug subjects.

The experimental approach, in contrast to the questionnaire approach, attempts to compare drug subjects with schizophrenic subjects on specific quantitatively precise tests like reaction time, digit span, the Stroop color word test, etc. There is a considerable literature on this subject, most of which again reveals equivocal results. For example, schizophrenics and LSD subjects both show somewhat slow reaction time (Shakow, 1963). In such tests the preparatory interval, that is, the time from which the subject is signalled that the reaction time will soon be required, may be fixed or varied. Shakow has shown that schizophrenics show a defect in the ability to take advantage of previous information to establish or maintain certain sets, and so their performance deteriorates with a variable preparatory interval. Wikler *et al.* (1965) have shown that LSD did not differentially affect performance between regular and irregular preparatory intervals. Keeler (1967) has obtained similar results with psilocybin. The results, then, show a similarity between schizophrenia and the drug-induced states if the preparatory interval is fixed, but show differences if the interval is varied. In tests of memory, cognition, and distractibility, similarities and differences both appear. Clearly, the problem has not been resolved by this approach.

Still another problem in the assessment of the relevance of the chemically-induced psychoses with schizophrenia has to do with tolerance. It is clear by now that tolerance develops to LSD, psilocybin, and mescaline, and that with some agents even cross tolerance develops. Tolerance develops not only in normals but also when the compounds are given to schizophrenics. In the latter case the psychotomimetic effects superimposed upon the schizophrenic condition disappear when the compound is continuously administered (Chessick *et al.*, 1964). If, then, schizophrenia is maintained by the continuous production of a psychotomimetic agent, why does tolerance not develop? It is, of course, possible that tolerance might not develop for the elusive endogenous agent we seek. It is also possible that tolerance in man may be a cyclic affair like in Koella's goats. And, finally, it is quite conceivable that our hypothetical toxic agent may not be produced all the time, but only intermittently under special stresses. Under such conditions tolerance might never develop. Again, we are lacking evidence on these points.

In the face of repeated failures to establish clearly the relevance of the chemical psychoses, and equally to establish a metabolic etiology or even biochemical correlates of schizophrenia, we must not only persist in the search with more sensitive and more refined tools, but it is also worth considering whether we are asking the right questions and making the right comparisons. For example, we generally tend to compare acute psychotomimetic reactions with chronic schizophrenia. This may be an error and perhaps we should compare acute drug states with acute schizophrenia and chronic drug states with chronic schizophrenia. Bowers and Freedman (1966) have examined acute psychoses and feel that the resemblance of very acute schizophrenia to the psychedelic experience may be quite great. I have no hard data to support this but do have a similar impression.

Comparison of the two chronic states is difficult, not only because we have no baseline about the pre-drug state of the subjects, but we also tend to make the social judgment that only potential schizophrenics would become chronic acid heads. Whether or not such judgments are correct, we cannot ignore the accumulating evidence that adverse drug reactions like persistent or recurring hallucinosis long after the drug has been discontinued may offer some clue to the schizophrenic process. We also tend to forget that the psychotomimetic experience might be very different if the subject did not know he was receiving a compound that would produce unusual experiences. A few reports of the accidental ingestion of LSD by children and anecdotal reports of people who took LSD without knowing it suggest that it is a terrifying experience that might closely resemble an acute schizophrenic reaction. There are also persistent rumors that psychotomimetics have been administered to naive troops in the Army with devastating results. Whether or not this is the case remains a military secret.

We must also consider the possibility that the model of schizophrenia which calls for the continued presence of a toxic metabolite is incorrect, and that such an agent may precipitate the illness which then continues autonomously. There is, of course, no direct evidence that this view is correct, but it is compatible with the findings that schizophrenics are at least as physically healthy as the population at large and that continued hospitalization for the illness for 50 years or more is by no means uncommon. It is somehow more difficult for me to imagine that such chronic patients have a metabolic defect which results in the continued production of an endogenous psychotomimetic, than to feel that they "leaned to schizophrene." Perhaps they adapt to an exceptionally stable environment with a set of psychotic psychological defenses that keep them free from stress. Severe emotional stresses might once again produce toxic metabolites in the fashion that I alluded to previously. If these surmises are correct, it might be a wiser strategy to focus in metabolic research mainly upon acutely ill and fresh cases. It would also be a wise strategy in the search for anti-psychotic drugs to do most of the testing on acute patients.

Finally, we cannot rule out the possibility that the appropriate model may be in the deficiency area. Such a model is unpopular with chemists because it is more difficult to pinpoint a substance which is absent when it should be present than to determine the presence of something unusual. Nonetheless, something resembling a deficiency model comes close to the position of those psychologists and psychiatrists who feel that unusual features of the early psychological environment may be the predominant factors in the etiology of schizophrenia. Advocates of "megavitamin" therapy like Hoffer and Pauling also use the deficiency model.

It is quite apparent that there is insufficient time to adequately discuss the use of these agents in therapy. I stated previously that at first glance the use of agents which produce a transient psychosis for therapeutic purposes would seem to be absurd. Yet, in so difficult a field as psychotherapy, where both the processes and the results are hard to clarify, it is conceivable that it is not. Their use for mystical experiences and religious conversions among primitive peoples is well known. More than a hundred years ago Moreau administered hashish to medical students so that they might gain insight into themselves and their mentally ill patients (Moreau, 1845). Both professional and amateur proponents of the use of these agents claim that new insights are derived from the experience, defenses are altered, and this may lead to personality and behavior reorganization. The subject has been reviewed on several occasions (Shepherd et al., 1968; Hollister, 1968; Abramson, 1967; Crockett et al., 1963; and Hoffer, 1965).

Technically, the drugs have been used for emotional abreactions, for facilitating insight psychotherapy and for producing an overwhelming psychedelic experience. Medically, they have been used in the treatment of psychoneuroses, chronic schizophrenics, depressions, alcoholism and psychopathology. Early in their use claims were made that the drug was the crucial variable; more recently it is the combination of drugs and psychotherapy with patients prepared by intensive psychotherapy and followed during the experience and after in psychotherapy which receives most attention. Frequently the drugs are used in those desperate situations where more conventional forms of treatment have failed. Significant success with such patients would be a very rigorous test of their value.

I am under the impression that the early enthusiastic claims for the effectiveness of psychotomimetic drug treatment have become more modest. In much of its use, as with psychoneurotics and psychopaths, where the criteria for efficacy are changes in personality, assessment is very difficult. In alcoholism, where a clear index of progress is a measurable reduction in drinking, the results are hardly spectacular, and favorable results have even been denied (Smart and Storm, 1966). Regardless of theoretical considerations, the value of these agents in therapy will stand or fall on the basis of carefully controlled clinical studies which can only come slowly.

REFERENCES

Abramson, H. A. (Ed.): *The Use of LSD in Psychotherapy and Alchoholism,* New York: The Bobbs Merrill Company, 1967.
Bleuler, M.: Comparison of Drug Induced and Endogenous Psychoses in Man. In P. B. Bradley, R. Deniker and C. Radouco-Thomas (Eds.), *Proceedings of the First International Congress of Neuropsychopharmacology,* Amsterdam: Elsevier, 1958.
Bowers, M. B., Jr., and Freedman, D. X.: Psychedelic experiences in acute psychoses. *Arch. Gen. Psychiat. 15:* 240, 1966.
Brune, G. G. and Himwich, H. E.: Biogenic Amines and Behavior in Schizophrenic Patients. In J. Wortis (Ed.) *Recent Advances in Biological Psychiatry, Vol. 5,* New York: Plenum Press, 1963.
Chessick, R., Haertzen, C. and Wikler, H.: Tolerance to LSD-25 in schizophrenic subjects. *Arch. Gen. Psychiat. 10:* 653, 1964.
Crockett, R., Sandison, R. A. and Walk, A. (Eds.): *Hallucinogenic Drugs and Their Therapeutic Use,* London: Lewis, 1963.
Friedhoff, A. J.: The Metabolism of Dimethoxyphenylethylamine and Its Possible Relationship to Schizophrenia. In John Romano (Ed.) *The Origins of Schizophrenia,* Amsterdam: Excerpta Medica Foundation, 1967.
Friedhoff, A. J. and Hollister, L. E.: Comparison of the metabolism of 3,4-dimethoxyphenylethylamine and mescaline in man. *Biochem. Pharmacol. 15:* 269, 1966.

Heath, R. G. and Krupp, I. M.: Schizophrenia as an immunologic disorder. *Arch. Gen. Psychiat. 16:* 1, 1967.
Hoffer, A.: D-lysergic acid diethylamide (LSD): A review of its present status. *Clin. Pharmacol. Therap. 6:* 183, 1965.
Hollister, L. E.: Drug-induced psychoses and schizophrenic reactions, a critical comparison. *Ann. N.Y. Acad. Sci. 96:* 80, 1962.
Hollister, L. E.: *Chemical Psychoses,* Springfield, Ill.: Charles C. Thomas, 1968.
Keeler, M. H.: Similarities and differences in set and attention between the psilocybin reaction and schizophrenia. *Int. J. Neuropsychiat. 3:* 434, 1967.
Kety, S. S.: The Hypothetical Relationships Between Amines and Mental Illness: A Critical Synthesis. In H. E. Himwich, S. S. Kety and J. R. Smythies (Eds.) *Amines and Schizophrenia,* Oxford: Pergamon Press, 1967.
Linton, H. B. and Langs, R. J.: Empirical dimensions of the LSD-25 reaction. *Arch. Gen. Psychiat. 10:* 496, 1964.
Moreau, S.: *Du Hachisch et de L'Alientation Mentale Etudes Psychologiques,* Paris: Fortin, Masson, 1845.
Rinkel, M. and Denber, H. C. B. (Eds.): *Chemical Concepts of Psychosis,* New York: McDowell, 1958.
Sachar, E. J., Mason, J. W., Kolmer, H. S. and Artiss, K. L., Psychoendocrine aspects of acute schizophrenic reactions. *Psychosom. Med. 25:* 510, 1963.
Shakow, D.: Behavioral deficit in schizophrenia. *Behav. Sci. 8:* 275, 1963.
Shepherd, M., Lader, M. and Rodnight, R.: Therapeutic Uses of Psychotomimetic Drugs. In *Clinical Psychopharmacology,* London: English Universities Press, Ltd., 1968.
Smart, R. G., Storm, T., Baker, E. F. W., and Solursh, L.: A controlled study of lysergide in the treatment of alcoholism. *Quart. J. Stud. Alcohol 27:* 469 (1966).
Smythies, J. R.: Introduction. In H. E. Himwich, S. S. Kety and J. R. Smythies (Eds.) *Amines and Schizophrenia,* Oxford: Pergamon Press, 1967.
Tanimukai, H., Ginther, R., Spaide, J., Bueno, J. R. and Himwich, H. E.: Occurrence of bufotenin in the urine of schizophrenic patients. *Life Sci. 6:* 1697 (1967).
Thudicum, J. W. L.: *A Treatise on the Chemical Constitution of the Brain,* London: Baillière, Tindall and Cox, 1884.
Turner, W. J. and Merlis, S.: Effect of some indolealkylamines in man. *Arch. Neurol. Psychiat. 81:* 121, 1959.
Wikler, A., Haertzen, C. A., Chessick, R. D., Hill, H. E. and Pescor, F. T.: Reaction time, "mental set," in control and chronic schizophrenic subjects and in post-addicts under placebo, LSD-125, morphine, pentobarbital and amphetamine. *Psychopharm. 7:* 423, 1965.

DISCUSSION

DR. DEMENT: In the autobiographies of schizophrenic patients written during periods of remission, there are descriptions of clear-cut abnormalities often existing years in advance of first overt clinically recognized psychotic episodes. One may think of some kind of metabolic or toxic or whatever other process you like starting either at birth, or developing insidiously, or occurring in episodic fashion which distorts the learning experience of the individual to a greater or lesser extent as he matures. These distortions could affect the important family and social interactions which, when disturbed, would seem in retrospect to be the primary pathogenic process.

DR. LIPTON: If I understand your question correctly, I see no incompatibility at all between the concept of a genetic diathesis and pathogenic environmental experience. The evidence is equally good or bad for both positions, and I feel it is necessary to integrate them into an interactive relationship. The problem is precisely how to do this.

Let me try to illustrate my position by using an analogy which might some day be put into an experiment. Suppose we were to try to teach a child to play a violin. We would use all possible tactics to motivate him by reward or punishment. Suppose we gave him a treacherous fiddle on which to learn to play. The instrument would be highly unreliable in pitch, tone, and volume, and would give several unpredictable sounds if played conventionally. I would imagine that the child, if sufficiently motivated, could soon learn to play simple tunes by making quick adjustments in his fingering and bowing in order to compensate quickly for the instrument's deviousness. But, if we made the music more and more difficult, there would come a point at which he would quit, smash the violin, and avoid the teacher, or at least be furious with him. Let us call this the equivalent of the psychotic break.

Suppose at this point we handed him a Stradivarious and said, "Now play." What problems would we face? I imagine we would first have to convince him that the new instrument was reliable, and that the teacher was also. If this were done, and he were remotivated, I think he might still play very badly because all of the habits which he had picked up in trying to deal with the unreliable instrument would become impediments which would have to be undone. If he could relearn at all it would probably take a long time. I would guess that he would never play as well as he might have had he not been exposed to the initial trauma.

I think something of this sort goes on in schizophrenia. The potential patient is born with a poor instrument, or has terrible teachers, or both. When the tunes of life are relatively uncomplicated, as in childhood and latency, he may play fairly well. When they get complicated with new impulses and new social roles after puberty, the instrument and earlier habits may be inadequate and a psychotic break ensues. If now the biological instrument were fully repaired—if we had a penicillin equivalent for schizophrenia—is it reasonable to think that we would suddenly have a virtuoso of living? I doubt it. Slow and painful re-education would still have to go on, just as it probably would have to in the case of the violinist. This is why I feel that even if we had a miracle drug we might not recognize it except in very acute cases or with less than global instruments.

DR. DEMENT: I would like only to make a clarifying remark. What I am talking about in terms of life-long abnormality, present already at birth is well illustrated in the book *I Never Promised You a Rose Garden* (Hannah

Green, World Publishing Co., Cleveland, 1964). We must answer the question: What is the true psychotic process and when does it really start? Is psychosis, in effect, present in terms of short, unnoticed episodes of greater or lesser abnormality? These episodes—you may call them squeaks and squawks if you like—might be genuine intrusions *from within* impinging upon the perceptual apparatus and resulting in distortion of the real world from an early age. The early strangeness of the eventual schizophrenic may be the individual's effort to learn to live with this internal noise. This sort of process would not be obvious in an infant. If it was not too intense, it might remain hidden even in a child but, as you say, when one gets to the level of life that requires greater virtuosity, one just cannot function. There is a beautiful laboratory model of internally generated intrusions onto the perceptual apparatus. This is the PCPA (*p*-chlorophenylalanine) cat where the PGO (pontine-geniculo-occipital) spikes of REM sleep occur in the waking state and do distort perceptual behavior.

DR. MANDELL: You said that the suggestibility of a patient with an LSD psychosis was distinctly different from that of a schizophrenic. I'm not sure everyone would agree with that. If you can make contact with a schizophrenic, they're almost compulsively, imitatively suggestible; they are so sensitive to the characteristics, suggestions, and models of the therapist that their ego boundaries fuse with yours.

The second point you made about the capacity for interpersonal contact is perhaps also not a feature discriminating schizophrenics from LSD psychotics. Schizophrenics are clinging and sucking. The therapist may become massively important to these patients.

DR. LIPTON: Dr. Mandell makes the point that, *if contact can be made,* the schizophrenic is hypersuggestible and eager for interpersonal contact. He therefore questions the validity of my statements about these behaviors as discriminants between the schizophrenic and the subject with a drug-induced psychosis. The crucial phrase is *if contact can be made*. The drug subject seeks it; the schizophrenic guards against it. Furthermore, contacts with a schizophrenic are very sensitive and tenuous, and his defensive posture is quickly re-established. Here, too, the drug subject differs. He seeks contact even to the point of seducing others into sharing his experience.

DR. FREEDMAN: I'm not sure what Dr. Mandell meant about Freud being right or wrong, since he's always both. I think that what he's talking about is the nature of the psychotic transference. If you look very carefully at the kinds of leaning on, merging with, but ignoring the physician that occurs in an LSD situation (by "ignoring" I mean not really regarding), it's very much like a psychotic transference. I think this whole field gets confused because the question is, what do you want to make this a model of? And for my money, LSD is a good way not to study necessarily a biochemical sequence which might in itself be relevant to clinical disorder, but it is as useful a way as hypnosis to study mechanisms and sequences in behavior; and if this is done systematically and well, I believe you can get some notion as to the sequence of symptom development that might be important in paranoid conditions. I think what Dr. Dement is talking about is important. How are these things related clinically? Our inability to predict which of these disturbed children is going to be schizophrenic later on disturbs me, as pitted against the genetic data that Heston first produced, and which the National Institute of Mental Health has picked up and begun to study with Kety, Rosenthal and others.

And those data are very convincing: there is a population at risk. And the question is: What is inherited? Is it a way of integrating and modulating perceptual input, as Silverman would spin the story? Is that the way it is inherited?

We would need two days of deliberation to discuss this accurately. So, I will end up by saying that I think on the whole that some of the acute schizophreniform psychoses look very much like many LSD experiences. Before we worry about Hollister's study (which I thought was a well done although bad one because he compared chronic schizophrenics with LSD users), there is the whole issue of idiosyncrasy in schizophrenia. This is always the way you distinguish it from an organic syndrome. You notice the very private, idiosyncratic kinds of references and symbols that a person demonstrates who has lived a long time with this way of thinking and who now is a schizophrenic. This is, perhaps, a distinguishing factor. Well, you can't hope to reproduce a psychosis in eight hours that might take a lifetime to develop. But you could, I think, begin to tease apart what is alike in LSD states and what is different, such as, let's say, the family relationships of a schizophrenic who has learned to communicate, though perhaps in irrational, ways.

That dimension of schizophrenic behavior could be distinguished from dimensions which might be more interesting to the biologist or the neurophysiologist. I think this could be done if we sort these things out. But we're going to get into trouble if we don't at least distinguish primary from secondary effects. I think that is the source of most of the variability in LSD research reports. The primary effects in LSD are very much like those in the acute psychosis. There's a loosening of association, a change of boundaries, whether you're talking about perceptual boundaries, boundaries of the self, cognitive structures, etc. It's a multi-potential, fluid state, and I think its outcome depends on a variety of other "secondary" circumstances.

DR. STEIN: With regard to your analogy about the schizophrenic playing a permanently damaged fiddle, could such a model account for the lucid intervals that schizophrenics sometimes are reported to have?

DR. LIPTON: I take it that what you're talking about is the curious phenomenon illustrated, for example, by the schizophrenic who sits mutely in a corner for twenty years and then when a fire breaks out in his dormitory, leads the fire brigade, puts out the fire and then goes back to his corner for the next twenty years. I have no ready explanation for that.

DR. STEIN: Well, what I was referring to is the idea of disorder of association in schizophrenics, the presumption being that schizophrenics somehow form associations in a different way than normals do. So basic a defect in mechanism does not seem to me to be compatible with the observation that schizophrenics may have lucid intervals. One gets the impression, rather, that there is a good deal of normality in the basic mechanisms of association, and that schizophrenic symptoms result from some other source.

DR. LIPTON: We must be careful not to get trapped in poor semantics. Few schizophrenics are totally irrational. Even in regressed wards one can see them watching television, performing mechanical tasks and even doing arithmetic or crossword puzzles. It is primarily in areas that are emotionally charged that one sees the loosened associations.

DR. KORNETSKY: One of the problems could be that there are no toxic endogenous substances or metabolites in the schizophrenic. Or maybe everyone has approximately the same amount of these "endogenous toxins" but in the normal there is some selective tolerance to the substances that for some reason does not develop in the schizophrenic.

DR. LIPTON: That may be. It would be very tough to test.

DR. LUDWIG: Yes. I was very impressed with your paper, Dr. Lipton. After thinking about what you have said, and after some of the notes I have made, I'm more convinced than ever that it is difficult to know for sure whether LSD produces a schizophrenic-like state.

I have a few other comments to make.

In terms of using the models that you talked about, the toxin model, the deficiency model, the enzyme starting process model, you brought up the matter of odor in schizophrenic patients. That would perhaps correspond to the toxin model. However, in our work with schizophrenic patients, if we look at it from a deficiency point of view, we find that the odor is due to the *lack* of soap, and it's amazing how the odor can disappear with an occasional shower.

DR. LIPTON: Well, I didn't have time to go into that. It's been established that soap will remove some of the odor and so will antibiotics. I'm simply giving a report of a highly unusual compound, and one I'm willing to bet is correct chemically. Even if it were an artifact that came from lack of soap, where would it come from? I wonder about that.

DR. LUDWIG: I had a few other comments.

A couple of things intrigued me. One is that when LSD was first used, the expectation was that this was a psychotomimetic drug, and it was interesting that people experienced schizophrenic-like symptoms at the time. However, as people began raising doubts about a psychotic-like effect of the drug, a whole variety of other experiences began developing. I'd like to re-emphasize Dr. Freedman's point about the multipotential nature of the state and its fluidity. In our work with LSD, we have seen anything ranging from states that resemble acute schizophrenia to very pleasant states. On the other hand, in our work with acute and chronic schizophrenics, we have seen many instances of psychedelic-like experiences with them, and also very frightening experiences.

What I'm saying is that many of the criteria which you say distinguish the LSD state from the schizophrenic state may not really hold up. To conclude anything from the studies that have been done on comparisons between the schizophrenic and the LSD-induced state you have to know what the expectations of LSD subjects were. You also have to know what kind of schizophrenics you're talking about. For example, most of Shakow's studies, most of the questionnaire studies with schizophrenics, and the reaction time studies have only applied to the more cooperative schizophrenics. Those are the ones who will participate. You have left out a bulk of schizophrenics who really don't get involved, or from whom you can't gather questionnaire data. If you do get a response from them, you can never really be sure it's a veridical response or one they really feel.

DR. OSMOND: These questions of models are always very interesting. The natural history of schizophrenia has been much neglected. It is a highly recoverable illness, and always has been so. It seems that about a third of those afflicted by it get well spontaneously. Some of them seem to get very well and remain that way. It was therefore unfortunate, to put it mildly, that in his classical studies Kraepelin took those who did not recover as typical examples of the illness which he came to call *dementia praecox*. This produced a picture of a hopeless illness which did not appear nearly so hopeless in pre-Kraepelinian times. Like Nolan D. C. Lewis of Columbia in the 1940's, John Conolly of Hanwell, England in the 1840's recognized that one might be ill for a few months, a few years, sometimes for a whole lifetime. The designation and description of *dementia praecox* made a great difference to the medical and social climate, and one that did not help the ill at all. I don't think it is always understood that however pleasant new and unusual experiences may be for a short time, if these put you out of touch with others for a long time, as they are bound to do if not shared by them, then these pleasant experiences may easily become frightening and distressing. I have asked many intelligent young schizophrenics about this and a number of them agreed that at first they were exhilarated and delighted. As Blake put it, "There is a joy in madness that only madmen know." I do not agree with the cruder interpretations made of the subtle notions produced by men such as Bateson, Jackson, Laing, etc. that schizophrenics are always rejected. What I suspect happens is that the sick person's tempo, their speed of perceiving, thinking, moving, feeling, etc., is so different from that of well people that the signalling system between the sick and the well goes askew. They are then bound to feel rebuffed, especially since very few of them know exactly what perceptual changes have assailed them, and hardly any understand what the consequences of such changes are likely to be. So long as they are living at a different tempo and have different perceptions, so long will they continue to be rebuffed. In such circumstances many people withdraw. It seems to me to be in essence a rather simple mechanical process. If you are unable to pick up the social signals from the people around you, or to signal back to them in an appropriate manner, you are going to feel hurt, and, being hurt, unless you are extremely good natured, you are then going to strike out, and as you see it, defend yourself; then you get hurt again. After that you either withdraw and become alienated or become a great nuisance to society and have to be expelled.

Regarding Dr. Ludwig's point about soap and water and the smell of schizophrenia, I think perhaps we should remember this: as a smoker, he is not well equipped for picking up the delicate and, to some, delightful schizophrenic odor. In well washed patients it is by no means an unpleasant smell, but resembles the smell of ripe, perhaps over-ripe apricots combined a certain muskiness. I have had staff members who were very good at picking up this smell and would predict relapses by means of it. Rats, too, I believe, have been trained to do just this. Smokers are liable to be insensitive to these matters and you will recall that physicians were especially sensitive to odors in the days before cigarette smoking was common. In those days the nose was a valuable, essential, and frequently used diagnostic and prognostic instrument. There are still physicians who use it that way today.

DR. FREEDMAN: Thank you, Dr. Osmond, for bringing matters of taste to this discussion.

I make one note for the record, and that is that I think you will find that really keen psychological examination of so-called recovered schizophrenics is perhaps the least studied area in schizophrenia.

DOET (2,5-DIMETHOXY-4-ETHYLAMPHETAMINE) AND DOM (STP) (2,5-DIMETHOXY-4-METHYLAMPHETAMINE), NEW PSYCHOTROPIC AGENTS: THEIR EFFECTS IN MAN

Solomon H. Snyder, M.D., Herbert Weingartner, Ph.D. and
Louis A. Faillace, M.D.

*Departments of Pharmacology and Psychiatry,
The Johns Hopkins University School of Medicine,
Baltimore, Maryland 21205*

INTRODUCTION

The psychedelic drugs embrace a large number of compounds of widely varied structures, including the phenylethylamine, tryptamine, amphetamine and lysergic acid classes, which, however, produce strikingly similar subjective effects. Despite the similar effects of the psychedelic drugs as well as the cross tolerance that exists among them, differences in the nuances of subjective effects occur among the different drugs. Such differences include many reports that mescaline produces a more sensual experience than does LSD. There are also variations in onset and duration of action. Thus, dimethyltryptamine has a duration of action of only one hour, while the effects of LSD last about 8 to 10 hours.

Shulgin (1964) has synthesized a number of methoxylated amphetamine derivatives, several of which are hallucinogenic. Some of these compounds, including MMDA (3-methoxy-4, 5-methylenedioxyamphetamine) as well as MDA (3,4-methylenedioxyamphetamine), tend to produce psychotropic effects with minimal perceptual distortion (Shulgin, 1964; Shulgin *et al.,* 1967). One of the compounds synthesized first by Shulgin, DOM (2,5-dimethoxy 4-methylamphetamine) has been used extensively by "hippie" populations and informally designated "STP." In a number of experiments we have examined the effects of DOM and of its ethyl homologue, DOET (2,5-dimethoxy-4-ethylamphetamine) (Fig. 1) in normal control subjects. Although in low doses

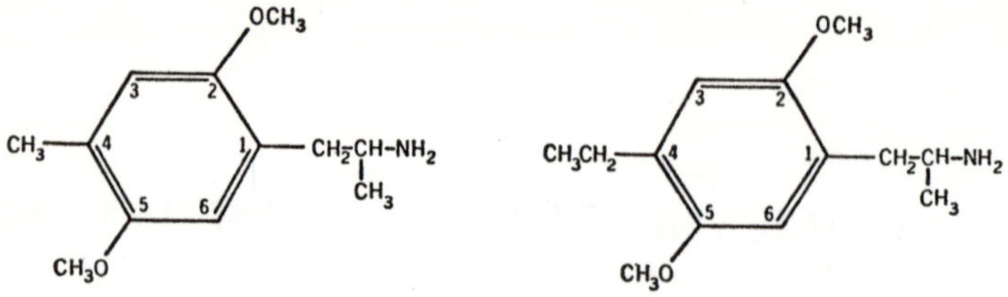

2,5-DIMETHOXY-4-METHYLAMPHETAMINE (DOM)   2,5-DIMETHOXY-4-ETHYLAMPHETAMINE (DOET)

FIG. 1. Structures of DOM and DOET.

these compounds produce similar effects, there are notable differences in dose-response characteristics.

METHODS

The subjects for both the DOET and DOM studies were male volunteers aged 21 to 35 obtained through the Financial Aid office of the Johns Hopkins University. Applicants were screened by an interview with an experienced psychiatrist and by the administration of the Minnesota Multiphasic Personality Inventory (MMPI), and applicants with a history of extensive drug use or evidence of borderline or psychotic emotional disturbances were rejected.

COMPARISON OF DOET AND AMPHETAMINE

In our initial study, the effects of DOET were contrasted with those of d-amphetamine. Subjects were admitted twice to the research ward of the Johns Hopkins Hospital with a two week interval between sessions. They were informed that they would receive on separate occasions d-amphetamine or DOET, a test drug which might produce "psychological effects."

DOET (1.5 mg as the hyrochloride) or d-amphetamine (10 mg as the sulfate) were given orally at 9:00 A.M. in a double blind design to subjects (Ss) who had fasted since the preceding midnight. Ss spent the drug day in their hospital room with a research assistant in a relaxed neutral atmosphere not designed to elicit any particular emotional set. On the evening prior to receiving the drug they were administered tests of free associations and their reproductions, free recall of random and organized words, and ranking of associations. These tests were readministered 2, 4 and 6 hours after receiving the drug.

Semistructured interviews were tape recorded at varying intervals, and transcripts of these interviews were scored blindly with respect to features which might be expected to characterize the experience of either drug. Subjects were also administered a self-rating subjective drug effects questionnaire (Katz, Waskow and Olsson, 1968) consisting of 240 items. This questionnaire is a comprehensive scale which measures the various aspects of perceptual, mood and somatic changes in subjects undergoing a drug experience. The scale was originally designed to measure the changes in Ss experience with low doses of LSD. The questionnaire contains several subscales, including a euphoria subscale, a dysphoria subscale and an LSD specific subscale.

Pulse rate, oral temperature, pupillary diameter and blood pressure were determined each hour. Urine was collected prior to drug ingestion and after 3, 6, 9 and 24 hours, and was refrigerated and assayed for unchanged DOET by a specific spectrophotofluorometric method. In this method, DOET is extracted from an alkaline urine solution saturated with salt into a mixture of heptane and isoamyl alcohol. After back extraction into 0.1 N H_2SO_4, the native fluorescence of DOET is measured (activation wave length 290mμ; fluorescent wave length 350mμ). This method can detect as little as 50mμg of DOET and is specific for the unchanged compound (Snyder and Sangavi, in preparation).

Subjective experiences: The most notable effects of DOET were a feeling of mild euphoria and enhanced self-awareness. Subjective effects were first noted about one and one half hours after drug administration and peaked in 3 to 4 hours, subsiding 5 to 6 hours after drug administration (Table I.). DOET and amphetamine shared certain subjective effects. Thus, with both drugs there were reports of euphoria and feeling "talkative." Other effects clearly differentiated these compounds. Seven out of 10 *d*-amphetamine sessions produced better than normal ability to concentrate, while 8 out of 10 DOET sessions were associated with subjective difficulty in concentrating. Only after DOET were there reports of "feels high," "reports insight," "notably pleasant experience," "aware of body image," "impatient with tests," "time passes slowly," "washed-out after drug," "thoughts faster than words," and "visual effects." The visual effects under DOET consisted only of closed eye imagery evoked upon the suggestion of the research assistant that Ss close their eyes and describe whatever happens. Only with *d*-amphetamine was there any loss of appetite.

Some features of the drug experience are best illustrated by the following excerpts from transcribed interviews: Mr. K., who received amphetamine first, reported, "I'm concentrating more. I've just been focussing on

TABLE I

Subjective effects of DOET and d-amphetamine

Effect	Number of Subjects Reporting Effect	
	DOET	d-amphetamine
feels high	6	0
reports insight	4	0
notably pleasant experience	7	0
aware of body image	5	0
impatient with tests	4	0
difficulty in concentrating	8	0
better concentration (than normal)	0	7
talkative	7	6
thoughts faster than words	6	0
visual effects	4	0
euphoric	6	4
time passes slowly	2	0
time passes quickly	0	1
"washed out" after drug	2	0
feels especially alert	2	6
loss of appetite	0	3

Transcripts of tape recorded interviews with subjects under DOET or d-amphetamine were graded blindly for the presence or absence of each effect. Data are presented as the number of subjects reporting the presence of an effect. Ten subjects received DOET and d-amphetamine on two separate occasions.

those cards and attending to the questions asked . . . I find this annoying. It isn't the way I like to be." On DOET, Mr. K. said, "I am more likely to have interesting or new associations of ideas. The other drug [d-amphetamine] helped concentration but wasn't relaxing, and didn't help me to associate at all except in a very limited sense. . . . A number of things are closer to the surface than they would normally be [on DOET] . . . I was tremendously suggestible today."

Mr. O. received DOET first and reported, "I can skip readily from one thing to another . . . but if something gets my attention I can get very involved and really focus. . . . I am more aware of myself . . . gee, I am smiling a lot." While on d-amphetamine he observed, "No, I am not noticing more about myself this time. . . . This time I haven't done any deep thinking. . . . I am able to concentrate more."

Physiological changes: DOET produced pupillary dilation in 8 out of 10 Ss with effects more prominent 4 hours after the drug (Table II). However, there were no marked changes in pulse rate, blood pressure or oral temperature with either drug.

TABLE II

Physiological effects of DOET and d-amphetamine

Parameters	2 Hours		4 Hours		6 Hours	
	DOET	AMPH	DOET	AMPH	DOET	AMPH
Pupillary Diameter						
No. of Ss with dilation	8	1	8	0	4	0
Mean dilatation (mm)	+1.1	+0.2	+1.4	+0.1	+1.1	0
Blood Pressure (Systolic)						
No. of Ss with increase > 20 mm Hg	0	2	0	1	0	0
Mean change (mm Hg)	+5.0	+8.0	+6.0	+4.0	+4.0	+2.0
Blood Pressure (Diastolic)						
No. of Ss with increase > 20 mm Hg	0	0	0	0	0	0
Mean change (mm Hg)	+2.0	+6.0	+3.0	+3.0	+2.0	+2.0
Pulse Rate						
No. of Ss with increase > 20/min	0	0	2	0	1	0
Mean change	+2	+3	+7	+5	+4	+5
Temperature (oral)						
No. of Ss with increase > 2° F	0	0	2	0	0	0
Mean change (° F)	+0.4	+0.2	+1.0	+0.5	+0.7	+0.1

Ten subjects each received DOET (1.5 mg) and d-amphetamine SO_4 (10 mg) on separate occasions.

Urinary excretion of DOET: In the 24 hours after administration of DOET, excretion ranged from 103 to 657 µg with a mean of 365 µg, so that between 10% and 40% of the ingested dose appeared in the urine as the unmetabolized compound. The rate of urinary excretion of DOET (Fig. 2) was greatest during the second three hour period, coinciding with the peak of subjective drug effects. If urinary DOET concentration reflects brain concentrations, this would suggest that the psychological effects of this drug are closely related to the presence of the unchanged compound, as has been shown for LSD (Aghajanian and Bing, 1964). The increased excretion of DOET in the second three hour period also suggests a retarded gastrointestinal absorption of the drug.

Drug effects questionnaire: This measure was administered to Ss on the evening prior to drug treatment as well as 2 and 4 hours after DOET and *d*-amphetamine. Both DOET and *d*-amphetamine increased the euphoria scores (Fig. 3) (p < .05 for 4 hours scores as compared to pre-drug scores

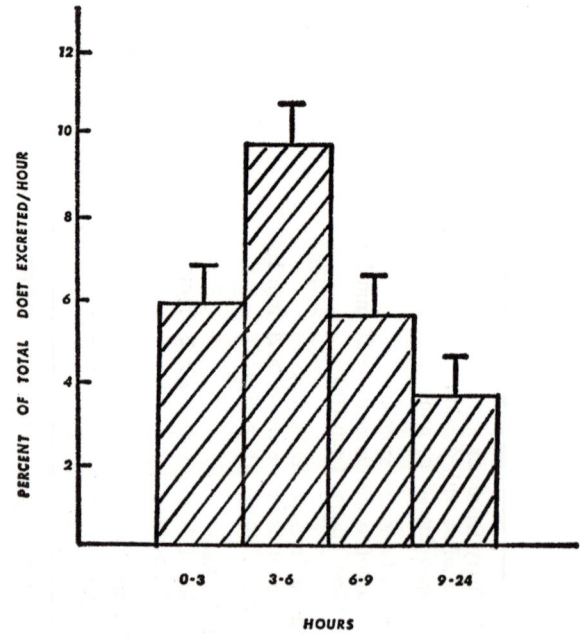

FIG. 2. Urinary excretion of unchanged DOET. Urinary excretion of DOET per hour in each collecton period was calculated as the percent of the total DOET excreted in the first 24 hours after drug administration. Bars and vertical lines show the mean and S.E.M. respectively for 10 subjects.

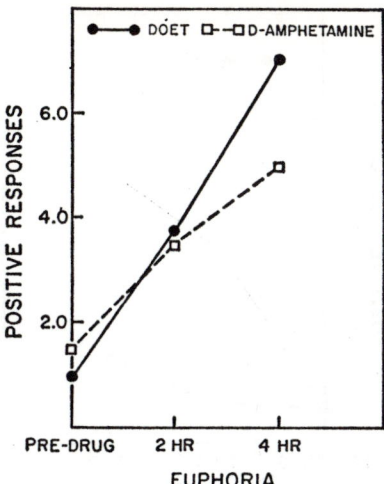

FIG. 3. Effect of DOET and d-amphetamine on the euphoria sub-scale of the drug effects questionnaire. Each point is the mean number of positive responses from 10 subjects.

by the t test for differences between correlated means). These data agree with the interview information which indicated that both drugs produced a mild euphoria. Only DOET produced an increase in LSD specific symptoms (Fig. 4) ($p < .05$ for 4 hour scores as compared to pre-drug scores by the t test for differences between correlated means). However, the LSD scores for the DOET Ss were considerably lower than those produced by 50 μg of LSD (Katz, Waskow, and Olsson, personal communication).

In summary, low doses of DOET consistently produced subjective effects, including a mild euphoria and feelings of enhanced self-awareness, without producing any perceptual or cognitive distortion. This dose of DOET could be clearly distinguished from the effects of 10 mg of d-amphetamine.

Ss receiving DOET were administered several tests to evaluate certain intellectual functions. In one task Ss were presented single stimulus words and asked to rank 7 other words in order of how closely they seem related to the stimulus words. Ranking of these words by an S was scored as correlations between his rankings and the rankings of the same words based on normative data (Snyder et al., 1968). Both at baseline and after DOET and d-amphetamine the Ss effectively ranked associative words to their stimuli according to their free associative strength in normative data. The correlation of Ss rankings and the ranking of the same words based on their associative response strength to the stimuli used to generate them was $R = 0.50$

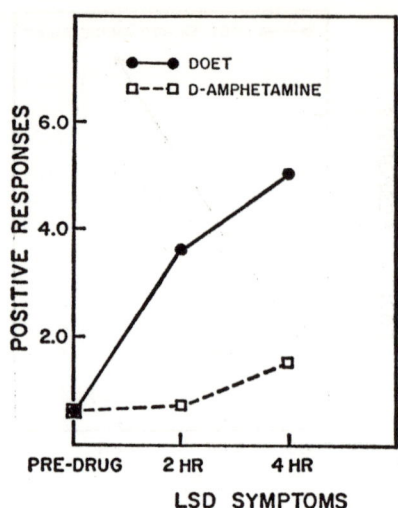

FIG. 4. Effect of DOET and d-amphetamine on LSD symptoms sub-scale of the drug questionnaire. Each point is the mean number of positive responses from 10 subjects.

($p < .01$), indicating that neither DOET nor d-amphetamine impaired performance on this task. Ss receiving DOET and amphetamine were also administered tests of free recall of words and showed no impairment in free recall of organized word sets (Snyder et al., 1968).

EFFECTS OF LOW DOSES OF DOM AND WATER PLACEBO IN NORMAL SUBJECTS

DOM has been identified by chemists at the U.S. Food and Drug Administration as the active ingredient in tablets of "STP," an hallucinogenic drug used by "hippie" populations. STP was reported in the lay press to produce hallucinogenic episodes lasting up to 72 hours; its effects were *accentuated* by chlorpromazine, a drug which *decreases* the effects of other psychedelic agents. In a pilot study (Snyder et al., 1967) we had examined the effects of varying doses of DOM in normal control Ss. Doses of 2.0 mg were barely perceptible. Doses between 2 and 3 mg produced subjective effects similar to those produced by 1.5 mg of DOET. Doses greater than 5 mg were hallucinogenic. The duration of action was similar to that of LSD, about 6 to 8 hours, with no reports of prolonged effects. In several Ss, chlorpromazine attenuated the effects of DOM.

In order to examine the effects of low doses of DOM in a more controlled study, the following experiment was performed. Ss were hospitalized on the John Hopkins research ward in a design similar to the experiment contrasting DOET with d-amphetamine, except that they were hospitalized only once and received only one drug treatment. In a double blind design, 6 Ss received water, 4 Ss received 3.3 mg of DOM and 2 Ss received 2.7 mg of DOM (all doses computed as the hydrochloride).

As in the study with DOET and d-amphetamine, interviews with Ss were tape recorded, Ss were administered free association tests and urinary excretion of DOM was determined. Blood pressure, pulse rate, pupil diameter and oral temperature were recorded each hour.

DOM was determined in the urine by a technique which was essentially the same as that used for the measurement of unchanged DOET. DOM had the same fluorescent spectrum as DOET and produced a fluorescence of the same intensity as DOET.

Data from the two dosages of DOM were consolidated, since statistical analysis indicated that there were no significant differences between the two drug dosages and because of the small number of Ss.

On the drug effects questionnaire, DOM produced an increase in the LSD-like symptoms (Fig. 5) ($p < .05$) similar to the score obtained by the

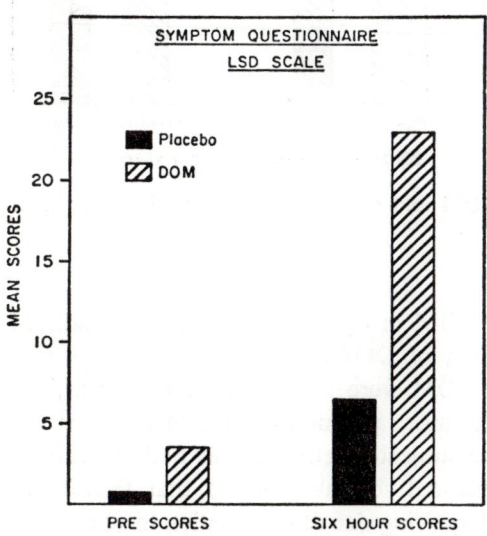

FIG. 5. Effects of DOM and water placebo. Each bar represents mean scores for 6 subjects.

Ss receiving 1.5 mg of DOET. There was a significant increase in both the euphoria and dysphoria scales (Fig. 6) for DOM as compared to placebo ($p < .05$). Interestingly, both drug and placebo groups showed significant increases ($p < .05$) in dysphoria symptoms from their pre-test scores. Apparently, both groups became somewhat uncomfortable in the hospital, complaining of a certain amount of physical symptoms during the 6 hour testing period.

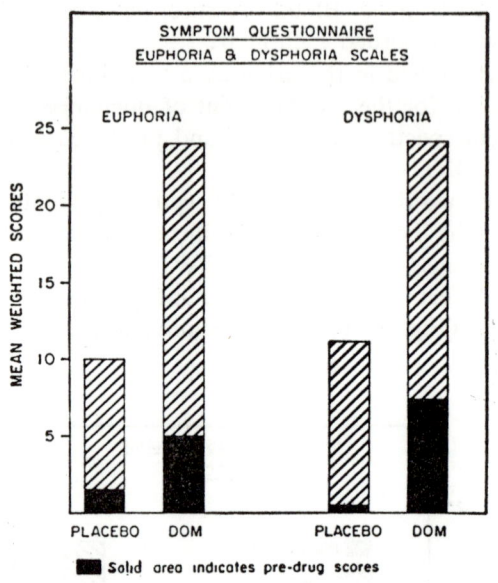

FIG. 6. Effect of DOM and water placebo. Each bar represents mean scores for 6 subjects.

In summary, DOM in doses of about 3 mg produced effects similar to the effects of 1.5 mg of DOET. Since, in an earlier study (Snyder *et al.*, 1967), 2.0 mg of DOM were barely detectable by Ss, it would appear that DOET is somewhat more potent than DOM in terms of the minimal dose required to produce subjective effects. This finding accords with the observation of Uyeno (personal communication) that DOET was almost twice as potent as DOM in impairing size discrimination in squirrel monkeys.

The subjective effects of the two dose levels of DOM resembled those of DOET and were distinguishable by blind analyses of tape transcripts from placebo. These effects had a time course similar to those following DOET, with onset after 1 to 1½ hours, a peak effect at 3 to 4 hours and subsidence by 5 to 6 hours. As with DOET there were no hallucinogenic or psychotomimetic effects. The only perceptual effects were "closed eye imagery" occurring in 3 of the 6 Ss. As with DOET, DOM did not produce a significant change in blood pressure, pulse rate or oral temperature, but did produce a slight pupil dilation.

The time course of DOM excretion resembled that of DOET except that there was not as pronounced a peaking of urinary DOM during the 3 to 6 hour collection period, as had occurred for DOET. Also, between 5 to 10% of the ingested dose of DOM was excreted during the 24 hours after drug administration, considerably less than the excretion of DOET.

In the experiment contrasting DOET with amphetamine, Ss under the effects of DOET had shown no impairment in the structured intellectual task of ranking free associations or in the free recall of organized word sets. To evaluate such functions with DOM, Ss were administered serial learning tasks in which they were asked to learn a list of 8 random words read to them. Learning trials were continued until Ss produced one perfect list, *i.e.,* repeated all 8 words in the order that they were presented. Equivalent lists were read to the Ss prior to the drug administration 2, 4 and 6 hours after DOM. Strikingly, the Ss who received DOM learned the list in significantly fewer trials than did those who were administered placebo (Snyder *et al.,* 1968). The improved performance by the DOM Ss was maximal 4 hours after drug ingestion, coinciding with maximal subjective effects and peak urinary excretion of unchanged DOM. Thus, as with DOET, small doses of DOM did not impair cognitive functions and may have resulted in improved performance.

Although DOM did not produce any gross perceptual changes, the possibility of subtle effects on simple visual perception was examined in tasks requiring the judgment of horizontal and vertical line lengths at short exposure. Ss receiving DOM or water were required to judge the length of horizontal and vertical lines at 1/100 sec exposure (Snyder *et al.,* 1968). There were no differences in performance of this task between Ss receiving DOM or placebo, indicating that DOM did not impair simple visual perception. The effects of DOM on the perception of more complex stimuli, thematic apperception cards at short intervals, will be discussed below.

THE EFFECTS OF VARYING DOSES OF DOET IN NORMAL SUBJECTS

In the study contrasting DOET and *d*-amphetamine, 1.5 mg of DOET had produced a mild euphoria and subjective feelings of enhanced self-awareness in the complete absence of hallucinogenic or psychotomimetic effects.

This suggested that DOET may differ from related compounds in failing to produce perceptual and cognitive distortion in doses which nonetheless produced noticeable subjective effects. To determine if DOET was in fact unique in its spectrum of psychological effects, we studied a wide range of doses of DOET in normal control Ss.

In this study, subject selection, hospitalization on the research ward and experimental setting were the same as in the two previous studies with DOET and DOM, respectively. Ss were admitted to the research ward on one occasion and received DOET in doses varying from 0.75 mg to 4.0 mg as the hydrochloride dissolved in distilled water, or received distilled water alone orally at 9:00 A.M. after fasting since the preceding midnight. Dosages were as follows: 4 Ss received water; 2 Ss received 0.75 mg; 2 Ss received 1.25 mg; 2 Ss received 2.0 mg; 2 Ss 2.5 mg; 2 Ss 3.0 mg; 2 Ss 3.5 mg, and 2 Ss received 4.0 mg. Ss spent the day that they received the drug in their hospital room with a research assistant in a relaxed, neutral atmosphere not designed to elicit any particular emotional set. The research assistants were blind to the drug or dose administered, as were the Ss. Interviews were tape recorded and their transcripts analyzed blindly, as in the study with DOET and amphetamine. Ss were administered tests of visual discrimination of light intensity and tests of weight discrimination. They were also administered tests of free association that Ss had received in the other two studies, as well as the same test of perception of tachistoscopically exposed thematic apperception cards as had been used with DOM. Pulse rate, blood pressure, oral temperature and pupil diameter were determined each hour.

Subjective effects were first noted about 1½ hours after drug ingestion, were most prominent after about 3 to 4 hours, and subsided at about 5 hours. They were similar in character to those observed in the study with DOET and amphetamine, and included a relaxed feeling which, in higher doses, was associated with some nervousness or restlessness, a tendency to be talkative and a sensation that thoughts were coming faster than words (Table III). There were also some reports of difficulty in concentration, although these did not appear to be dose related. Under DOET Ss felt light headed and were very much aware of their body image. Out of 14 Ss receiving DOET, only 2 reported any visual effects, and these consisted solely of closed eye imagery. Moreover one of the Ss receiving water reported similar effects.

The lowest dose of DOET employed was readily distinguished from placebo (Table IV). The total subjective effects scores for the Ss receiving lowest doses of DOET were 7 times greater than those of Ss receiving placebo. The total subjective effect scores of Ss receiving medium and high doses were higher than those of Ss receiving lowest doses, although the difference was not statistically significant. In no Ss was there any evidence of perceptual

TABLE III

Subjective effects of varying doses of DOET

Effect	Placebo (H_2O) (n = 4)	Low dose (0.75–1.0 mg) (n = 4)	Medium dose (2.0–3.0 mg) (n = 5)	High dose (3.5–4.0 mg) (n = 4)
high	0	0	1.20(3)	1.00(2)
pleasant	0.25(1)	0.50(1)	1.20(2)	1.25(2)
unpleasant	0	0.25(1)	0.80(2)	0.25(1)
difficulty concentrating	0	0.75(2)	1.80(3)	0.50(1)
talkative	0	1.00(2)	1.20(2)	1.25(2)
thoughts faster than words	0	0.75(2)	0.60(1)	0.50(1)
visual effects	0.25(1)	0.25(1)	0.40(1)	0.00
"nervous" or restless	0	0.25(1)	0.60(1)	1.50(3)
euphoric	0	0.25(1)	0.80(2)	0.75(1)
relaxed	0	0.75(2)	1.00(2)	0.50(1)
light-headed	0.25(1)	1.25(4)	1.40(3)	2.25(4)
aware of body image	0.25(1)	1.00(3)	1.80(5)	1.50(3)

Transcripts of tape recorded interviews with subjects receiving different doses of DOET or placebo were graded blindly for each effect. Scoring was as follows: 0 = no effect at all; 1 = slight effect; 2 = moderate effect; 3 = marked effect. Data are presented as the mean score per subject. Numbers in parentheses indicate the number of subjects reporting the presence of an effect.

TABLE IV

Total subjective effect scores of subjects with varying doses of DOET

Group	Subjective Effect Scores ± S.E.M.
placebo	1.00 ± 1.00[a] (4)
low dose (0.75–1.0 mg)	7.00 ± 1.41 (4)
medium dose (2.0–3.0 mg)	12.80 ± 3.43 (5)
high dose (3.5–4.0 mg)	11.25 ± 2.97 (4)

[a] Differs from all drug dose levels $p < .02$.

Transcripts of tape recorded interviews with subjects receiving different doses of DOET or placebo were graded blindly for different subjective effects detailed in Table I. Scoring was as follows: 0 = no effect at all; 1 = slight effect; 2 = moderate effect; 3 = marked effect. Data are presented as the mean score per subject for all effects. Numbers in parentheses indicate the number of subjects in each group.

distortion or cognitive impairment. Thus in doses 5 times greater than the dose at which subjective effects could be clearly discerned, DOET was neither hallucinogenic nor psychotomimetic.

On the tasks of discriminating lights of different intensities and weights of different masses, there was no impairment irrespective of the dose of DOET. This indicates no impairment of perceptual discrimination. Effects of varying doses of DOET on perception of thematic apperception cards exposed for short intervals will be discussed below.

At none of the doses of DOET was there any change in systolic or diastolic blood pressure, pulse rate or oral temperature. There was mild pupil dilation with effects most prominent at 4 hours.

EFFECTS OF DOET AND DOM ON THE PERCEPTION OF THEMATIC APPERCEPTION CARDS

In the three studies described above, a large number of psychological tests were administered. Of these, tests of the perception of tachistoscopically exposed TAT cards were administered both with DOM and DOET, and indicated a differential response to the two drugs. Accordingly, the performance of Ss in the three different experiments in the tasks will be discussed together.

Eight thematic apperception (TAT) cards were projected as slides for a period during which Ss were asked to give a different associative label to each slide. The slides were then reprojected in different, random orders, successively at 1/100 sec, 1/25 sec and 1/10 sec exposures, and Ss were required to label the cards with their initial associations. All procedures, including choosing labels during long exposure time and attempting to reproduce them at short exposures, were performed prior to drug ingestion and 2, 4 and 6 hours afterwards. Ss were asked to guess if they were unsure of which stimulus had been presented. This task was administered to Ss in the DOM study and in the study using varying doses of DOET, but was not used in the study contrasting DOET and amphetamine.

In the DOM study, Ss receiving DOM mislabelled stimuli more frequently than did Ss receiving placebo (Fig. 7). This effect was maximal at 4 hours, corresponding to the time of peak subjective effects. The differences in performance between Ss receiving DOM and those receiving placebo were greatest with shortest exposure times. This difference in mislabelling tended to disappear as viewing time was increased. It is striking that DOM caused impairment in labelling TAT cards, since it had not impaired perception of line length. The TAT cards are complex stimuli that presumably contain emotionally meaningful material, while the horizontal and vertical lines are not emotionally meaningful. This suggests that DOM altered performance in the TAT tasks by affecting the associative organization of perceptual organization without affecting "simple" visual perception.

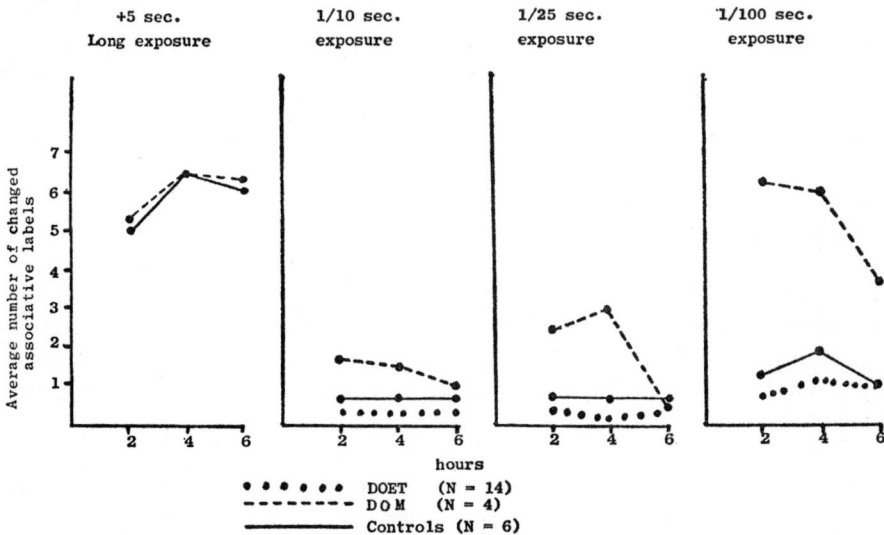

FIG. 7. The effect of DOM, DOET or water placebo on associations to thematic apperception test (TAT) cards exposed for varying time periods. Data for varying doses of DOET were combined.

In the study with varying doses of DOET, the drug had no effect on the perception of TAT cards (Fig. 7) regardless of the dose employed. The highest doses of DOET employed (4.0 mg) were higher than the absolute dose of DOM used. Moreover, if DOET is more potent in terms of threshold for subjective effects, 4.0 mg of DOET would be equivalent to a dosage of DOM considerably higher than 3.0 mg. These considerations suggest that DOET differs significantly from DOM in its paucity of disorganizing effects on perception.

SUMMARY

We have studied the effects of DOM and DOET in normal control subjects. In one study the effects of DOET were contrasted with those of *d*-amphetamine, while in the others the effects of varying doses of DOET or DOM were contrasted with those of a water placebo. Our results indicate that over a 5-fold range of dosage, DOET is able to produce significant subjective effects, the most prominent of which are a mild euphoria and enhanced self-awareness. These occur in the absence of hallucinogenic or psychotomimetic effects. At 5 times the minimal perceptible dose of LSD or other psychedelic drugs, marked hallucinogenic or psychotomimetic changes are usually observed. This would indicate that DOET differs qualitatively in its spectrum of psychological effects from most other "psychedelic" agents. Indeed, it is possible that in terms of its subjective effects, DOET ought not to be classified along with the other psychedelic agents. Despite a chemical resemblance to amphetamine, the effects of DOET are distinctly different from those of amphetamine and were distinguishable in a double blind experiment.

DOM has previously been shown (Snyder et al., 1967) to be hallucinogenic and psychotomimetic in doses exceeding 5 mg. In doses of about 3 mg. its subjective effects were similar to those of DOET. However, in a task requiring the labelling of tachistoscopically presented thematic apperception cards, DOM produced impaired performance, while DOET in higher doses was without effect. This suggests a difference in the effects produced by the two drugs. Although extensive dose-response data is not available on DOM, it appears that 2.0 mg is about the minimal perceptible dose (Shulgin, personal communication; Snyder et al., 1967), while doses greater than 5.0 mg tend to be hallucinogenic. This suggests that the hallucinogenic-psychotomimetic threshold for DOM is considerably closer to the minimal perceptible dose than is the case for DOET. Indeed, there is yet no evidence that DOET is in fact hallucinogenic. The ability of DOET to produce mild euphoria and enhanced self-awareness in the absence of cognitive or perceptual distortion suggests that it may be of therapeutic utility in psychiatry.

This research was supported in part by U.S. Food and Drug Administration Contract 68.8 and NIGMS Grant FR-35. Solomon H. Snyder is a recipient of NIMH Research Career Development Award 5-K03-MH-33128.

REFERENCES

Aghajanian, G. K. and Bing, O. H. L.: Persistence of lysergic acid diethylamide in the plasma of human subjects. *Clin. Pharmacol. Ther.* 5: 611–614 (1964).
Clark, H.: The prediction of recall in simple active sentences. *J. Verb. Learn. Verb. Behav.* 5: 99–106 (1966).
Jenkins, J. J. and Palermo, D. S.: *Word Association Norms.* University of Minnesota Press, Minneapolis (1963).
Katz, M. M., Waskow, I. E. and Olsson, J.: Characterizing the psychological state produced by LSD. *J. Abnorm. Psychol.* 73: 1–14 (1968).
Shulgin, A. T.: Psychotomimetic amphetamines: methoxy-3,4-dialkoxyamphetamines. *Experientia* 20: 366–369 (1964).
Shulgin, A. T., Sargent, T. and Naranjo C.: The chemistry and psychopharmacology of nutmeg and of several related phenylisopropylamines. *In: Ethnopharmacologic Search for Psychoactive Drugs,* edited by D. H. Efron, p. 202. U.S. Government Printing Office, Washington, D.C. P.H.S. Publication No. 1589 (1967).

Shulgin, A. T., Sargent, T. and Naranjo, C.: Structure-activity relationships of one-ring psychotomimetics. *Nature 221:* 537–540 (1969).

Snyder, S. H., Faillace, L. and Hollister, L.: 2,5-Dimethoxy-4-methyl-amphetamine (STP); a new hallucinogenic drug. *Science 158:* 669–670 (1967).

Snyder, S. H., Faillace, L. A. and Weingartner, H.: DOM (STP), a new hallucinogenic drug and DOET: effects in normal subjects. *Amer. J. Psychiat. 125:* 357–364 (1968).

DISCUSSION

DR. STEIN: Do you have D- and L-isomers of DOM and DOET? Is there any difference?

DR. SNYDER: No, we don't, but you can ask Dr. Shulgin about that.

DR. SHULGIN: I know of three separate experiments in three separate laboratories. There seem to have been efforts made to resolve them into D- and L-components. All three have failed so far.

DR. LUDWIG: I am interested in possible clinical applications. What are your thoughts about this in terms of treating minor types of depression? I refer to DOET specifically.

DR. SNYDER: The use of DOET in depression seems to be an interesting possibility. The first concern would be that DOET should have a reasonably high therapeutic index, so that untoward psychotropic effects do not occur at doses close to the therapeutic levels.

From our studies in normal control subjects, we feel that DOET might also be useful as an adjunct to psychotherapy since it produced an enhancement of self awareness.

DR. DOMINO: In view of the fact that you obtained dose-effect curves with DOET, I was a little disappointed you didn't do the same with amphetamine. You implied a basic difference. Do you think that really is valid?

DR. SNYDER: I don't know. I hope I wasn't trying to imply that it was different from amphetamine in dose-response characteristics at all.

The only point I was making about the dose-response data with DOET was that we were very impressed that with a dose that was five times greater than a dose which produced definite subjective effects, DOET still was not psychotomimetic or hallucinogenic. In this way DOET seemed to differ from other psychedelic drugs.

DR. DOMINO: Is there any difference between DOET and amphetamine? I think this is an important point.

DR. SNYDER: Yes, in the double-blind comparison of DOET and amphetamine they were clearly distinguishable, both in subjective effects and in their effects on the performance of several psychological tests.

Our own impression is that there is a real difference between amphetamine and DOET. The principal subjective effect of DOET is one of feeling more relaxed, open to new insight while fully lucid. It's a very different type of effect from what is conventionally reported with amphetamine.

DR. DOMINO: My point was you only used one dose, 10 mg., and to be fair you would have to run dose-effect curves with amphetamine as well.

CHILDREN'S REACTIONS TO PSYCHOTOMIMETIC DRUGS

Lauretta Bender, M.D.

*Consultant in Child Psychiatry,
New York State Department of Mental Hygiene
Creedmoor State Hospital, Queens Village, New York 11724*

In this paper I shall discuss some of my rather extensive experiences with both amphetamine (Benzedrine®) and LSD in children.

I started as a child psychiatrist in the early 1930's in the Bellevue psychiatric children's wards with children under the age of 13. At that time the post-encephalitic disorders following the epidemic of encephalitis were still observable. Those were the model for the concept of the hyperkinetic child, or the brain-driven child. That concept has remained until today, although I was convinced very early that the hyperkinetic child is not a child who has a problem with increased motor activity, or with increased physical energy, or with increased impulses, but rather that it is a problem of perceptual disorganization.

I came to these conclusions from my use of the Visual Motor Gestalt Test (Bender, 1938) and many other kinds of perceptual tests, such as the block design and the weight evaluation test in the Stanford-Binet Scale, and particularly the body image test in the drawing of a man.

The hyperkinetic child is one who has difficulty in organizing his perceptual experiences, in getting a body image concept and in getting, therefore, a self-image concept. Consequently, his restlessness is due to searching and seeking movements which lead him to contact the world about him in every way that he can, by moving about, by grasping things with his hands, or by biting, sucking or tasting with his mouth. Such behavior, of course, is quite distracting to the child himself and may prove to be destructive and aggressive.

The child who is hyperkinetic on the basis of cerebral pathology is seen to be a child with maturational lags; his behavior is immature, disorganized, and not goal directed. We do not wish to reduce the amount of activity but rather to enhance the pattern of activity, including a goal, and maturation. Thus, organization of behavior should be both cross-sectional and longitudinal.

At that time we were seeking a medication that would help with these children. Bradley and Bowen (1940, 1941) had used amphetamine in large doses of 20, 30, 40 and 50 mg per day in children, and claimed that it was useful in the hyperkinetic child with organic brain disease.

We were also interested in finding a drug that would help us with the sexually stimulated children, of which we had a number at that time. Paul Schilder (1938) had found in his psychoanalytic practice that if amphetamine was given to an adult who was under pressure to finish writing by a deadline, for example, it would be effective for the purpose given, but would also lead to a suppression of sexual interests and capacities; it was, therefore, not particularly liked by many such people.

And we were also concerned about children, particularly Negro boys, who were poor achievers, were not learning, and were, one might say, "sleeping in the noonday sun." That is, they tended to sleep in any situation of stress or boredom. They reminded us of cases of narcolepsy. Consequently, we used amphetamine for these problems.

When we gave amphetamine in the doses that Bradley recommended, we found that many children reacted with autonomic nervous system disorders, pallor and vomiting, and became very distraught, breaking windows, etc. Therefore, we lowered the dose and started out with a routine in which we gave 5 mg one morning, 10 the next, and 15 the next, then 20, and then stabilized the daily dosage at that level. For children under seven years we halved this dosage routine, while some robust children tolerated and benefited by doubling it. This is a routine which I have now used for these many years.

Occasionally there are children who still exhibit autonomic nervous system disorders and some tendency to sleeplessness, loss of appetite, and weight loss. This will pass off in a few days, or, at the most, in 10 days to two weeks. If one is patient and persists with the drug, one can get most children to tolerate it very well.

This drug will affect the children in such a way that they are relieved of a great deal of tension and anxiety, have a better learning capacity, and get along much better, both with peers, teachers and other authoritative figures. They feel more highly valued, better loved, better appreciated and more capable of doing things, and they advance more rapidly in the learning processes. If we arranged tutoring, a good school program, or any therapeutic or remedial program that the child needed, the child would advance.

The sexual problems simply melted away. Excessive sexual drives and preoccupations in a prepuberty child gradually disappeared. The child quit talking about them, then denied them and soon forgot them, or became amnestic for them. This is a process which happens normally in children, but the drug facilitates it. The hyperkinetic child becomes quieter because his behavior pattern is better organized and directed towards the normal goals of childhood, *i.e.*, learning and experiencing life.

We have been able to give this drug for weeks, months, and in some cases two and three years. We have never seen anything in the way of an amphetamine psychosis. Furthermore, and even more interesting, anything in the way of tolerance is rarely seen, so that it did not become ineffective, and it was not necessary to increase the dose. Also the drug can be stopped without getting any kind of withdrawal symptoms or effects. Whatever the child had gained would have grown into his system or built into his developmental pattern, and he would not regress to his former behavior.

For years before the new psychotropic drugs became available, the amphetamines were our most effective drugs in the modification of behavior in children with problems.

Recently a very interesting paper by Keith Connors (1966) of the Johns Hopkins University has reported the effects of d-amphetamine (Dexedrine®) on rapid visual discrimination and motor control in hyperkinetic children under mild stress. He used sophisticated test procedures and concluded that motor control was in no way affected, and that there were more organized perceptual responses in rapid visual discrimination together with an improvement in clinical symptomatology and school performance in a number of test measures.

Connor's conclusions confirm my experiences and convictions that the hyperkinetic child's basic problem is one of organization of perceptual experiences, and that the amphetamines are effective in modifying the behavior of children by facilitating perceptual organization.

That children never get a schizophrenic-like psychosis from amphetamine is partly due to the fact that childhood schizophrenia is not like adult schizophrenia. Children with schizophrenia do not experience hallucinations of the projected type like adults, but only of the introjected type. Children hear voices inside their head or other parts of the body, feel that they originate inside themselves and do not feel persecuted by them. Children get projected hallucinations in some toxic delirious states or in some neurotic situations, but not in schizophrenia. I have never known of a child to experience hallucinations of any kind because of amphetamine medication.

We also used, as the years went by and new drugs came in, all of the antihistamines, reserpine, meprobamate, energizers, phenothiazines and anticonvulsants (Bender and Nichtern, 1956; Bender and Faretra, 1961) and found that these drugs in general do not sedate children, except temporarily, that they do not quiet them down in the sense of quieting down motor over-activity, but that they help them to organize their behavior, to pattern it more completely and to maturate more satisfactorily. Occasionally a large dose is given intravenously to control a major disturbance in a child. Children rarely get side effects with the drugs. The psychotropic drugs can be given in larger doses to children than to adults. We do not find any difficulty in stopping the drugs since children rarely show withdrawal symptoms.

My experience with LSD has been since 1961 at the Children's Unit of Creedmoor State Hospital (Bender et al., 1962). I started in 1961, when Paul Hoch was Commissioner of the Department of Mental Hygiene in New York. He was very much opposed to the use of LSD to produce psychotic episodes as a method of therapy, and we had some difficulty in getting him to let us use the drug on children, until we convinced him that we did not want to use it because of its known psychotomimetic effects, but because it was known to inhibit serotonin, and as an agent, to quote Brodie (1958) which would cause "arousal and increased responsiveness to sensory stimuli, preponderance of sympathetic activity and increased skeletal and muscle tone and activity."

These are the basic features which I think define schizophrenia in childhood. In childhood schizophrenia, all boundaries are lost, not only of the psychological and personality experiences, but also those of the visceral functions, autonomic nervous system, vascular tone, muscular tone and perception.

It was hoped that the LSD would be effective in correcting these disorders. We started out with it very carefully because of the two warnings that we had: one, that the children would become disturbed, and the other, that repeated use of the drug would lead to tolerance. So we gave it once a week in small doses, 25 μg intramuscularly, to prepuberty children, 5 to 11 years of age. Two children between 10 and 11 years of age did become panicky and anxious; we immediately stopped the effects of the drug in these two children with sodium amytal. None of the other children became disturbed. They all showed a tendency to become "high" and lively. Where they were pale and blue-lipped before, they developed a bright, pink color, eyes were bright, and they looked up. They tried to make a contact with us for expressions of affection, and to engage in motor play. These were mute, autistic, schizophrenic children. And they showed a general improvement in well-being, appearance, and lift in mood.

We worked with these children, gradually increasing the dose and the frequency until we were giving 150 μg per day orally in two divided doses morning and evening, and continued this for weeks, months, and in some cases for a year or two. We meanwhile were making all kinds of psychological, clinical and biological studies.

We gave this first to young, autistic children, and we found that we were able to get an improvement in their general well-being, general tone, habit patterning, eating patterns and sleeping patterns, and we could raise the Vineland Social Maturity score, which is the behavior evaluation score. In a few children we got some more vocalization, although not actually any improvement or increase in language as such (Bender et al., 1962; 1963). We soon gave it also to older autistic children and got somewhat less beneficial effects, since these were more chronic, and complicated with more organicity in some cases.

We then gave LSD in the same doses to non-autistic schizophrenic boys 6 to 12 years of age. They were intelligent and verbal and could be tested psychologically and in psychiatric interviews (Bender et al., 1963). They were selected because they had typical schizophrenic psychosis, with flying fantasies and identification and body image difficulties, loose ego boundaries, introjected objects and voices and bizarre ideologies. They had obvious anxiety and labile vaso-vegetative functions. After administering LSD to these children we found results contrary to those reported in adults. These children became more insightful, more objective, more realistic; and in a short time they became frankly depressed for reality reasons. They noted they were in the hospital, that they were away from their family, and that they had had "crazy" ideas before.

These were children who were not subjected to special psychotherapy but only to our usual activity program. They all benefited sufficiently so that those who did have a place to go were in some months able to return to their homes and community schools.

We also tried LSD on two adolescent boys who were mildly schizophrenic (Bender, 1966a). These were boys whom we had known for many months. When we gave the first dose of 100 μg of LSD orally, Dr. Faretra and I sat opposite the boys for two hours, encouraging them to talk and to draw. Within a half hour they began to report distortions in visual experiences, such things as claiming that we were grimacing at them, smiling at them, and making faces at them, that the other boy's face was turning green, that the lines in their corduroy pants were getting too numerous and were moving around, and that the pencils they were using were getting rubbery. These by and large represented fluidity or motility in visual experiences that they really had. There were no hallucinations.

They became disturbed to the extent that they said we were experimenting on them. In two or three hours this passed off, and the next day we put them back into their group activity after repeating the dose; they had no trouble that day as long as they were in their own group and away from close observation of the psychiatrist.

We continued these boys for some months on 150 µg in two divided doses daily. One of them benefited very much, and was able to go home and return to school, although he has since returned as a disturbed adult schizophrenic.

The other one had been tried many times out of the hospital in foster homes, without success. After some months he complained that we were experimenting on him with the drug and trying to keep him from getting out of the hospital. We discontinued the drug. That was not because of the drug but because of the boy's attitude toward it, based on his own psychopathology.

We also used methysergide (UML, Sansert®) in daily doses of two or three 4 mg space tabs. This is a methylated derivative of LSD which is used to prevent migraine headaches. We found that it had effects similar to LSD on schizophrenic children.

Gloria Faretra and I (1965) did a study, using the Funkenstein Test on the autonomic nervous system, of a series of children. We were able to show that LSD, methysergide and psilocybin have a normalizing effect upon the labile plastic autonomic system characteristic of schizophrenic children.

We used LSD on 89 children from January 1961 to July 1965, when Sandoz no longer made it available for research purposes. We were unwilling to apply to N.I.M.H. for supplies at that time because of the reports of chromosome damage in LSD users. We immediately started examining the chromosomes of the children who had received LSD and methysergide, although it was up to two years after termination of the drugs. We were not able to confirm that there was chromosome damage in any of those children that we had examined (Bender and Sankar, 1968).

We hope to go back to using LSD because we have found that it is one of the most effective methods of treatment we have for childhood schizophrenia. It tends to normalize the labile, boundaryless physiological, perceptual and psychological functions in schizophrenic children, and helps them to a more normal physiological, psychological and social adjustment.

REFERENCES

Bender, L.: *A Visual Motor Gestalt Test and Its Clinical Use.* Monograph No. 3. American Orthopsychiatric Association, New York (1938).

Bender, L.: Post-encephalitic behavior disorders in childhood. In: *Encephalitis, A Clinical Study,* Josephine Neale, editor, chapt. VIII, pp. 361–385. Grune & Stratton, New York (1942).

Bender, L.: D-Lysergic acid in the treatment of the biological features of childhood schizophrenia. *Dis. Nerv. Syst. 27:* 39–42 (1966a).
Bender, L.: The treatment of childhood schizophrenia with LSD and UML. In: *Biological Treatment of Mental Illness,* edited by Max Rinkel, editor, pp. 463–491. L. C. Page & Co., New York (1966b).
Bender, L. and Cottington, F.: The use of amphetamine sulphate (Benzedrine) in child psychiatry. *Am. J. Psychiat. 99:* 116–121 (1942).
Bender, L. and Sankar, D. V. S.: Chromosome damage not found in leukocytes of children treated with LSD-25. A letter to *Science 159:* Jan. 10, 1968.
Bender, L. and Faretra, G.: Organic therapy in pediatric psychiatry. *Dis. of Nerv. Syst. Monog. Suppl. 22:* 110–111 (1961).
Bender, L., Faretra, G. and Cobrinik, L.: LSD and UML treatment of hospitalized disturbed children. In: *Recent Advances in Biological Psychiatry,* J. Wortis, editor. *5:* 84–92 (1963).
Bender, L., Goldschmidt, L. and Sankar, D. V. S.: Treatment of autistic schizophrenic children with LSD-25 and UML-491. In: *Recent Advances in Biological Psychiatry,* J. Wortis, editor. *4:* 170–177 (1962).
Bender, L. and Nichtern, S.: Chemotherapy in child psychiatry. *N.Y. State J. of Med. 56:* 2791–2795 (1956).
Bradley, C. and Bowen, M.: School performance of children receiving amphetamine (Benzedrine sulphate). *Am. J. Orthopsychiat. 10:* 782 (1940).
Bradley, C. and Bowen, M.: Amphetamine (Benzedrine) therapy of children's behavior disorders. *Am. J. Orthopsychiat. 11:* 92 (1941).
Brodie, B. B.: Interaction of psychotropic drugs with physiologic and biochemical mechanisms in the brain. *Mod. Med.,* Aug. 1, pp. 69–80 (1958).
Connors, C. K.: The effects of Dexedrine on rapid discrimination and motor control of hyperkinetic children under mild stress. *J. Nerv. Ment. Dis. 142:* 429–433 (1966).
Faretra, G. and Bender, L.: Autonomic nervous system responses in hospitalized children treated with LSD and UML. In: *Recent Advances in Biological Psychiatry,* J. Wortis, editor. *7:* 1 (1965).
Sankar, D. V. S., Broer, H. H. and Cates, N.: Studies on biogenic amines and psychoactive drug actions with special reference to LSD. *Trans. N.Y. Acad. Sci. 26:* 369–376 (1964).
Schilder, P.: Psychological effects of Benzedrine sulphate. *J. Nerv. Ment. Dis. 87:* 584 (1948).

DISCUSSION

DR. WEST: You say you started out with a dose in the small children of 25 µg of LSD per week. You gave them one dose a week, and the effects that you noted—

DR. BENDER:—Only lasted a few hours.

DR. WEST: But then you said you went up to 150 µg per day?

DR. BENDER: Yes. We increased it gradually to test its safety, and to avoid disturbances. Finally we gave 150 µg daily in two divided doses. We saw no evidence of anything that was called tolerance, unless you speak of tolerance in terms of the fact they did not become disturbed as adults do.

They showed no evidence of tolerance in terms of the effects upon the stabilizing or normalizing of the autonomic nervous system and general well-being.

Ongoing biochemical studies by Dr. Sankar showed a binding of serotonin and histamine and freeing of epinephrine. This progressed for some weeks, tended to level off to a plateau and continued on a plateau thereafter, indicating some tolerance (Sankar et al., 1964).

Another study (Bender 1966b) was done by several of the doctors (D. Winn, J. Dowling, G. Dooher) involving six pairs of matched prepuberty schizophrenic boys who received the usual dose of LSD. From the first day, they watched them carefully, asking for every possible subjective reaction, as well as doing psychiatric interviews on selected psychological, sensory and neurological tests. They did find that some children were mildly disturbed the first day, and could find in half of the children some kind of sensory disorder. In all but two, this disappeared by the second day. And in one it lasted as long as 10 days, but beyond that there was no further disorder.

So, there is evidence that there are disturbances that occur the first day, which you can play down if you leave the child in the usual routine. Or you can emphasize them if you look for them very carefully. As for the tolerance to the physiological effects, this appears, from laboratory evidence, about the end of the third or fourth week, and then reaches a plateau. Clinically, changes are seen to continue for months and are integrated into a more healthy and mature level in the development of the child.

DR. FREEDMAN: Did you have a large pupil with LSD?

DR. BENDER: Yes. The pupils were examined during the time we did the Funkenstein Test, and on many other occasions, and in two-thirds of the children they showed large pupils after the first dose.

DR. FREEDMAN: And did that occur after every dose, or do they get tolerant?

DR. BENDER: Some children, but not all, became tolerant to that.

DR. FREEDMAN: Of course, the definition of tolerance has to do a great deal with correlates with autonomic tolerance. That is, tolerance to mydriasis, and tolerance to mental effects in man. It may be that they showed tolerance in that respect.

DR. BENDER: Yes.

DR. HOLMSTEDT: There's one thing here which I find disturbing. You say that you get as good effects with methysergide, and that it produces no hallucinations whatsoever.

DR. BENDER: Well, so it is sometimes said. Actually, it is known to be an hallucinogen, although not as strong as LSD. It has also been used by some "hippies" in California. I am a migraine headache sufferer and have found it a very effective preventive. But I assure you that I experienced perceptual, especially visual, distortions when I first started the medication and when I make a mistake and take a double dose.

DR. MANDELL: I know of some differing data, Dr. Bender, and it perhaps has to do with the diagnostic heterogeneity of your population. Dr. Simmons at U.C.L.A. used the Rimland Scale criteria for autistic children and, on the basis of your work with Dr. Faretra on LSD, tried this on autistic children three times a week. He found, in general, only a little bit of drug induced an increase in activity. In general, after several treatments, the U.C.L.A. group saw no more increase in tendency to talk, to relate, or to make contact. Studying this group over several months, they failed to duplicate your findings. But, on the other hand, it may have been some function of the heterogeneity of your group of children versus this rather homogeneous group that they were working with.

DR. BENDER: I thing Rimland's Scale is a pretty rigid scale, and I suspect many of his cases are also organic as well as schizophrenic, or perhaps only organic. Also, you only gave LSD three times a week. We gave it daily.

DR. LEHRER: Dr. Bender, when you first started with amphetamine, I assume that it was the racemic amphetamine

DR. BENDER: We never use Dexedrine (d-amphetamine) because in the city and state hospital Benzedrine is the drug that is available, and we soon learned to use it so well we had no reason for shifting over to Dexedrine. I have known some doctors who in their private practice used Dexedrine, and they claimed they didn't get as good results.

DR. LEHRER: I was wondering whether some of the vomiting and other concomitants may not have been due to the *levo* component?

DR. BENDER: Well, that may have been.

DR. GESSNER: Dr. Bender, could you tell us whether you sometimes used methysergide together with LSD?

DR. BENDER: We never used them both at one time on the same patient. We used them on different patients, and there were times when we shifted from methysergide to LSD because methysergide did occasionally have side effects, *e.g.,* causing ergot effects in the vascular system, especially of the legs. We had that in three or four of the children, and consequently changed them over to LSD. Also, we had to give up LSD earlier than methysergide. So, some of the children that were getting LSD were continued on methysergide. We never gave both drugs at the same time to one child.

DR. GESSNER: I asked my question simply because Sai-Halasz had reported methysergide to potentiate the effects of hallucinogens (Sai-Halasz, A.: *Experientia, 18:* 137–138, 1962).

DMT (N,N-DIMETHYLTRYPTAMINE) AND HOMOLOGUES: CLINICAL AND PHARMACOLOGICAL CONSIDERATIONS

Stephen Szara, M.D.

Section on Psychopharmacology, Division of Special Mental Health Research, National Institute of Mental Health, St. Elizabeths Hospital, Washington, D.C. 20032

During the past 13 years we have been working on the biochemistry and pharmacology of the various N-alkylated tryptamine derivatives, both in man and in animals.

Interest in the possible hallucinogenic activity of N,N-dimethyltryptamine (DMT) stems from the report by Fish, Horning and Johnson (1955) who found DMT, together with bufotenin, in snuff powder prepared by Haitian natives from *Piptadenia peregrina* seeds which the natives used in their religious ceremonies to produce mystical states of consciousness.

In 1956 the hallucinogenic action of bufotenin was reported by Fabing, but no information as to whether DMT had similar psychotropic activity was available. We prepared DMT by chemical synthesis and tested its activity on animals and humans. It was found that it produced symptoms similar to those caused by mescaline and LSD and which lasted for a surprisingly short period of time (45 min-1 hr) after intramuscular injection of about 1 mg/kg of the drug (Szara, 1956).

The hallucinogenic activity of N,N-diethyltryptamine (DET) was first reported in 1957 (Szara, 1957), and a more systematic study was reported later by us (Szara, *et al.*, 1966) and independently by Boszormenyi *et al.* (1959).

Speeter and Anthony (1954) reported that N,N-dipropyltryptamine (DPT), another tryptamine derivative, produced observable effects in dogs. The similarity in chemical structure between DPT (Fig. 1) and other hal-

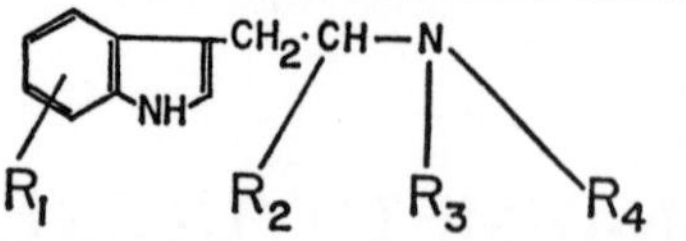

Compound	R_1	R_2	R_3	R_4	Psychotropic dose
1 Tryptamine (T)	-H	-H	-H	-H	500 mg ?
2 DMT	-H	-H	-CH$_3$	-CH$_3$	60 mg i.m.
3 DET	-H	-H	-C$_2$H$_5$	-C$_2$H$_5$	60 mg i.m. or p.o.
4 Dipropyl-T	-H	-H	-C$_3$H$_7$	-C$_3$H$_7$	60 " " "
5 Diallyl-T	-H	-H	-C$_3$H$_5$	-C$_3$H$_5$	60 " " "
6 α-methyl-T	-H	-CH$_3$	-H	-H	20 mg p.o.
7 α-ethyl-T	-H	-C$_2$H$_5$	-H	-H	20 mg p.o.
8 Psilocybin	4-OPO$_3$H$_2$	-H	-CH$_3$	-CH$_3$	15 mg p.o.
9 Bufotenin	5-HO-	-H	-CH$_3$	-CH$_3$	16 mg i.v.

FIG. 1. Simple derivatives of tryptamine with psychotropic activity.

lucinogenic tryptamine derivatives and its reported effects in animals suggested that this compound might be capable of producing hallucinogenic effects in humans.

One of the major problems in evaluating hallucinogenic compounds is the absence of an effective placebo which could mimic some of the effects of these drugs, such as physical symptoms and mood changes, without producing the psychedelic effects.

On the basis of animal experiments and some human metabolic data we came to the conclusion that the 6-hydroxylation of the indole ring of the hallucinogenic tryptamine derivatives might be an important pathway for the metabolism of these compounds (Kalir and Szara, 1963). We prepared a series of compounds substituted at the 6-position. One of these synthesized compounds, 6-fluorodiethyltryptamine (6-FDET), was observed to produce autonomic symptoms and mood changes in humans without producing the characteristic perceptual and thinking disturbances usually seen with psychotomimetic drugs. From this initial data, we postulated that 6-FDET might be useful as an active placebo in clinical studies.

In order to test the hypothesis that DPT is another effective hallucinogenic drug, and to confirm the previous work that 6-FDET is an active placebo, a double-blind pilot study was undertaken at Saint Elizabeths Hospital. This research project set out to measure psychological, biochemical and physiological effects produced by DPT and 6-FDET as compared to the related chemical compound, DET, a potent, known hallucinogenic compound, in the same experimental subjects (Faillace, Vourlekis and Szara, 1967).

Twelve chronic, non-psychotic, alcoholic, hospitalized patients volunteered to participate in the program. They all were in good physical condition without evidence of organic deterioration, schizophrenia or manic depressive illness. They ranged from 29 to 48 years of age, with a mean age of 38.2. The length of hospitalization prior to treatment varied from one month to five years. All had been drinking heavily for over ten years. All had had multiple arrests for alcoholism. Prior to treatment, all the subjects had an extensive medical work up which included CBC, BUN, glucose, thymol turbidity, alkaline phosphatase, cephaline flocculation, SGOT, SGPT, EKG and EEG. Thus, they were considered to be in excellent physical health. The subjects were informed about the nature of the drug experience; however, they were not informed of the possibility of receiving an active placebo in one or more of the sessions.

Several questionnaires have been devised to measure the subjective effects of LSD-25 in humans. However, the 74 item questionnaire by Linton and Langs (1962; 1964) was selected because it contained a wide range of perceptual, cognitive, affective and somatic items. The main focus of the questionnaire is on the subject's altered state of consciousness. Linton and Langs also classified the major dimensions of the subjective effects of LSD-25 into four empirical scales: Subscale "A" contains items related to impaired attention and loss of inhibition; subscale "B" deals with feelings of unreality, of having lost control and with paranoid ideation; subscale "C" deals mainly with body image changes and certain somatic symptoms; finally, subscale "D" contains questions dealing with overt anxiety and related somatic symptoms.

The Rockland-Pollin (RP) scale (Rockland and Pollin, 1965) consisting of 16 items, was used to record observable psychotic behavior by assessing mental status data. Two psychiatrists scored the patients independently on this scale before the drug session and at the termination, but before the subjective questionnaire was answered. The RP scale is grouped in three main categories: (1) general appearance and manner (6 items); (2) affect and mood (4 items); and (3) content of thought and thought processes (6 items). This instrument was chosen because it was originally derived partly from observing the effects of DET on normal individuals.

The double-blind design allowed each patient to receive DET, DPT and 6-FDET at least once, with one of these drugs given in two different dosages (0.7 and 1.0 mg/kg) intramuscularly. In our patient population, seven subjects received each drug at the 1 mg/kg dose in a random design.

The evaluation of the results is based on data obtained from testing the seven patients of our series who each received 1 mg/kg of DPT, DET and 6-FDET during their second or subsequent drug session. The data from the first session were not used because the results from these sessions would be highly influenced by the patient's initial anxiety. Since this kind of experience is unique for most individuals, data obtained from the first session would be most biased and could not be reliably compared to subsequent sessions.

We shall examine this problem a little later, but first let me show you some of the results of these comparisons (Fig. 2).

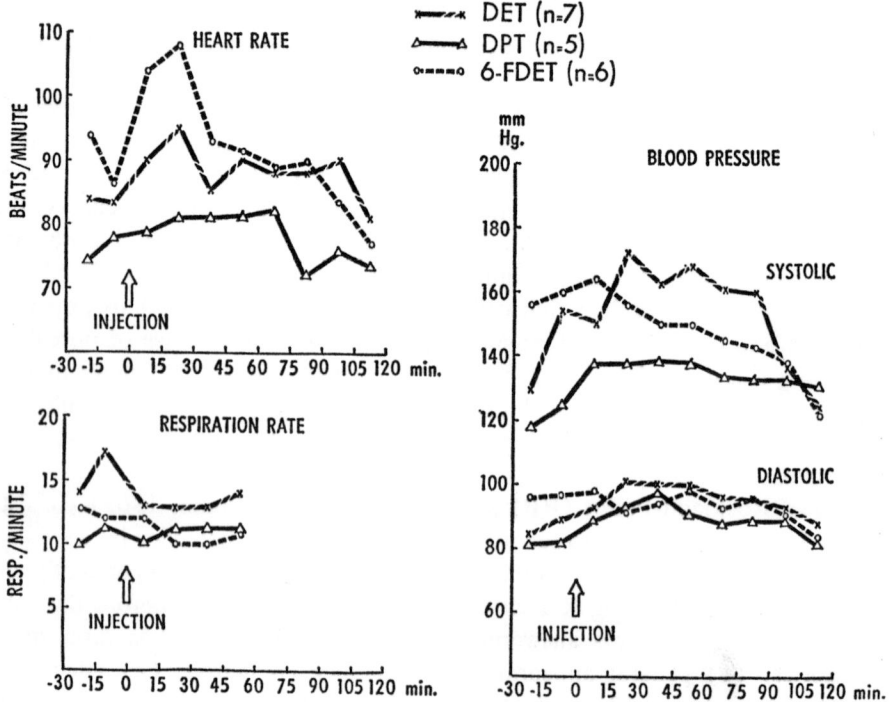

FIG. 2. Time course of autonomic changes produced by three psychotropic tryptamine derivatives in man.

The time course of autonomic changes produced by these three compounds shows that all three produce a slight increase in heart rate and blood pressure, returning to normal within two hours (Szara et al., 1967).

The psychological effects, which were evaluated by the two scales already mentioned, are summarized in Tables I and II.

TABLE I

Significance of difference between pre-drug and drug scores—Wilcoxon Matched Pairs Signed Rank Test; P Values[a]

	Subscales				Rockland-Pollin Scale
	A	B	C	D	
DET	< 0.05	< 0.05	< 0.02	< 0.02	< 0.05
DPT	< 0.02	< 0.02	< 0.02	< 0.02	< 0.05
6-FDET	N.S.	N.S.	< 0.02	< 0.02	N.S.

[a] For drug schedules and other experimental details, see text.

Table I summarizes the significance of the difference between the pre-drug and drug scores as measured by the Wilcoxon Matched Pairs Signed Rank Test. Both DET and DPT show a significant difference between pre-drug and drug scores on all the subscales of the Linton and Langs questionnaire. However, with 6-FDET, subscales A and B show no significant difference.

TABLE II

Summary of Friedman's Two-Way Analysis of Variance By Ranks for subjective and objective scales.[a]

Scale		P value
Linton and Langs	subscale A	< 0.001
	” B	< 0.005
	” C	< 0.02
	” D	N.S.
Rockland-Pollin		N.S.

[a] For experimental details see text.

Table II shows Friedman's Two-Way Analysis of Variance comparing the difference between pre-drug and drug scores of the three compounds for each patient. Only subscale D, concerned primarily with somatic symptoms, shows no significant difference when comparing the three drugs.

The Wilcoxon Signed Rank Test for measuring the significance of difference between pre-drug and drug scores of the RP Scale showed a significant difference ($p < 0.05$) for DET and DPT. However, there was no significant difference for 6-FDET. Friedman's Two-Way Analysis of Variance comparing the scores on the RP Scale for the three drugs showed a difference ($p < 0.1$) between the drugs which was not considered to be statistically significant.

The data presented here tend to affirm the assumption that 6-FDET produces some of the same physical and mood changes as the known hallucinogen, DET, and the new hallucinogen, DPT. These changes produced by 6-FDET are indistinguishable from the changes produced by the two hallucinogenic compounds in the same patients. From the results presented, which must be viewed cautiously because of the small sample, 6-FDET appears to be an effective placebo and warrants further study.

I would like to direct attention to a point mentioned earlier, namely that the psychological data from the first session were not used because of the possibility of distorting the evaluation with the effects of anxiety generated by the novelty of the first experience.

There is no question in anybody's mind who has ever taken an effective dose of a hallucinogen that the experience is new in many ways at the perceptual, emotional and cognitive levels, and at subsequent occasions, if the drug is taken repeatedly, this novelty value of the experience is diminished. Since novelty is an important aspect of the experience, it is expected that the first and subsequent experiences will differ from each other.

There are also a number of observations which suggest that even after a single drug experience, in many subjects there is a more or less long lasting aftereffect which might have physiological and/or biochemical as well as psychological origin.

The Spring Grove group refers to this aftereffect as the "psychedelic afterglow" which seems to appear quite regularly in patients after the LSD session, lasts sometimes for weeks, is characterized by a greatly reduced anxiety level and, psychologically, by a "shifting of the emotional center towards loving and harmonious affections" and "a seemingly enhanced capacity and disposition to enter into close interpersonal relationships and a sort of generalized benignity of outlook" (Kurland and Unger, 1969).

W. H. McGlothlin, S. Cohen and M. S. McGlothlin (1967) have found a significant increase in a passivity test at 2 weeks after a single LSD experience, indicating increased preference for "quiet receptivity, contemplation and humble obedience" as opposed to "group action, progress through realism and physical interaction." There were some less spectacular changes in other psychological measures at 6 month follow-up time (Marlow-Crowne Social Desirability Scale, and in Rosenzweig's Picture Frustration test, this last measuring the manner in which aggression is expressed). These same authors have also found a significant drop in galvanic skin response to a stress situation, which seems to confirm the clinical observation of the Spring Grove group about the reduced anxiety level during the period of the "afterglow."

In our own study the repeated administration of the hallucinogenic tryptamine derivatives at weekly intervals for 5 weeks allowed us to make a comparison between the first and the subsequent reactions at the psychological and at the biochemical levels. (Only two later sessions were followed by electrophysiological recordings, so we cannot make comparisons at this level.)

Various items at the Linton and Langs Scale were clearly different between the first and all the subsequent sessions. No statistical evaluation is feasible, since only 5 subjects received hallucinogenic drugs as the first dose, but the clinical impression was that the bodily symptoms were different when the drug was first taken from all subsequent sessions.

At the psychological level, however, it was fairly general that items referring to sense of time, passage or stopping of time, were answered negatively at the first session, while at all the subsequent sessions there was a marked change in these subjective time sensations. On the other hand, positive answers to some other items (feeling silly, awareness of changed judging ability, etc.) seemed to be more pronounced at the first session than in the subsequent sessions.

At the biochemical level, none of the routine medical laboratory tests showed pathological changes when the before and after specimens of blood and urine were examined. However, in the more specific area of metabolizing hallucinogenic drugs, we did find a subtle but significant change after the first exposure to a particular drug.

Before presenting these results, let us review briefly the pathways involved in the metabolism of the alkylated tryptamine derivatives (Fig. 3).

Table III shows the average 24 hr excretion values for the unchanged drug, for the apparent 6-hydroxy bases and for the apparent 3-indoleacetic acid (3-IAA) after the administration of each of the three drugs.

Please note the differences between the DET and DPT line in the unchanged and 6-hydroxy-base column. The 3-IAA values were essentially

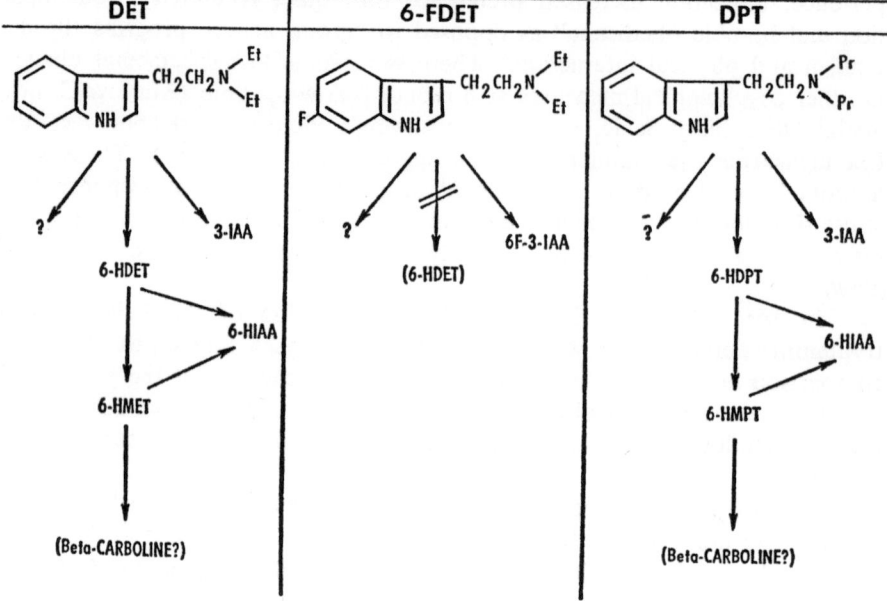

FIG. 3. Metabolic pathways for three psychotropic tryptamine derivatives.

the same for both drugs, but for 6-FDET the apparent 3-IAA (actually 6F-3-IAA, but indistinguishable by the method used) was significantly higher.

Breaking up the data in a different manner would enable us to see whether the metabolism at the second exposure to a drug was significantly affected by the first exposure one or two weeks earlier (Table IV).

TABLE III

Metabolism of tryptamine derivatives in man; 24 hour excretion values expressed as percent of administered drug

Drug	n	Drug excreted as		
		Unchanged	6-hydroxy base (apparent)	3-IAA (apparent)
DET	15	3.68 ± 2.24	4.04 ± 2.05	14.5 ± 5.9
DPT	20	1.04 ± 1.05	.76 ± .33	13.1 ± 8.6
6-FDET	12	2.86 ± 1.94	(.33 ± .23)	33.8 ± 13.1

Data are expressed as the mean percentage of the administered dose ±S.D.

TABLE IV[a]

Drug	DPT (n = 8)		DET (n = 5)	
Exposure	1st	second	1st	second
unchanged	.92 ± .19	.96 ± .34	4.48 ± .94	3.80 ± .82
as 3-IAA	12.2 ± 2.0	14.8 ± 3.2	12.3 ± 1.2	17.1 ± 2.7
as 6-hydroxy base	.81 ± .14	.73 ± .10	3.64 ± .75	4.53 ± .94

[a] Data are expressed as the mean percentage of the administered dose found ±S.E.M.

In this last table the DPT values were not significantly different when the values for the first day or for a larger exposure to the drug were compared.

In case of DET however (in 5 subjects) the unchanged drug excreted after a later exposure was significantly lower, while the excretion of the metabolites which were measured in this case were higher than at the first exposure to DET ($p < .05$, Wilcoxon test).

Since we could account for only a fraction of the administered drug in the 24 hr urine of the patients, these data have to be interpreted with extreme caution. We don't know what happens to the rest of the administered compounds. In animals these metabolites account for more than 90% of the administered drugs, and we did not have the opportunity yet to study the fate of the radioactive labeled hallucinogenic drugs in man.

It seems to be safe to conclude from the presented data that a first exposure to some hallucinogenic drugs does affect the metabolic machinery of the human organism in the direction of increased metabolism. Enzyme induction comes immediately to our mind as a possibility, but the data do not allow us to propose this as the only possible explanation.

Whether or not this biochemical change is related to some long term psychological and physiological effects cannot be ascertained. We can only suggest that the clinical significance of the "psychedelic afterglow" (Kurland and Unger, 1968), the increased reactivity of chronic "acid heads" to low intensity light stimuli (Blacker et al., 1968) and the increased psychological responses to marihuana after the first exposure (Weil, 1968) seem to be strong enough impetus for a continued search for biochemical and physiological correlates of long lasting effects of hallucinogenic drugs.

REFERENCES

Blacker, U. H., Jones, R. T., Stone, G. C. and Pfefferbaum, D.: Chronic users of LSD: the "acid heads." *Amer. J. Psychiat.* 125: 341–351 (1968).

Boszormenyi, Z., Der, P. and Nagy, T.: Observations on the psychotogenic effect of

N,N-diethyltryptamine: a new tryptamine derivative. *J. Ment. Sci. 105:* 171–181 (1959).
Fabing, H. D. and Hawkins, J. R.: Intravenous bufotenine injection in the human being. *Science, 123:* 886–887 (1956).
Faillace, L. A., Vourlekis, A. and Szara, S.: Clinical evaluation of some hallucinogenic tryptamine derivatives. *J. Nerv. Ment. Dis. 145:* 306–313 (1967).
Fish, M. S., Johnson, N. M. and Horning, E. C.: Piptadenia alkaloids—indole bases of *P. peregrina (L.) benth.* and related species, *J. Amer. Chem. Soc. 77:* 5892–5895 (1955).
Kalir, A. and Szara, S.: Synthesis and pharmacological activity of fluorinated tryptamine derivatives. *J. Med. Chem. 6:* 716–719 (1963).
Kurland, A. A. and Unger, S.: The present status and future direction of psychedelic LSD research, with special reference to the Spring Grove studies. Paper presented at the 7th Annual Meeting of the American College of Neuropsychopharmacology, San Juan, Puerto Rico, December 18–20, 1968.
Linton, H. B. and Langs, R. J.: Subjective reactions to lysergic acid diehylamide (LSD-25). *Arch. Gen. Psychiat. 6:* 352–368 (1962).
Linton, H. B.: Placebo reactions in a study of lysergic acid diethylamide (LSD-25). *Arch. Gen. Psychiat. 6:* 369–383 (1962).
Linton, H. B.: Empirical dimensions of LSD-25 reaction. *Arch. Gen. Psychiat. 10:* 496–485 (1964).
McGlothlin, W. H., Cohen, S. and McGlothlin, M. S.: Long lasting effects of LSD on normals. *Arch. Gen. Psychiat. 17:* 521–532 (1967).
Rockland, L. H. and Pollin, W.: Quantification of psychiatric mental status. *Arch. Gen. Pyschiat. 12:* 23–28 (1965).
Speeter, M. E. and Anthony, W. C.: The action of oxalylchloride on indoles: a new approach to tryptamines. *J. Amer. Chem. Soc. 76:* 6208–6210 (1954).
Szara, S.: Dimethyltryptamine: Its metabolism in man; the relation of its psychotic effect to the serotonin metabolism. *Experientia, 12:* 441–442 (1956).
Szara, S.: The comparison of the psychotic effect of tryptamine derivatives with the effects of mescaline and LSD-25 in self-experiments. In: *Psychotropic Drugs,* edited by S. Garattini and V. Ghetti, pp. 460–467. Elsevier, Amsterdam (1957).
Szara, S., Rockland, L. H., Rosenthal, D. and Handlon, J. H.: Psychological effects and metabolism of N,N-diethyltryptamine in man. *Arch. Gen. Psychiat. 15:* 320–329 (1966).
Szara, S., Faillace, L. A. and Speck, L. B.: Metabolic and physiological correlates of the psychological reaction to three short-acting tryptamine derivatives. In: *Neuropsychopharmacology,* edited by H. Brill, p. 1115. Excerpta Medica Foundation, Amsterdam (1967).
Weil, A. T., Zinberg, N. E. and Nelsen. J. M.: Clinical and psychological effects of marihuana in man. *Science, 162:* 1234–1242 (1968).

DISCUSSION

DR. WEST: This interesting paper is now open for discussion.

DR. SHULGIN: I believe some years ago in a book by Garattini mention was made of the N,N-dibutyltryptamine. Do you know of any subsequent work that has been done?

DR. SZARA: I have tried it. It's psychopharmacologically inactive, at least in doses of one mg/kg, although the other three compounds which were discussed here were active.

There are several more compounds which belong to this tryptamine series which have been synthesized and tested in animals, and they probably are active in humans. One of these is the pyrrolidine derivative of tryptamine, which is probably active; I had a personal communication from Dr. Smythies in San Juan before Christmas who said that this is an extremely active compound. He must have tested it in humans. We have only animal data on it.

Another compound has an oxygen in the ring and it may be called morpholinotryptamine. This compound in animals shows some activity, but we don't have any human data on it.

DR. SHULGIN: Did you mean the 5-membered pyrrolidine or the 6-membered piperidine?

DR. SZARA: 5-Membered pyrrolidine. A series of them was synthesized by Nogradi, by the way.

DR. FREEDMAN: What effects have they in animals?

DR. SZARA: They cause hyperactivity in mice.

DR. FREEDMAN: I think Dr Smythies studied it only in rats. He has a very nice test.

DR. USDIN: Do you have any intention of trying to go on and get a third and fourth experience with people who had used DET, to find out if there has been any enzyme induction?

DR. SZARA: If it is long-lasting, you mean? Some of these people are still around in the hospital and could be tested.

By the way, these subjects were alcoholics for years, and they were really skid row alcoholics; we had followed them for two years. In one year, we had four or five who showed improvement in terms of drinking behavior or getting a job and finding their way outside the hospital. But after a two-year follow up we had only three of these subjects who actually improved. So, we still have some of them in the hospital, and we could actually study them.

DR. USDIN: You suggest that the differences in the amount of 3-indoleacetic acid formed from DET may depend on enzyme induction. Are these differences significant? I feel that it might be useful to repeat this experiment at even a later time, when the enzyme induction would be more obvious and the changes in metabolite level more pronounced.

DR. SZARA: We had only two or three occasions when we gave the same drug to the same subjects, so we didn't have much opportunity to find out what happens to these measures on repeated administration.

DR. LEHRER: In how many patients was there a decrease in excretion of, say, indoleacetic acid when the average showed an increase?

DR. SZARA: I would have to go back to the data. I think two of them showed reduced amounts, and all the ten others showed increases.

DR. HOLMSTEDT: I have a comment and also a couple of questions.

The isolation of bufotenine and dimethyltryptamine by Fish, Johnson, Horning and Stromberg from the seeds of *Piptadenia peregrina* was made, I think, 15 years ago. They had a sample of seeds grown in Puerto Rico, and it so happens that the amounts of these well known tryptamines vary with location, soil, and season. This sample, which is still available (I have analyzed it myself since), happened to contain bufotenine and dimethyltryptamine, whereas other samples of *Piptadenia* that I have analyzed so far contain as the main component 5-methoxy-N,N-dimethyltryptamine and small amounts of dimethyltryptamine.

Now, my questions are the following: Some years ago you attached particular importance to 6-hydroxylation, and you were of the opinion that the 6-hydroxylated product was essential for the psychotomimetic effect. Do you still have this opinion?

DR. SZARA: Well, I'm not attaching as much significance to this. Let's put it this way. I maintain that 6-hydroxylation may still be rather relevant, a view based mainly on the clinical finding that there is a compound, 6-fluorodiethyltryptamine, which cannot be hydroxylated and does not produce hallucinations.

DR. HOLMSTEDT: Neither does 6-hydroxydimethyltryptamine.

DR. SZARA: No, it doesn't. It may be involved in a way which is unexplained. It might be in intermediate for a carboline derivative. So, it is really still an open question.

DR. HOLMSTEDT: Did the 6-hydroxylation have any bearing on the data that you presented in Table 4?

DR. SZARA: No. At least in these particular subjects, the rate of 6-hydroxylation did not change significantly. The rate went up a little on the second exposure to DET, but it was not significant (Table 4).

DR. HOLMSTEDT: The third question is, how do you determine these metabolites?

DR. SZARA: For the indoleacetic acids we used the Weissbach method (H. Weissbach *et al.*, *J. Biol. Chem.*, 234: 81–86, 1959). It's a colorimetric method.

DR. HOLMSTEDT: Then you have to separate them by some kind of extraction or chromatography?

DR. SZARA: Correct. The extraction precedes the colorimetric determination.

DR. HOLMSTEDT: That is, the colorimetric method may not give you the right answer unless you are very sure about your separation.

DR. SZARA: Certainly, we have to find the best solvent system and pH to extract these compounds in their proper solvents.

PSYCHOSIS INDUCED BY THE ADMINISTRATION OF d-AMPHETAMINE TO HUMAN VOLUNTEERS

John D. Griffith, M.D., John H. Cavanaugh, M.D., Ph.D. and
John A. Oates, M.D.

*Departments of Psychiatry and Pharmacology
Vanderbilt University School of Medicine, Nashville, Tennessee 37203*

INTRODUCTION

At this conference there has been a discussion of the LSD psychosis, a discussion of the schizophrenic psychosis and some debate as to whether there is much or little in common between the two. We shall not pretend to resolve this debate except to point out that it is the consensus of most investigators that the psychosis produced by such hallucinogens as LSD and mescaline can be rather easily differentiated from schizophrenic reactions (Jacobsen, 1963; Hollister, 1968; MacDonald and Galvin, 1956).

On the other hand, there are numerous published case reports which suggest that patients who are treated with drugs such as ACTH, corticosteroids, disulfiram or amphetamines may sustain a psychosis that can be indistinguishable from acute parnoid schizophrenic reactions. Indeed, the psychosis caused by these drugs can be so deceptive that it is not unusual for these patients to be confined in mental institutions and treated as schizophrenics until a history of drug use is obtained. Clinical comparisons of this group of drug-induced psychoses and schizophrenia also emphasize a similarity. Independent studies (Connell, 1958; Bell, 1965; Weiner, 1964) of amphetamine-induced psychoses led these authors to conclude that it is difficult to differentiate between a schizophrenic patient with a history of amphetamine use and an amphetamine user hospitalized for a psychosis. Angst (1956) has reviewed the literature pertaining to disulfiram psychosis and makes it clear that these cases can be symptomatically indistinguishable from schizophrenia. Finally, Adams (1966) has remarked on the similarity between endocrine and functional psychoses. This mass of clinical data has caused a number of investigators including Kety (1960; 1967), Rome (1950) and Adams (1966) to suggest that studies of these psychoses, observed so frequently in clinical medicine, might well throw light on possible biochemical abnormalities present in schizophrenia. Curiously, however, a controlled evaluation of the psychotomimetic effects of these agents has not been made.

One reason for this neglect is that many authors have felt that the psychoses induced by amphetamines, disulfiram or corticosteroids are examples of rare, adverse drug reactions which occur—quite possibly—only in borderline psychotics. Others dismiss these drug-induced psychoses as a result of such drug side effects as sleep deprivation and avitaminosis, or as mere examples of an acute brain syndrome which is no more remarkable than delirium tremens. However, when one of us (Griffith, 1966) was persuaded by the then Governor of Oklahoma, Henry Bellmon, to conduct a field study on illicit amphetamine drug traffic, it was learned that if addicts took large doses of d-amphetamine or desoxyephedrine long enough, they would almost certainly experience a psychosis. Also, the predrug personality of these amphetamine addicts did not seem to fit clinical descriptions of borderline psychotics. For these reasons it appeared to us that amphetamine might be a more predicable psychotomimetic substance than isolated clinical case reports might indicate. A controlled study of this drug was undertaken to determine the importance of such factors as sleep deprivation, barbiturate use or prepsychotic personality.

METHODS

Rare examples of amphetamine hypersensitivity have been reported in the medical literature (Zalis and Parmley, 1962). For this reason, drug-naive subjects were not used in this initial study. Instead, subjects were accepted as volunteers who had previously self-administered large doses of d-amphetamine without serious consequences and who denied a history of amphetamine psychosis or symptoms of schizophrenia. Four adult males, ages 25–33, met these criteria; for ethical reasons, they were informed as to the possible hazards of the study and were unpaid. An independent psychiatrist considered the subjects to be of normal intelligence, exhibiting no organic brain disease, and showing no psychiatric disorder greater than a personality trait disturbance. One subject was an alcoholic. All were considered capable of rendering informed consent.

Each subject was hospitalized on a psychiatric ward for not less than six weeks to insure a drug-free interval. Each was carefully examined by an internist to rule out any health problem, especially impairment in cardiac, renal, hepatic or thyroid function. One week before drug administration each patient was assigned to a private room on a research ward and was allowed some freedom of movement and casual entertainment such as television, books, radio, telephone and occupational therapy. A liquid placebo was administered and control observations carried out during this phase.

At the beginning of the drug period, each subject was given 10 mg of d-amphetamine intravenously to determine the effect of acute administration. After this initial dose, 5 to 10 mg of d-amphetamine sulfate solution was administered each hour, if tolerated. Tolerance to amphetamine was determined by changes in supine blood pressure, pulse rate, oral temperature and ECG which were monitored at hourly intervals. Subjects were given a 100 mEq sodium diet per day, and were required to consume minimum amounts of food and fluids. A psychiatrist stayed at the subject's bedside continuously.

The effect of amphetamine on each subject's mental status was determined by a number of methods: (1) narratives written by psychiatrists who maintained the patient under continuous observation; (2) audio tape recordings of mental status interviews which were later rated by a psychiatrist who was not aware of the sequence of the interviews or the drug dosage; (3) evaluation by one psychiatrist who saw the patient at least four times a day and knew the drug dosage; (4) a symptom check list of questions designed to rate changes in affect and paranoid thinking; (5) retrospective descriptions of the psychosis by the subject; (6) clinical psychological tests (Holtzman Inkblot Technique, Ravens Progressive Matrices, House-Tree-Person Drawings, and Tien Organic Integrity Test) given during the control period and immediately after the psychosis (patients, while paranoid, would not permit administration of the tests); (7) perceptual tests (size estimation, two-flash fusion, word association and Muller-Lyer Illusion) which were obtained each day during the control period, during drug administration and two days following drug administration.

Concomitant with this evaluation of the psychotomimetic effects of amphetamine, the effects of this drug on the pressor responses to tyramine and norepinephrine were evaluated, as was the conversion of ^{3}H-amphetamine to amphetamine metabolites. The details of the results of these studies will be reported in a separate communication.

RESULTS

Subjects tolerated the administration of amphetamine for one to five days before experiencing a psychosis (see Table I).

TABLE I

Tolerance of oral doses of d-amphetamine as shown by temperature, blood pressure, ECG change, and occurrence of psychosis

Subject no.	Total dose in mg. of d-amphetamine prescribed 8 A.M.–8 A.M.					Maximum supine blood pressure	Maximum oral temp. °C	ECG abnormalities
	Day 1	Day 2	Day 3	Day 4	Day 5			
1	95	125	120	135	170[a]	150/100	37.9	OCC PVC's × 6 hrs.
2	60	155	165	130	190[a]	164/110	38.1	rare PVC's
3	130	120[a]	—	—	—	160/100	37.9	none
4	100	20[a]	—	—	—	140/94	37.9	none

[a] Psychosis occurred.

Because the symptoms manifested by subject no. 3 were not at first very clear-cut (ideas of reference, followed by quick denials), administration of amphetamine was continued for an additional nine hours. This subject then became very psychotic and exhibited residual symptoms for three days. The other subjects were psychotic only one to five hours.

The sequence of symptoms preceding the psychosis and the type of psychosis elicited was remarkably similar in all subjects.

Initially, subjects seemed mildly euphoric, although they minimized this on direct questioning and in their symptom check lists. This euphoria was accompanied by a hypersensitivity to the pressor effects of tyramine. Once the cumulative dose exceeded 50 mg, however, they then became depressed in that they talked less, spent more time in bed, were irritable, showed less interest in television and people, complained because they were required to eat and drink, and were extremely hypochondriacal. During this phase, however, the subjects were quite lucid, showed considerable modulation of affect, and related to the attending psychiatrist in a clinging, dependent manner.

Several hours before the onset of a florid psychosis, the subjects would become quite taciturn, withdrawn, and would defend against attempts to find out what they were thinking. From time to time they would ask questions about people or objects in the room, but then refuse to give reasons for their questions. During this prepsychotic phase they would appear to relax for a few minutes, be less defensive, but still refuse to answer questions. Patients told us later that they were experiencing paranoid ideas that could be dismissed with some effort as unreal.

The onset of a florid psychosis was usually quite abrupt. Previously taciturn subjects would begin to discuss frankly paranoid ideas openly and with conviction. Two withdrew to their rooms and objected to being under constant observation. All felt that they were in real and immediate danger. The mildest and most transitory episode was experienced by the first subject, who imagined that his ex-wife had hired an assassin who was on his way to the room. Except for this delusion, he was in good contact with his surroundings. After one hour he became more comfortable and began to discuss his paranoid ideas as having been a product of his imagination.

Another patient, while watching television, turned off the set and the light in the room and sat up in bed. He then explained that "everyone knows that electricity travels slower in the dark than in the light" . . . that a "giant oscillator" in the ceiling was sending rays which controlled his thoughts and caused his skin to tingle. He also claimed to be able to tell who was being controlled by the "giant oscillator." When asked why he thought these ideas, he replied, "I know this is part of the experiment and I am willing to go through with it, but I should have been told . . ."

Ideas of reference were quite common. The patient just described felt that he was being discussed on television even though his description of the program content was not distorted. Another patient felt he was being photographed from behind a mirror. When encouraged to examine it himself—and seeing that there was no camera there—he said "it must be in the ceiling then." Subjects also expressed their distrust by an unwillingness to complete or a need to normalize their symptom check lists.

True visual hallucinations were not seen; that is, patients did not see "things that were not there." However, they were very prone to attach personal significance to familiar objects. For example, one subject saw an exit sign which he felt had been placed there as a message for him to leave the hospital. Neither were auditory hallucinations prominent, although patients would wonder if poorly heard conversations might be about them. One subject reported olfactory hallucinations and another complained of intensification of odors. No evidence of thought disorder was observed. The psychotic phase was accompanied by a hyposensitivity to the pressor effect of intravenous tyramine.

Psychological tests employed clinically to identify psychotic reactions (Holtzman, H-T-P) and to identify brain damage (Bender-Gestalt, Ravens

Matrices, Tien OIT) were essentially unchanged from control observations. It should be pointed out, however, that subjects would not permit testing while paranoid. Perceptual tests, for all practical purposes, furnished little statistically significant data in this small series of subjects.

DISCUSSION

This study indicates that the administration of large doses of d-amphetamine can precipitate a paranoid psychosis in non-psychotic individuals without causing appreciable alterations in sensorium or orientation. Neither do factors such as sleep deprivation, health, nutrition, barbiturate use, or acute brain damage appear essential in the evolution of this symptomatology. Whether only patients with a personality disorder will respond with a psychosis when given amphetamines is a question this study cannot answer. However, accidental poisonings and similar case histories suggest that a personality defect is not an essential factor.

At least one author has suggested that the amphetamine psychosis might be a drug withdrawal phenomena (Young et al., 1961). At first glance it might appear that this study rules out drug withdrawal also; however, only the first two patients were given d-amphetamine "around the clock," and then only for the first three days. It is interesting that all subjects sustained a psychosis following short periods of drug withdrawal and while their vital signs were returning to normal.

The amphetamine psychosis seen in this study resembles paranoid schizophrenia in that subjects exhibited paranoid ideation, ideas of reference, personality alteration and affect change without appreciable intellectual disorganization or alteration of consciousness. It should be noted, however, that none of the subjects exhibited a thought disorder, a symptom fairly unique to schizophrenia. Neither were true auditory or visual hallucinations reported. In paranoid schizophrenia, however, thought disturbance and true hallucinations are relatively uncommon as compared with other types of schizophrenic reactions.

Although the amphetamine psychosis might be viewed as a state of hyperstimulation caused by the drug, this explanation is unlikely as the sole mechanism, since it was observed that the subjects were depressed. We suggest, as an alternative hypothesis, that the CNS symptoms caused by large-dose administration might be the result of central norepinephrine depletion. This depletion might occur either by direct release of norepinephrine or by substitution of norepinephrine by amphetamine or an amphetamine metabolite.

This hypothesis is consistent, at least, with effects noted in the peripheral nervous system.

SUMMARY

The medical literature leaves little doubt that several common drugs such as the corticosteroids, disulfiram and amphetamine may induce a psychosis that can resemble a functional psychosis such as schizophrenia. For this reason, d-amphetamine was tested as a psychotomimetic in four human volunteers. All subjects sustained a paranoid psychosis after receiving large doses of d-amphetamine for one to five days. None of the subjects exhibited alteration of consciousness, disorientation or a blatant thought disorder, nor were true visual hallucinations seen.

A surprising finding was that subjects on large doses of d-amphetamine appeared depressed. This is in sharp contrast to the elation and hyperactivity demonstrated by subjects receiving small doses of d-amphetamine acutely.

The authors speculate that the psychosis may be the result of a depletion of central norepinephrine stores by either amphetamine or one of its metabolites.

REFERENCES

Adams, R. D., and Hope, J.: Schizophrenia, paranoia, puerperal and endocrine psychoses. In: *Principles of Internal Medicine,* 5th ed., edited by T. R. Harrison et al. McGraw-Hill, New York (1966).
Bell, D. S.: Comparison of amphetamine psychosis and schizophrenia. *Brit. J. Psychiat.* 111: 701–707 (1965).
Connell, P. H.: *Amphetamine Psychosis.* Maudsley Monograph No. 5. Maudsley, London (1958).
Griffith, J. D.: A study of illicit amphetamine drug traffic in Oklahoma City. *Amer. J. Psychiat.* 123: 560–569 (1966).
Hollister, L. E.: *Chemical Psychoses.* Charles C Thomas, Springfield, Illinois (1968).
Jacobsen, E.: The clinical pharmacology of the hallucinogens. *Clin. Pharmacol. Therap.* 4: 480–503 (1963).
Kety, S. S.: Recent biochemical theories of schizophrenia. In: *The Etiology of Schizophrenia,* edited by D. D. Jackson, pp. 120–145. Basic Books, New York (1960).
Kety, S. S.: The hypothetical relationships between amines and mental illness; a critical synthesis. In: *Amines and Schizophrenia,* edited by H. E. Himwich, S. S. Kety and J. R. Smythies, pp. 271–277. Pergamon Press, New York (1967).
Kety, S. S.: The hypothetical relationships between amines and mental illness; a critical synthesis. In: *Amines and Schizophrenia,* edited by H. E. Himwich, S. S. Kety, and J. R. Smythies, Jr., pp. 271–277. Pergamon Press, New York (1967).
Macdonald, J. M., and Galvin, J. A.: Experimental psychotic states. *Amer. J. Psychiat.* 112 (2): 970–976 (1956).
Rome, H. P., and Braceland, F. J.: Use of cortisone and ACTH in certain diseases: psychiatric aspects. *Mayo Clin. Proc.* 25: 495–497 (1950).

Weiner, I. B.: Differential diagnosis in amphetamine poisoning. *Psychiatric Quart.* 38: 707–716 (1964).

Young, G. Y., Simson, C. B., and Frohman, C. E.: Clinical and biochemical studies of an amphetamine withdrawal psychosis. *J. Nerv. Mental Dis.* 132: 234–238 (1961).

Zalis, E. G. and Parmley, L. F., Jr.: Fatal amphetamine poisoning. *Arch. Int. Med.* 112: 60–64 (1963).

DISCUSSION

DR. SULSER: In species where amphetamine is converted to *p*-hydroxyamphetamine and *p*-hydroxynorephedrine, the decreased blood pressure responses to the indirectly acting tyramine after chronic amphetamine administration could be explained by release of the "false" transmitter *p*-hydroxynorephedrine. *p*-Hydroxynorephedrine has been shown to accumulate in the cat after amphetamine administration and to fulfill the criteria of a "false" transmitter. I wonder whether these amphetamine metabolites have been identified in man?

DR. GRIFFITH: Yes, two metabolites, *p*-hydroxyamphetamine and *p*-hydroxynorephedrine were identified by J. Cavanaugh and J. Oates in the urine of these patients.

A VOICE: What were the observations on the sleep of the subjects, and if you had any, what changes, if any, occurred when the latter two subjects became psychotic?

DR. GRIFFITH: The subjects were not sleep deprived during the control periods, as demonstrated by their sleep EEG's. Two subjects had a psychosis after being sleep deprived for only one night. That is, they did not go to sleep that night and had a psychosis the next day. The other two subjects, after going without sleep for one day, would then sleep in short bursts of three hours or so and would average about eight hours of sleep every 24 hours. We would like to have had EEG's during the psychotic phase but the patients would pull the electrodes off when they became psychotic.

DR. OSMOND: Connell had some excellent reports on people who popped amphetamine inhalers into coffee and took, I believe, about 180 mg of these substances that way. Do you recall this?

DR. GRIFFITH: Yes, I observed patients who would take 150 mg at one sitting from an inhaler. That product is now off the market.

DR. KOPIN: I was intrigued by the difference in the dosage that was required to elicit the psychosis. In one case it was about 100 to 200 mg, and in the other was 500 to 800 mg. I was wondering if there is any difference in the urinary pH of these patients. The rate of amphetamine excretion and detoxification is related to urinary pH. It would be interesting if there was a good correlation between the total dose you had to give and the urinary pH.

DR. GRIFFITH: We were interested in 24-hour urines and dumped them into hydrochloric acid. We did not measure the pH of individual urines except as spot checks.

The other reason we didn't do it is that we were administering the drug up to tolerance levels, so if the patient could take more, he would get more.

DR. HOLMSTEDT: Then, Dr. Mandell added to the reputation Sweden already has with regard to movies and politics. We also have recently had an epidemic of amphetamine abuse, and this led the Swedish representative at the World Health Organization to suggest that amphetamine be banned or put under the same restrictions as the opiates.

With regard to dosage, I am informed by the people who study this in Sweden that they have observed cases of injections of up to 1000 mg i.v.

DR. GRIFFITH: Sweden's reputation for intravenous amphetamine abuse is not isolated. It has also been reported in epidemic proportions in the U.S. (Kramer, J. C., *J.A.M.A. 201:* 89, 1967), and in the U.K. (Hawkes, D., *et al.*, Addiction Research Center, Maudsley Hospital, London, in press).

DR. MANDELL: Your experiment, I think, may shake one of the statements formalized in Connell's monograph on amphetamine psychosis in which he proposed that a predisposing character disorder in a male is necessary to produce an amphetamine paranoid psychosis. So, the first question is: do you feel that your data contradict Connell's conclusion? Second and partially related to Dr. Kopin's question, since amphetamines are anorexigenic agents and starvation leads to an acid urine, does this bias your amphetamine excretion data?

DR. GRIFFITH: Individuals with weak egos may be more susceptible to the psychotomimetic effects of amphetamines than others; however, I believe (more on the basis of accidental poisonings than my study) that a fragile personality is not essential to the psychosis. Personality theories of amphetamine psychosis do not explain, either, why these cases are almost always paranoid. Lastly, both Ellingwood and I have noted that schizophrenics are not as susceptible to the psychotomimetic effects of amphetamines as others. We occasionally checked urine pH and these ranged between 5 and 7. The subjects were required to eat, so that I doubt that much ketosis occurred. However, variation in amphetamine excretion could have played a part in subject sensitivity to the drug. On the other hand, it should be understood that by giving amphetamine in small, frequent increments the drug most surely will accumulate. Measures of blood amphetamine levels bear this out.

DR. WASER: In the general opinion of psychiatrists today, is amphetamine psychosis or LSD psychosis more similar to schizophrenia? This is very important for projected biochemical studies in man.

DR. GRIFFITH: Most psychiatrists consider LSD psychosis to be rather easily differentiated from schizophrenic reactions. On the other hand, it can be a very difficult matter to differentiate between schizophrenics and those with an amphetamine psychosis. Connell was the first to point this out and to suggest that amphetamine psychosis might be an appropriate study model for schizophrenic psychosis.

DR. DEMENT: A problem I cannot resolve in my mind is why do drug abusers continue to use drugs when it is no longer reinforcing; when it no longer causes significant euphoria. Indeed, we have interviewed two individuals in the Haight-Ashbury district of San Francisco who used intravenous methamphetamine, and if they could not get a drug they would inject blood, tap water, a fantastic list of things. The idea is that even though the effect lasted only a second or two, they would get a flash, and that in itself apparently was sufficiently reinforcing.

DR. GRIFFITH: You raise an interesting question that no one has answered satisfactorily. Our subjects reported that the use of amphetamine under clinical conditions was unpleasant. Perhaps there are rewards for drug use that we have not yet identified.

DR. GESSNER: Reinforcing Dr. Waser's point, I understand that psychiatrists have difficulty in diagnosing intoxication due to bromides from pathology derived from endogenous processes. Has anyone worked on this?

DR. FREEDMAN: I think they do directly distinguish them now. It's often by physical and clinical clues. I have done it, and residents have done it.

DR. GESSNER: Without analyzing for bromide levels?

DR. FREEDMAN: You pick them up, whether it's history, clues, the skin, etc.; something catches your attention. Very few people ever pay attention to this idiotic diagnostic process that we go through in the clinic, but while we often do miss organics, we often pick them up. For example, if you ask a man, "Well, how did you spot that?" It's often something in the gestalt that's missing that tips you off. So, I wouldn't say it's that much of a masquerader.

DR. GRIFFITH: I wonder if I might ask a question. An English investigator reported that five manic patients received amphetamine and dropped their mania. We tried it in one patient in which he gave up his manic symptomatology. Is there any other experience on this subject?

DR. DOMINO: I don't have any. However, I have two questions. The first is, did you notice any repetitive stereotyped behavior in your amphetamine-induced psychoses?

DR. GRIFFITH: No.

DR. DOMINO: The second one is, is there such a phenomenon as amphetamine withdrawal psychosis?

DR. GRIFFITH: Patients who are undergoing withdrawal from large doses of amphetamine are characteristically depressed, irritable, and drowsy. However, one generally does not think of them as psychotic. Amphetamine withdrawal psychosis has been reported, but there is the problem of differentiating such a psychosis from either an underlying schizophrenic process or a concomitant barbiturate or alcohol withdrawal syndrome.

DR. FREEDMAN: I think there's one comment worth noting, that in the second phase of LSD after the acute TV show in the head is over, you can get a lot of these symptoms that sound to me very much like the presymptoms of the amphetamine psychosis: isolation, ideas of reference, the feeling that one is in the center of things.

And if one wanted to study LSD from a new standpoint, then look at this second phase of the LSD reaction, and you'd have a different order of behavioral phenomenon and maybe different biochemical changes.

DR. STEIN: I was wondering, is the amphetamine psychosis treatable with chlorpromazine?

DR. GRIFFITH: Yes. These patients are quite sensitive to chlorpromazine and chlorpromazine is almost a specific treatment for the illness. In fact, if a patient begins discussing his symptoms as unreal a few hours after a single dose of chlorpromazine, then one has presumptive evidence that he is dealing with an amphetamine psychosis.

DR. KOPIN: What do you mean when you said that these patients were more sensitive to chlorpromazine?

DR. GRIFFITH: Well, they become drowsy on 5 or 10 mg.

DR. LUDWIG: How about the effects of barbiturates? I have treated a couple of patients who have been amphetamine addicts, and they almost always treat themselves with barbiturates. I would suspect that barbiturates, if anything, are perhaps more specific for amphetamine psychosis than chlorpromazine. At least the patients themselves have arrived at this way of handling the drug effects from amphetamine. What are your thoughts?

DR. GRIFFITH: Amphetamine addicts prefer to use barbiturates with amphetamines, during both the acute and chronic phases of drug use. I have observed amphetamine addicts in the field who have had access to both drugs and observed that barbiturates do not terminate the psychosis. The patients may sleep for a while, but when they awake, they are psychotic again.

DR. KORNETSKY: How similar is this psychosis to the withdrawal psychosis of barbiturates? One of the effects of abrupt withdrawal of barbiturates is a physiological rebound. Functions that are depressed are enhanced, and vice versa.

DR. GRIFFITH: Paranoid symptoms are seen in barbiturate withdrawal psychosis. However, these are poorly systematized and are easily changed by suggestion. This is not usually true for schizophrenia.

DR. KORNETSKY: This paranoid feature is seen with abrupt withdrawal of barbiturates.

DR. GRIFFITH: Even there it is very short-lived. In other words, first they are afraid of some imaginary thing they see. Then they are afraid of the doctor, then the nurse, but they switch almost while you are talking with them.

DR. LEVINE: Dr. Griffith, I was very impressed that four out of four patients developed this psychosis. I was wondering, had they had amphetamine psychosis before? Was this a criterion for including them, or were they just amphetamine users before? Were there any patients that you did try and in whom you could not induce a psychosis?

DR. GRIFFITH: The four patients reported here gave a history of amphetamine use, but denied a history of psychosis or amphetamine psychosis. We studied two more patients. Both of these had given a history of amphetamine psychosis prior to the study. One became psychotic on 60 mg of amphetamine. The other patient received up to 100 mg of amphetamine a day, but did not exhibit psychotic behavior. It is quite possible that if we had increased this patient's dose as we did with the first four he too might have experienced a psychosis.

DR. LEVINE: One patient out of six, then, did not develop a psychosis, even though you went to the limit?

DR. GRIFFITH: No, we didn't go to the limit on the one who did not develop the psychosis. We backed off from it. We were just trying to get metabolic data.

DR. AGHAJANIAN: You mentioned that chlorpromazine was very effective in treating amphetamine psychosis. What dose did you use?

DR. GRIFFITH: I usually give a test dose of 10 mg of chlorpromazine to determine if the patient is not unduly reactive to the drug. If the patient does not become unduly sedated on this dose, I will keep doubling every 6 hour dose until the patient is finally receiving 26 mg a day.

DR. AGHAJANIAN: I find that very interesting. We have been looking at some cells in the midbrain reticular area that are activated by amphetamine, and we see an extraordinary response to chlorpromazine. After very small doses of chlorpromazine (0.5 mg/kg), these cells drop down to their original rates almost immediately, *i.e.,* within two or three minutes.

DR. FREEDMAN: It makes you wonder again about that small dose of chlorpromazine (30 mg/kg) that blocks LSD in the rat behavior tests.

DR. AGHAJANIAN: It doesn't block LSD, by the way.

DR. FREEDMAN: You haven't tried it in all the neural systems yet. You never know.

EFFECTS OF MARIHUANA SMOKING ON SENSORY THRESHOLDS IN MAN

Donald F. Caldwell, Ph.D., Steven A. Myers, M.D. and
Edward F. Domino, M.D.[1]

Lafayette Clinic, Detroit, Michigan 48207

INTRODUCTION

I should begin by explaining my peculiar position. I am a neuropsychopharmacologist interested in the role of neurotransmitters in mental health and disease, talking at a clinical session about marihuana and using the techniques of an experimental psychologist. The research I would like to present has been the consequence of several different interests among three investigators. First, there are increasing community pressures concerned with the psychiatric and social problems of marihuana use, particularly with the home grown and Mexican varieties. Second, the paucity of current behavioral research on marihuana "effects" led Dr. Myers (psychiatry), in collaboration with Dr. Caldwell (psychology) and myself (pharmacology) to submit a protocol for the study of the psychological and pharmacological effects of marihuana smoking in man. Third, Dr. Efron of the Psychopharmacology Research Branch of the National Institute of Mental Health suggested that I initiate some studies with marihuana and its derivatives as part of the collaborative Neuropsychopharmacology Research Program at the University of Michigan and the Lafayette Clinic. Dr. Efron was probably unaware that he "struck a sensitive chord" because of our previous collaborative research on marihuana derivatives with Drs. Seevers and Hardman at the University of Michigan. We hope to publish the results of this research soon. Much of the psychological data on the effects of marihuana smoking in sophisticated users

---

[1] Presented by E. F. Domino.

to be described herein will appear in a more extensive publication in the future. I would like to discuss at this time some of our findings to date.

It is well known, as we heard from Dr. Holmstedt quoting the descriptions of hashish intoxication by Beaudelaire and others, and from the personal experiences of Dr. Sim, that marihuana, hashish or its extracts seem to enhance subjectively auditory and visual perception.

However, Morrow (1944) was unable to demonstrate any significant alteration in auditory acuity or musical aptitude, as measured by the Galton Whistle and the Kwalwasser-Dykema Tests, respectively, in subjects who were under the influence of various natural and synthetic marihuana preparations. Similarly, Williams et al. (1946) observed no marked alterations in musical talent, as measured by the Seashore Test, in subjects smoking crude marihuana. Three of twelve subjects, however, were felt to demonstrate a definite enhancement of auditory acuity while in a state of marihuana intoxication. Recently Weil et al. (1968) reported their findings on the physiological and psychological effects of marihuana. Our study should be considered complementary to theirs.

The tetrahydrocannabinols (THC) have long been considered responsible for the pharmacological effects of marihuana. Adams and Baker (1940) synthesized a THC which possessed marihuana activity. Lowe (1944) has written an extensive review of investigations reporting the cannabinols as the active principles in hemp. In the search to identify the exact structure of the active compound, both l-Δ^9-trans-THC (Gaoni and Mechoulam, 1964) and l-Δ^8-trans-THC (Hively et al., 1966) were found to occur in hashish. The marihuana activity of Δ^9-THC has recently been demonstrated in man (Isbell et al., 1967). This is believed to be the first demonstration of such activity of a THC of known chemical structure. The possibility of a conversion by heat of Δ^9-THC to a Δ^8 isomer (Taylor et al., 1966) has been disputed (Claussen and Korte, 1967). Amaral Vieira et al. (1967) obtained pharmacologically active extracts from dried hashish heated to 600° C.

In an attempt to gain a better understanding of the effects of marihuana on auditory and visual systems, we believed that a logical first step would be to determine whether intoxication with the drug measurably alters these primary sensory functions. A demonstration of facilitation or inhibition (as measured by threshold changes) for either of these sensory systems would call for a thorough investigation of the specific factors involved. A failure to demonstrate significant alterations may imply a need to investigate the influence of other psychological, sociological or physiological factors which may be operative in the perceptual phenomena reported by marihuana users.

METHODS

Male subjects were selected from among university students who responded to a request for volunteers to participate in a study involving the use of marihuana. They were asked to donate their time free without any compensation whatsoever. We were literally deluged by many volunteer users of marihuana who were anxious to show scientists there was something to the "pot story."

Final selection of these subjects was made following interviews with a psychiatrist. Subjects were in good physical condition who were experienced users of marihuana, but not of other drugs. Informed consent was obtained following the procedures outlined by the Lafayette Clinic Committee on the Conduction of Human Research. The control and experimental groups consisted of ten subjects each who reported previous pleasurable experiences with marihuana.

Measurements of auditory and visual sensory thresholds were obtained in both the pre-drug and post-drug states. The control subjects did not smoke marihuana, but alfalfa. Some of our experienced pot smokers were surprised that the alfalfa was similar to marihuana in taste and smell. In our experience naive subjects may have great difficulty telling active marihuana from alfalfa.

The following experimental design was utilized:

Control group	*Experimental group*
Pre-test C_1 (alfalfa)	E_1 (alfalfa)
Post-test C_2 (alfalfa)	E_2 (marihuana *ad libitum,* to subjective "high")

A comparison of the mean changes in sensory thresholds between C_1 and C_2 was a measure of practice effect during testing. A comparison of the mean change in E_1 *vs* E_2 and C_2 *vs* E_2 was a measure of the effects of marihuana.

Data were analyzed by parametric statistics when appropriate. Where data distributions were not normal, appropriate non-parametric statistics for related samples were to be used (*i.e.,* McNemar Test, Wilcoxon Matched-Pairs Signed-Ranks Test).

All test measurements were accomplished with the subject in a sitting position in a totally dark, sound proof, air conditioned room. Any subject vocalizations were monitored by the experimenter in adjacent quarters through an intercom system. Each subject began testing at either 6 P.M. or 9 P.M.

and remained under observation at the hospital overnight. Control subjects were instructed to smoke one alfalfa cigarette by deep inhalation within a period of 10 to 15 minutes. After resting for 15 minutes, pre-drug testing began. The control group smoked the first and second alfalfa cigarettes at approximately hourly intervals during which the sensory tests were made. The experimental drug group smoked one alfalfa cigarette followed an hour later by the marihuana on an *ad libitum* schedule until he reported feeling "high." The cigarettes contained 300 mg of crude marihuana. We obtained the crude marihuana through Dr. Scigliano and the courtesy of the N.I.M.H. *ad hoc* committee on marihuana. According to Dr. Scigliano, the material contained 1.312 percent Δ^9-THC.[1] A total percent cannabinol content was unavailable. Most of our experienced users reported the marihuana to be "good stuff." Heart rate was usually measured, and blood pressure occasionally, in order not to interfere with the psychological testing procedures. The following procedures were applied to all subjects during both the first and second cigarette test phases of the investigation:

A. Auditory threshold determination

The subject was fitted with a pair of stereo headphones which received an input from an audio oscillator in series with a step attenuator. The subject received, through one ear, a signal tone of constant duration (0.5 sec) and frequency (1000 Hz). Beginning at suprathreshold levels, the signal was attenuated in a graded serial order until the subject reported that he no longer sensed the tone. Attenuation of the signal was then gradually decreased until the subject again reported hearing the tone. The absolute tone threshold was then computed.

B. Tone amplitude differential threshold

The method of minimal change (Guilford, 1954) was used to determine the difference threshold (DL) for sound intensity. Each subject was asked to report whether the second member of a tone pair was "louder," "equal," or "quieter" when compared with the first, or standard, tone of the pair. Both the standard and comparison tones were 1000 Hz and 500 msec duration. The interval between the tones was 30 msec. All time sequences were electronically controlled. The procedure consisted of presenting the subject with a descending tone series in which the comparison tone was attenuated in 2 db serial steps from well above each subject's DL to that point where the subject reported the comparison tone as "quieter" in amplitude than the standard.

See Note added in Proof on p. 321.

Similarly, an ascending series was presented decreasing attenuation of the comparison tone in 2 db steps until the subject reported the comparison tone as "louder" than the standard. Upper (DL_u) and lower (DL_l) difference limens were obtained for each subject by the formula L_u-S and S-L_l, respectively. In addition, the mean differential thresholds (*i.e.*, $DL_u + DL_½$) and the point of subjective equality (*i.e.*, $L_u + L_½$) was computed for each subject.

C. Tone frequency differential threshold

The method of minimal change was used in determining the difference threshold for tone frequency discrimination. The procedure was the same as that outlined previously, with the exception that both standard and comparison tone were of the same amplitude and frequency. The comparison tone was changed in both ascending and descending series in 4.0 Hz steps.

D. Light intensity differential threshold

The method used to determine each subject's difference threshold for intensity discrimination of a neutral color white light differed from that for sound measurements. The subject was presented with two 2.5 cm diameter 6 V incandescent lights mounted in frost glass and horizontally separated by 43 cm. Light-to-subject distance was approximately 1.5 m. Two separate matching sequences were performed for a dim and bright light standard (2.40 foot candles and 4.80 foot candles, respectively). The comparison light was alternately varied between being brighter than or dimmer than the respective standard light. The subject's task upon each new paired presentation was to match as closely as was subjectively possible the comparison light with the standard. This was accomplished by means of a hand-held regulating toggle switch. Ten comparison values ranging in intensity from 1.12 to 4.80 foot candles and 2.80 to 7.00 foot candles were used for the dim and bright light standards, respectively.

RESULTS

Pharmacological observations

The technique for smoking marihuana differs markedly from that of smoking tobacco. In fact, with 5 naive subjects who inhaled like smoking tobacco, no subjective psychological effects were reported. The experienced marihuana smoker inhales deeply and allows cool air to pass with the smoke at the sides of his mouth. This apparently permits condensation of the tars in the alveoli. The trapped smoke is kept in the lungs and the exhaled breath is free of smoke particles. This procedure itself results in considerable alterations in heart rate.

The endpoint used for stopping smoking was when each subject achieved a marihuana "high." An observer cannot easily determine this endpoint with a casual physical examination. We would look at our subjects and they would look at us and say they were "high." They were aware of their surroundings and would converse in a normal manner. If left alone, the high would return, but leave with arousal induced by conversation, etc. This ability of afferent stimuli to alert the individual has been previously observed in our unpublished studies with Drs. Seevers and Hardman, and is a very important point for future research. Better blood pressure studies are also being planned, inasmuch as some THC analogues produce remarkable cardiovascular effects. Another interesting point is that our subjects were allowed to smoke up to two 300 mg marihuana cigarettes. In actual fact, they smoked a mean $\pm$ S.D. of 483.0 mg $\pm$ 92.9 to achieve a "high" and declined from taking more. Only one experienced some nausea and faintness sufficient to require putting his head temporarily between his legs.

Characteristically, a tachycardia is seen about the time the subject states he is "high." Some of these data are listed in Table I. It may be noted that the tachycardia occurs promptly and persists beyond 30 minutes. In some subjects a tachycardia was evident for several hours, but was greatest only immediately after becoming "high." It remains to be determined whether this tachycardia arises specifically as a result of the effect of marihuana or is a consequence of the technique of deep inhalation smoking. Since the tachycardia after smoking marihuana persists for such a long period, it is probable that this effect is related to the contents of the marihuana smoke. Reddening of the eyeballs or pupillary changes usually were not seen.

Psychological observations

It was difficult for the subjects to describe their "high." It was pleasant. Some described a floating sensation in slow motion. Many felt subjective improvement in the tests taken. The results of the group performance comparisons on the auditory and visual threshold tests were mostly statistically negative. Table II summarizes the mean tests scores for both the control and experimental groups for the first and second test periods for all measurements. Note that in the case of the auditory amplitude difference threshold test, the

TABLE I

Effects of alfalfa and marihuana smoking on mean heart rate in experienced marihuana users

Group	N	Before alfalfa	After alfalfa	Before alfalfa or marihuana	Mean HR ± S.E.			
					Minutes After			
					5	10	15	30
Control (alfalfa)	5	84.5 ± 2.0	84.3 ± 1.7	80.0 ± 1.7	73.9 ± 1.6[a]	74.0 ± 4.3[a]	73.8 ± 3.9[a]	72.6 ± 3.3[a]
Experimental (marihuana)	7	77.0 ± 1.8	75.5 ± 1.5	70.8 ± 1.4	90.1 ± 1.0[a]	87.3 ± 2.5[a]	84.3 ± 2.7[a]	80.2 ± 3.0[a]

[a] Statistically significant $P < .05$, paired comparison student t test. Note that although alfalfa smoking does not change the heart rate, over time there is a significant decrease. In contrast, marihuana smoking causes a dramatic increase in heart rate.

TABLE II

Lack of significant differences in mean performance scores for alfalfa and marihuana groups for visual and auditory discrimination measurements

Variables	First test session		Second test session	
	Control group (alfalfa)	Experimental group (alfalfa)	Control group (alfalfa)	Experimental group (marihuana)
I. Visual brightness test				
2.40 foot candle standard	2.25	2.51	2.21	2.46
4.80 foot candle standard	4.09	4.93	4.60	4.91
II. Auditory amplitude threshold test (decibels)				
difference threshold	1.46	1.71	0.94[a]	1.63[a]
point of subjective equality	14.56	14.40	14.59	14.41
constant error	−0.44	−0.66	−0.40	−0.63
III. Auditory frequency threshold test (cycles/sec)				
difference threshold	3.64	4.06	2.53	3.79
point of subjective equality	1001.67	1001.24	1000.88	1000.05
constant error	+1.67	+1.24	+0.88	+0.05
IV. Auditory threshold test (decibels)	75.11	73.83	75.87	76.74

[a] $t = 3.25$, $P < .01$. Note that the threshold was increased for the second test session for the marihuana subjects when compared to the second test controls. All other test results were not significantly different.

threshold was increased for the second test session for the marihuana subjects when compared with the second test controls. However, in all other tests the differences between the alfalfa and marihuana groups were not significant. These negative findings may be due to the fact that only small amounts of Δ^9-THC were inhaled for a subjective "high" or that the psychological tests used were insensitive. That a subjective "high" on marihuana causes minimal physiological changes attests to the small doses of active THC used in these studies.

ACKNOWLEDGMENT

This research was supported in part by the Michigan Neuropsychopharmacology Research Program, University of Michigan and Lafayette Clinic, grant MH-11846, U.S.P.H.S.

REFERENCES

Adams, R. and Baker, B. R.: Structure of cannabinol. VII. A method of synthesis of a tetrahydrocannabinol which possesses marihuana activity. *J. Amer. Chem. Soc.* 62: 2405–2408 (1940).
Amaral Vieira, F. J., Aguiar, M. B., Alencar, J. W., Seabra, A. P., Tursch, B. M. and Leclercq, J.: Effects of the organic layer of hashish smoke extract and preliminary results of its chemical analysis. *Psychopharmacologia* (Berlin) 10: 361–362 (1967).
Claussen, U., and Korte, u. F.: Über das Verhalten der Cannabes-Phenole beim Rauchen. *Tetrahedron Letters,* 2067 (1967).
Gaoni, Y. and Mechoulam, R.: Isolation, structure and partial synthesis of an active constituent of hashish. *J. Amer. Chem. Soc.* 86: 1646–1648 (1964).
Guilford, J. P.: *Psychometric methods.* New York, McGraw-Hill (1936).
Hively, R. L., Mosher, W. A., and Hoffman, F.: Isolation of trans-delta^6-tetrahydrocannabinol from marihuana. *J. Amer. Chem. Soc.* 88: 1832–1833 (1966).
Isbell, H., Gorodetzsky, C. W., Jasinski, D., Claussen, U., Spulak, F. V. and Korte, F.: Effects of delta^9-trans-tetrahydrocannabinol in man. *Psychopharmacologia* (Berlin) 11: 184–188 (1967).
Loewe, S.: Pharmacological study. In: *The Marihuana Problem in the City of New York; Mayor's Committee on Marihuana,* pp. 149–212. Jacques Cattell Press, Lancaster, Pa. (1944).
Morrow, R. S.: Psychological aspects. In: *The Marihuana Problem in the City of New York; Mayor's Committee on Marihuana,* pp. 285–290. Jaques Cattell Press, Lancaster, Pa. (1944). (Abstracted in: *The Marihuana Papers,* pp. 285–290. Bobbs-Merrill, 1966.)
Taylor, E. D., Lenard, K., and Shvo, Y.: Active constituents of hashish, synthesis of dl-delta^6-3,4-trans-tetrahydrocannabinol. *J. Amer. Chem. Soc.* 88: 367 (1966).
Weil, A. T., Zinberg, N. E., and Nelsen, J. M.: Clinical and psychological effects of marihuana in man. *Science 162:* 1234–1242 (1968).
Williams, E. G., Himmelsbach, C. K., Wikler, A., and Ruble, D. C.: Studies on marihuana and pyrahexyl compounds. *Public Health Reports 61:* 1059–1082 (1946).

DISCUSSION

DR. HOLMSTEDT: Dr. Domino, what were the changes in blood pressure after marihuana?

DR. DOMINO: Blood pressure was not routinely measured, since we were concentrating on sensory thresholds. A few that I took didn't show anything dramatic. This bothers me very much in view of what Dr. Sim said last night. I am planning to study this further. We don't have Dr. Leo Hollister in the audience. I would like to know of his recent observations.

DR. JOFFE: Dr. Hollister has told me that there was possibly a tendency towards a change in blood pressure. This is as far as he could go. I think what he meant was that there wasn't any change, and this is what Isbell reported.

DR. DOMINO: What about tachycardia?

DR. JOFFEE: Some tachycardia was seen, but not change in blood pressure.

DR. LEVINE: I think there is an orthostatic hypotension.

DR. DOMINO: We have no data on this, unfortunately. Our subjects were sitting in a chair during the entire procedure.

I was very impressed with the method of inhaling used by the subjects. I wondered about carbon monoxide intoxication or lack of oxygen as part of the picture. There is an art in the method of inhaling marihuana smoke. In fact, if you smoke like an ordinary tobacco smoker you will never get a "high." You have to smoke in such a way as to allow cold air to go along either side of the mouth to allow all of the resin to condense in the lungs. When you exhale, not a particle of smoke comes out.

DR. LEVINE: Did you notice any injection of the conjunctiva?

DR. DOMINO: We did not notice any.

DR. LEVINE: Did you look for it?

DR. DOMINO: We looked for it but not routinely. Once in a while we convinced ourselves that there was something there, but it wasn't very obvious. Dryness of the mouth was characteristic.

A very interesting observation, which I wish to follow up, was particularly dramatic in one of our subjects. The fellow had no patellar reflex whatsoever. But when he got high, he had an active patellar reflex. About three hours later when he came "down," the patellar reflex was again absent. This should be studied further because in animals one measures ataxia as an end point of tetrahydrocannabinol (THC) effects.

Again, the changes in the patellar reflex were not always apparent. With some there was no change at all. But I shall never forget this one subject.

The onset of the "high" was rapid. It usually lasted with decreasing intensity for a period of about three hours. We weren't quite sure about the total duration of the effect. Since it has been said that in some it lasts much longer than in others, we asked our subjects to stay in the hospital overnight.

As described in the formal paper, taking all of the subjects as a group, we found no objective changes in either visual or auditory threshold, or in their ability to discriminate between differences in either light or sound intensity. Yet, one of the 10 experienced users had a marked lowering of auditory threshold to the point that I felt he was guessing, and on occasion he would hear things when I really didn't turn on the switch. But in most cases he properly responded to a marked lowering of the sound. This was the exception rather than the rule. It is reminiscent of the work of Williams *et al.* in 1946 who had somewhat similar findings. We could not find any consistent and significant change in sensory thresholds. It may be related to the fact that our measures are not sensitive enough, or to the sterility of the environmental situation, to afferent arousal or to an inadequate dose. I feel that it is the latter. It's like studying LSD-25 at 10 to 20 μg doses rather than at 100 μg or more.

DR. WINTERS: Did these patients describe any after-effects? Any hangover?

DR. DOMINO: They did not describe any hangover.

I was amazed to discover that some of our medical students smoke marihuana not only on weekends but during the week as well. In fact, one of our subjects was studying pharmacology and preparing for an exam. He told me that he had previously smoked marihuana on the weekend and felt that he could concentrate better. This surely must be a subjective effect that is not a general phenomenon. However, one of the popular anecdotes about marihuana is an enhanced ability to concentrate or focus on part of the environment. Some of the subjects talked about concentrating on the sound of the air conditioning in the testing room. This is reminiscent of what Dr. Sim said last night.

In the small doses we used there was no obvious hallucinogenic effect. I have seen subjects under LSD-25 and phencyclidine. However, our subjects did not show an obvious hallucinogenic effect. Thus, our data with small doses of marihuana are similar to those of Weil *et al.* (1968). Of course, larger doses are reported to be markedly hallucinogenic.

DR. LEVINE: Is it possible, if you objectively measure the subject's ability to study under the influence of the drug, that what will be found is that they subjectively feel they can study better but that they actually perform no better or worse?

DR. DOMINO: I think this is true.

DR. FREEDMAN: I have never heard any pot smokers talk about *wanting* to concentrate or really be able to do intellectual work. It's a time-out period for them, a form of relaxation.

DR. DOMINO: I would agree with what you say. I'm only trying to highlight the fact that at least one medical student claimed to be able to function under marihuana, and I was impressed. Of course, this is anecdotal and needs further study.

DR. FREEDMAN: I, too, was just reporting anecdotes.

DR. LEHRER: In view of these reported experiences, including Dr. Sim's and the ones described by your users, I wonder whether absolute changes in threshold are as good a measure of the reported experience as the ability to pick a specific signal out of white noise. In other words, how well can they discriminate a signal from noise? And is that improved by marihuana? Do you have any data on that?

DR. DOMINO: No, we don't, but I think your suggestion is an excellent one.

DR. AGHAJANIAN: From Isbell's work one would predict that your subjects would not have hallucinations from one or two cigarettes because these hallucinations were dose-related and only occurred at considerably higher doses than would be obtained here. So, I think there is no conflict and no surprise.

DR. EFRON: I would like to bring to your attention a problem in connection with yesterday's comments of Dr. Sim and today's presentation of Dr. Domino. Dr. Sim reported the effects of "synthetic red oil" [see page 332] using two dosages: one very low and one quite high. The high dose he used on himself. Dr. Domino has reported the use of rather low doses. Besides this, Dr. Sim's material was different from that used by Dr. Domino. So, I don't know if one can compare their results. And this is probably the reason why Dr. Domino does not see the changes in orthostatic pressure that Dr. Sim has observed.

I would also like to ask a question: Dr. Domino is speaking about experienced smokers. What exactly does that mean? How much has one to smoke and for how long before he is considered an experienced smoker? I am asking this question for the following reasons: We now have much better pharmacological data about marihuana than previously, but practically all of them are rather an acute basis, and there is probably a big difference in the reaction to marihuana between acute and chronic users. I would like to know how many of Dr. Domino's subjects were chronic smokers of marihuana.

DR. DOMINO: In general, the users said they smoked marihuana off and on for at least a year. The "off and on" means weekends, etc.

One of them who said this, I suspect, was lying, in view of the fact that when he smoked his second marihuana cigarette he got very nauseated, which was not characteristic of the other fellows in the group. He acted as though this was a somewhat new experience for him, although when I questioned him he denied it.

DR. KORNETSKY: I would say that these studies certainly agree closely with the findings of Weil et al. (*Science 162:* 1234–1242, 1968).

DR. DIAMOND: I would like to suggest the possibility that changes measured in masked threshold might be due to the subject shifting his criterion value. The increased false-alarm rate accompanying the large drop in threshold in one of your subjects would seem to imply that his selectivity was shifted to a lower signal level, rather than indicate a change in sensitivity of his sensory apparatus.

DR. SHULGIN: I'd like to amplify a point that Dr. Efron mentioned. I think that besides the consideration of the difference in dose and dose response, attention should be paid to the origin of the material that is under investigation. In both the cases of Dr. Isbell and in the present study, the material was from natural sources. Dr. Isbell actually used an isomer of tetrahydrocannabinol that was isolated from the plant. In the case of the report yesterday by Dr. Sim, which describes orthostatic hypotension and a variety of other biological effects, he was working with synthetic isomers. So, on the basis of this and this alone, I think we could quite fairly say that the psychically active component of marihuana is not yet known.

DR. FREEDMAN: I have used the same compound that Isbell has, the Δ^9 isomer of tetrahydrocannabinol. In mice the drop in temperature and some of the other physiological functions look the same.

I have a question which I think is an important one, and I would like Dr. Efron to answer it. It sounds as if the Δ^9 and the Δ^8 isomers are the isomers which are now held to be the psychically active ones. Is this the case?

DR. SHULGIN: It didn't sound like that last night.

DR. EFRON: We are assuming that the Δ^9 or the Δ^1 compound, call it as you wish, is the active component of marihuana, and we base this on two facts: First, this is the compound that one finds predominant in the tetrahydrocannabinol fraction of the active resins of marihuana.[1] (Another active

---

[1] See: *Cannabis*. Report by the Advisory Committee on Drug Dependence. London, Her Majesty's Stationery Office, 1968; and Bicher and Mechoulam, *Arch. Int. Pharmacodyn. 172:* 24, 1968.

compound is $\Delta^{1(6)}$-tetrahydrocannabinol,[2] but this occurs in much smaller amounts than does the Δ^1.) Second, some experienced smokers, when they have used the Δ^1 compound on a blind basis, say, "I have the same feeling as I have during the smoking of marihuana."

DR. SHULGIN: From what source is this Δ^1 isomer that has the same effect?

DR. EFRON: I'm speaking about the synthetic compound.

DR. SHULGIN: I didn't know this work had been reported.

DR. EFRON: Yes, it was reported by Isbell, H., et al., (Gorodetzsky, C. W., Jasinski, D., Claussen, U., Spulak, F. V. and Korte, F. *Psychopharmacol.* (Berlin) *11:* 184, 1967). I would like to make an additional comment. I feel that we may have a similar situation as, for example, with digitalis. When the digitalis glycosides were isolated, it was the feeling that they could substitute for the extract of the whole plant and that one of them might be the active principle of digitalis. It was hoped that by using a pure glycoside one would always have a preparation of the same purity and potency. Then it was shown that different glycosides have different activities and that a mixture of them has a different activity than has an extract of the whole plant. The same may be true for marihuana. The activity of tetrahydrocannabinol may be different from the activity of the plant, but it still remains probably true that the principal active compound is the Δ^1-THC. Some additional efforts now are being made to synthesize other tetrahydrocannabinols and other components of marihuana. Again, I would like to stress the point that the tetrahydrocannabinol molecule is a very peculiar one in the sense that its activity depends very much upon the position of the double bond in the cyclohexene ring.

DR. TEUBER: I would like to point out a curious feature of our discussion. After we had listened to your account of these negative results, Dr. Domino, based on such a very thorough and beautifully documented search for behavioral effects, we turned very quickly from a discussion of the psychological methods to a searching and elaborate pharmacologic discussion. I found it instructive to listen to the questions about which compound could be the most potent ingredient in the crude drug, or how one could potentiate its effects—all this apparently on the assumption (which may be quite false) that if we only had a more powerful variant of the drug, auditory thresholds, as measured by Guilford's method, would have shown a change.

Why should we expect a change in ordinary sensory thresholds? Morrow (in the *LaGuardia Commission Report on Marihuana*) had already obtained

---

[2] The resins of *Cannabis sativa* also contain cannabidiol, cannabinol, cannabigerol, cannabichromene and cannabidiolic acid.

negative results with somewhat less refined psychophysical methods. I do not mean to imply that such negative results are unimportant; it was worthwhile to use laboratory methods for sensory testing still more refined than Morrow's to make absolutely sure, but now we have to ask: Where else do we look for behavioral effects which are undoubtedly present in the subjective reports? If we are dealing, in fact, with "psychotomimetic agents," we should certainly not expect the sort of threshold changes that 19th century methods in psychophysics would be able to bring out. These methods turn up equally negative results in most psychotic patients.

One possible way of going beyond these rather insensitive methods is to use the sort of approach intimated by Dr. Diamond: Instead of dealing with thresholds, in the classical sense, we might wish to apply modern theory, and try to get at a subject's criterion of guessing, his false-alarm rate, so to speak, as can be done in quite the same experimental setting as that used for your auditory threshold experiments. I am not sure that one would get positive results under drugs, but it seems to me a bit more likely than with ordinary thresholds.

Similarly, one could look for the rather special effects one gets on succesive comparisons of intensities or sizes of stimuli—the old concept of "time error" or "order error" in psychophysics (Köhler, 1923). With certain inter-stimulus intervals, the second of two equally intense stimuli tends to be overestimated, and there have been early claims that drugs may alter, or at least enhance, this normal effect.

In searching for adequate methods, one can actually go all the way back to one of the principal founders of psychopharmacology, that is, to Kraepelin (1896) who asked for the systematic application of psychological laboratory tests to psychotic patients, and, concurrently, to normal volunteers under the influence of various drugs. Out of this tradition came the work of Specht (1907) and others, including a publication on effects of alcohol on time-error function, which was published in an ambitious journal of experimental psychopathology, a journal that promptly became defunct after its first two issues (Lange & Specht, 1914–19). It seems still more likely to me that certain complex perceptual displays would bring out these subtle but important effects of drugs, such as some of the beautiful displays by Drs. Harmon and Julesz, earlier in this meeting, or the older figures with reversible perspective, or anything that requires the perceiver to impose a complex structure on the material presented, in contrast to ordinary threshold tests.

If you have a patient with a temporal lobe focus, and he says, "You know, I always know when I am going to get my attack. I look around the room and everything looks just right. All the lines are very precise. All the girls look prettier. All the men look extremely manly." Do I expect that his discrimination of the curvature of a nose or of a neck line is different? I think this is really on a different level—a tremendously interesting one—but a level that these old psychologic laboratory methods from the early years obviously do not reach.

It may be our fate that when two different teams march along, both quite sure of their progress, and they begin to build a bridge across the river between them, they always build it to where the other party has been, not to where it is! When psychologists do psychopharmacology, their pharmacologic methods tend to be obsolete and not always right, and when pharmacologists do psychologic tests, someone is sure to hand them some rather old tools that may not have been too sensitive in the first place. We can do better if we bring the behavioral methods and the pharmacologic ones to the same level of refinement.

DR. HOLMSTEDT: Is it then possible to advance in this field? I have been intrigued, having read both Milton Mezzrow and J. J. Moreau (de Tours), by the fact that musicians use so much marihuana, as do people listening. I have never smoked marihuana myself, unfortunately, but there is only one investigation with regard to music. You mentioned this old experiment with the Seashore test. I don't know what that is. Could you tell me if it is valid or not? Dr. Domino and Dr. Teuber, I'm sure, can elaborate.

DR. DOMINO: Dr. Teuber is the expert and should comment on its validity.

DR. TEUBER: It is a useful battery of standardized tests of musical ability, successive comparisons of snatches of melody, of rhythms, and things of that sort.

Yet I believe it would be better *not* to use the ordinary Seashore tests. Instead, we might consider the sort of variations introduced by Broadbent (1964) and Doreen Kimura, in Dr. Brenda Milner's laboratory; that is, to put different auditory stimulus sequences simultaneously into each of a listener's ears.

Again, there is no empirical basis for predicting that such "dichotic" methods of stimulating would be more sensitive to central changes under drugs, but the method can be pushed quite far. For instance, one can put one entire sentence into one ear and another into the other: the first sentence can be made ambiguous, syntactically, and the other sentence so that it "disambiguates" the first. One of our graduate students, Mr. James Lackner, is currently playing with this effect. It is quite amazing that normal adult listeners will tell you that they don't comprehend the "disambiguated" sentence under these conditions; they cannot even tell what language it is in. Yet it clearly affects the ambiguous sentence by "disambiguating" it.

There are many more of these complex tasks that are worth exploring; ultimately one may have to reach a level of behavioral reputation by norms, if one really wants to get at the central effects of certain drugs on human behavior.

I am reminded of a most instructive psychopharmacologic study—quite a simple one—done in England. A number of drivers were asked to drive trucks or some other large vehicle through parallel rows of stakes, slalom fashion, before and after alcohol intake. As I recall the outcome, there were remarkably few differences in driving skill between the men under alcohol and those without alcohol, yet a real separation of the two groups appeared when the stakes were put so close together that the width of the vehicle exceeded the width of the passage. The moment that was done, the sober subjects refused to continue the test, and those under alcohol drove cheerfully over the stakes! I submit that last test really tapped a level we need to reach.

DR. LATIES: I can give you the source. It was done by Professor J. Cohen and his colleagues and they were driving a two-story London bus. (Cohen, J., Dearnaley, E. J. and Hansel, C. E. M. *Brit. Med. J.* 1438–1442, June 21, 1958). They used off-duty bus drivers and the bus was eight feet wide, and after a couple of shots of alcohol, the drivers attempted to go between stakes placed seven feet ten inches apart.

DR. DOMINO: I'd like to make an anecdotal statement regarding the experience of one of my colleagues who got "high" with marihuana while listening to the hippie, beat-type music which was placed on a cheap phonograph. The reproduction was rather terrible. When he became "high" the room was suddenly filled with the most grandiose symphonic orchestra there ever existed. In fact, it has scared me. I would suggest that pot-smoking can be terribly reinforcing, and that one should not use naive subjects.

DR. HOLMSTEDT: What kind of music was this?

DR. DOMINO: This was the usual teenagers beat music.

DR. WEST: It's called rock-and-roll.

DR. DOMINO: It's not rock-and-roll. That's in your generation and in mine. It's a monotonous repetitive beating-type music that might be called "progressive" or "acid rock."

Incidentally, that beat apparently slows down while under the influence of marihuana. Perhaps it would suggest another type of test to use incorporating some sort of a timing phenomena.

DR. MANDELL: I'm wondering if Dr. Domino's work doesn't reflect a social principle operating in doing psychopharmacological studies in man: the "dirtier," and I mean dirty in the sexual sense, the more sterile the design has to be. For example, if one is studying phenobarbital one would never think of using JND's.[3] One would insist on an imaginative design with implied important basic issues. But if one uses an agent that is of a highly questionable nature socially, one has to *demonstrate* Calvinism by retreating to a historically acceptable and well-established (though out-of-date) experimental methodology.

DR. WASER: I want to come back to the unknown substance which causes hallucinations in marihuana.

There is a difference. Dr. Sim told us he took his compound in castor oil, and all the others have smoked it. So, it is very probable that you have pyrolytic degradation to other compounds.

DR. DOMINO: I like what you say, Dr. Waser. Pyrolysis involves oxidation. There was an observation made accidentally by one of my graduate students, John Morrison, which bears looking into if we can get more Δ^9-THC. John gave 10 mg/kg s.c. to a rat on a fixed interval schedule. He found no effect whatsoever. He saved the remaining Δ^9-THC. After several weeks the solution was brown. Since Δ^9-THC is very scarce I had him inject it again. This time he got an amphetamine-like reaction in the same rat. This needs to be repeated, of course. But it does suggest the importance of oxidation of THC derivatives.

DR. JULESZ: I would like to comment along the same lines as Dr. Teuber did. I really feel that those processes which are as simple as sensory thresholds depend greatly on the modalities used because they are peripheral. Now, many of the phenomena I heard here are much more central. If they are much more central, then they are almost modality-independent.

Let me give you an example. If you present two brief impulses of sound, light, or tactile stimuli, and test for simultaneity, you will get very different thresholds for the three modalities. On the other hand, if you ask which of the two impulses came first, and try to measure the minimum stimulus duration, this is a much more difficult task, but it would seem to be identical for the different modalities. There is a great difference between these two perceptual tasks, *i.e.,* whether you ask for simultaneity or whether you ask for temporal order.

I just don't think that you can quantify your drug-induced phenomena until you use stimuli which are more complex than sensorium but less complex than cognition (for instance, when listening to a late Beethoven quartet). Thus, you may use the rich phenomenal repertoire of perception, instead of sensorium or cognition, which are the two extremes.

DR. SHULGIN: I think a comment is in order concerning Dr. Domino's discussion of a friend who had experiences with marihuana and who had

---

[3] *I.e.,* just noticeable differences.

experienced a very strong reinforcement with music. Therefore, Dr. Domino has questioned the use of naive subjects for experiments with marihuana. In the recent report by Andrew Weil that was mentioned he made a point of including naive subjects as part of his experimental program, which led to two rather interesting observations. The naive subjects were rather unexpectedly insensitive to the intoxicating effects of marihuana, as opposed to the experienced control that had a more learned response. If so, perhaps this should not be a serious reservation on your part. The other interesting observation was that one of the most difficult parts of his first experiment was finding eight inexperienced subjects in the Boston area.

DR. GESSNER: From descriptions of the effect of drugs such as tetrahydrocannabinol it would appear that a person under their influence is able to concentrate, or at any rate becomes concentrated on, some sound that he normally attaches little or no attention to; *i.e.,* what we might call background noise. On the other hand, I'm conscious that much of the time I am capable of, and do in fact have to screen out, all kinds of background sounds in order to listen to what is being said by, for instance, the people assembled here. In fact, it might even be rather difficult for a person like myself to concentrate under present conditions on a background noise such as rustling paper, although, in the absence of more meaningful sound stimuli, I think paper can be heard a very long distance away. I am impressed, however, that my ability to screen out background stimuli is lost if I have to listen to a tape recording of a conversation. I wonder if somebody could enlighten me somewhat as to the reasons for this phenomenon. I also wonder whether perhaps there is not some analogy between this phenomenon and the apparent ability of the person under the influence of a drug such as tetrahydrocannabinol to concentrate on background stimuli.

DR. HARMON: The reason for that stems from the spatial localization that one gets with binaural hearing. If you make a stereophonic tape rather than a monophonic tape recording, then you can discriminate separate sound sources easily. This relates to the "cocktail party effect" which permits you to look directly into the face of someone talking to you while listening to someone elsewhere in the room. The selective attention that you can bring to bear is postulated to reside in one's ability to shift to some differential delays in the two channels and then to compare signals.

In fact, electronic models have been made to simulate this cocktail-party effect, and they work rather well. This doesn't prove of course, that this is the way it happens physiologically. However there is some evidence that makes us tend to believe that similar operations may occur neurophysiologically.

You could, if you wish, make perfectly objective measures of such shiftable attention ability under the influence of various drugs. The results could readily be quantified by having two persons read unambiguous texts and by testing the listener for subsequent comprehension. By using various controlled angles and relative levels, detection (comprehension) likelihood could be predicted and used to derive measures of performance deterioration.

DR. DIAMOND: Dr. Julesz commented earlier on the superabundance of descriptive data that have evolved from numerous subjective reports of psychotomimetic drug effects and from equally numerous clinical observations made under loosely structured experimental conditions. It would certainly not be reasonable to expect major scientific gains from endless additions of raw phenomenologic material to an already fat corpus of soft data. I do not believe, however, that we can infer from this seeming superfluity of disjointed qualitative information that further attention to the phenomenology of drug-induced behavioral changes is unwarranted.

There are two reasons for this position. First, the set of descriptive data is endless and can never be complete. As in all other fields, what is observed and reported is a function of what is known, and adding critical observations to a swollen list may identify redundant and perhaps irrelevant data. Thus, obtaining more data may permit a reduction in its total mass and complexity.

A second reason for continuing work on a descriptive level is that advances in scientific knowledge are rarely accomplished by a continuous progression from simple observation to a formal theory. We do not proceed irreversibly from descriptive work (or experiments referred to as "Class B" by Brindley[4]) to rigorously designed psychophysical studies measuring the identity or non-identity of two sensations ("Class A" experiments) and then to basic chemical or physiological investigations of mechanisms followed by concise mathematical formulations. There is a constant looping back and interaction among all methodologic links in the chain. In particular, on the descriptive level, new observations suggest new hypotheses. Though one must be cautious about overreliance on the tentative hypotheses and concepts inferred from soft data, it is well known that they can point out new directions for productive work in the more exact sciences. Since this is recognized as one of the most important tasks of science, *i.e.,* to stimulate new research, one should not call a moratorium on additional clinical observations.

A corollary to this position is that the results of investigations seeking to examine psychophysical, neurophysiological and biochemical effects of drugs should be reported operationally. Premature, unjustified attempts to harden soft data by such techniques as verbal substitution of some well defined, easily measurable physical variable for a fuzzy set of introspective phenomena can

---

[4] Brindley, G. S.: *Physiology of the Retina and the Visual Pathway.* Edward Arnold, London, 1960.

lead to confusion. For example, suppose that an "hallucinogen" is known regularly to produce quantitative changes in the pattern of electrical activity recorded from a region of the nervous system. If a study determines that these electrophysiological effects are correlated with changes in levels of a certain metabolite, one is occasionally prompted by pressing practical (non-scientific) considerations to infer by transitivity that the biochemical alterations correlate with, and possibly provide a basis for, the behavioral effects. This should be guarded against, not because such speculations are *a priori* of no value, but because the behavioral effects—hallucinations in this case, are still imperfectly characterized.

Additionally, provisional models derived from any experimental data, soft or hard, may prove helpful. It should also be remembered, that a complex neuronal circuit representing some vague behavioral phenomenon is not necessarily more helpful than an informal model like the "squeaky violin" mentioned in another discussion at this meeting.

DR. OSMOND: I'd like to return to the problem about listening to music. I had a curious experience while taking *ololiuqui* when it was supposed to be an inactive substance and I was still not quite sure about it. (Later, it was proved to be quite active.) I was listening to music by Gesualdo, a nobleman of the Italian Renaissance whose works I usually find somewhat repugnant. This time, however, I really listened to the music and enjoyed it greatly. I have no doubt about that. And after listening to it since without *ololiuqui* it has continued to be of interest to me. I am not musical and normally this very complicated music is beyond me, but it was as if my perception of the music had in some way been altered or possibly reorganized, and this persisted afterwards. These complex things may not be very useful at the moment perhaps, but I think one day they may be.

DR. HOLMSTEDT: I would like to comment upon the means of administration of marihuana and THC.

It is well known that in cigarettes when you have alkaloids present, be it nicotine or atropine or something you add to the leaves, about 20 percent remains in the mainstream smoke; 80 percent is burned. In addition to that, of course, there can be changes during pyrolysis.

In this case it would mean, according to your analysis, that you had 1.3 percent, and you gave them no more than 600 milligrams of marihuana.

DR. DOMINO: That is correct. One can use the mean of 483 mg of cigarette smoked. Assuming all of the THC is absorbed, this means 6.34 mg of Δ^9-THC. Assuming 72 kg mean body weight, this means a dose of 88 μg/kg by inhalation. I think this is a low dose of Δ^9-THC and should be compared to Isbell's 50 μg/kg dose.

DR. HOLMSTEDT: Yes, but did you calculate for the 80 percent loss?

DR. DOMINO: No.

DR. AGHAJANIAN: Doesn't that depend on the volatility of the material?

DR. HOLMSTEDT: That's right, but between 18 and 20 percent of alkaloids are destroyed, according to experiments I made a long time ago, and also according to what the tobacco people report. Of course, this is not an alkaloid, and we must know how much THC passes over in the mainstream smoke.

The second thing is that it is common knowledge for a long time that if you smoke superficially, you retain the aerosol produced, amounting to less than 5%. If you inhale deeply and briefly hold your breath, you retain almost everything. It's equivalent to an intravenous injection.

And you say that those people took deep breaths while inhaling?

DR. DOMINO: Yes.

DR. HOLMSTEDT: Is that what marihuana smokers do all the time?

DR. DOMINO: Yes. It's quite an unusual and characteristic style.

DR. HOLMSTEDT: Then, if you have an accurate analysis of the contents in the mainstream smoke, you could easily tell how much they absorbed?

DR. DOMINO: Your points are well taken, Dr. Holmstedt. However, in Isbell's study they injected the material into cigarettes. I don't know what the nicotine content was. I believe that if you take our figures and those of Isbell (50 μg/kg), they are roughly similar. He also used a 250 μg/kg amount, which is quite hallucinogenic.

DR. EFRON: But why go to such a high dosage?

DR. HOLMSTEDT: Because it doesn't take into account how much is destroyed.

DR. LATIES: My only point insofar as Dr. Domino's data are concerned is that he simply used the criterion of "highness" and allowed the person to smoke until he got to that point. So, it is immaterial whether 80 percent was burned or not. The subject continued smoking until he reached a criterion.

DR. DOMINO: In our limited series of marihuana smokers, I was impressed that when they get "high," they don't want any more marihuana. I wonder if a larger dose would be unpleasant? By smoking, the subject seems to titrate himself to a very precise subjective level.

DR. SHULGIN: Specific comments are necessary on the potential fractionation of components in marihuana due to smoking techniques. In addition to potential oxidative pyrolysis, there is decomposition within the residue of the cigarette. Work in Switzerland, Germany, and Israel has shown that chemical reactions can occur in the course of smoking: both cyclization and decarboxylation can convert essentially inactive components to active ones.

DR. AGHAJANIAN: The way your studies were designed, your subjects couldn't possibly have had hallucinations because the end-point was decided to be just when they reached the "high." Now, in Isbell's study, the point at which hallucinations appeared was at two or three times the level that was required to just reach a "high." Thus, there was no possibility for you to see hallucinations.

DR. FREEDMAN: The other thing it should be compared with is Isbell's dose-response curve that he got with respect to pulse rate, which turned out to be a straight line. I, too, imagine it was due to the point that Dr. Aghajanian brought up in terms of design.

NOTE ADDED IN PROOF
(*Footnote to p. 302*)

This value for Δ^9-THC content was established about two years before the actual use of the material in this study and was referred to us by N.I.M.H. The same batch was assayed nine months after the study was completed by two different, independent laboratories using gas-liquid chromatography. One of the laboratories reported 0.51%, the other one 0.20% content of Δ^9-THC. Dr. Scigliano indicates that his data show the mean content of Δ^9-THC in this batch to be 1.2% over the past year. These methodological discrepancies must still be resolved.

Nevertheless, because the end-point of drug effect was a subjective high, our findings can still be considered applicable for this state. (E. F. Domino)

GENERAL DISCUSSION, SUMMARY

AND CLOSING REMARKS

GENERAL DISCUSSION

DR. EFRON: We will now have the general discussion. All aspects of our workshop may be discussed.

Dr. West will start the discussion.

DR. WEST: There is a story about two hippies who are sitting in Golden Gate Park. Both are high on "pot." A jet aircraft goes zooming overhead and is gone; whereupon one hippie turns to the other one and says, "Man, I thought he'd never leave!"

This conference is having the opposite effect upon me. All of a sudden it's almost over, and there were a number of things that I was hoping my friends, the chemists and pharmacologists, would straighten out for me; but that doesn't seem to have happened yet.

I'm particularly concerned because I feel there are many issues related to the marihuana problem that haven't been penetrated very deeply here in the last two days. I'd like to touch on them now in the hope that at the next conference Dr. Efron organizes we shall have more time to focus on this deeply troublesome problem. True, more data are needed; but I'd like to hear more speculation about some of these matters. I for one am very content to listen to the speculations of people who are as informed as some of those present.

There were a couple of points I wanted to make about the question of the effect of marihuana on auditory threshold and the hallucinogenic effects of the tetrahydrocannabinols.

One point has already been made about the dose relationship. Many marihuana smokers titrate their "high" to euphoria, avoiding higher doses. I feel that until one gets into higher doses one shouldn't expect to see significant or consistent hallucinogenic effects. In my clinical observations of people who have taken larger quantities of tetrahydrocannabinols, under two conditions have I definitely observed hallucinogenic effects.

One condition is where marihuana or hashish is eaten. The smoker's control of dosage by subjective cues does not obtain under these conditions. The subject may, in oral consumption, take a larger amount than he realized or planned. You can't titrate it when you eat it. You take it in and you experience more or less of a dose-related response depending on your gastrointestinal state, absorption rate, and other variables not under voluntary control.

The other hallucinatory circumstance was in the smokers of hashish. There is a fair amount of hashish now in this country. Many of the young people are smoking it in preference to ordinary marihuana: they have special pipes for it, and so on. Apparently, in smoking hashish, it is more likely that one will overdose oneself, passing the point of the ideal "high" that the more gradual process of marihuana cigarette smoking produces, leading to more profound phenomena including hallucinations.

Lincoln Clark has been studying a marihuana extract he calls "Clark's Elixir of Pot," which is probably very much like the red oil of Dr. Sim. Dr. Clark has been using audiometric techniques and he assures me (personal communication) that a number of his subjects show reliably lowered auditory thresholds while intoxicated with the extract. As you know, Dr. Clark is a very careful investigator. The lowering of a sensory threshold is a very exciting finding. In the light of Dr. Clark's observations we might be wise to reserve our judgment about whether marihuana intoxication merely produces a differential discrimination (as has been suggested here), or whether a significant effect can be observed on actual sensory information transport.

More refined measurements will be required, especially with higher doses of intoxicating substances, whether they be specific tetrahydrocannabinols, or whether they be extracts like Dr. Clark's, which undoubtedly contains a number of the different fractions that wouldn't be present in the purified substance, be it Δ^9- or Δ^1-tetrahydrocannabinol.

There are several more terribly important things that we have passed over; I want some of the chemists to help me with these problems.

First, I'm very interested in the unusual and peculiar phenomenon of the "experienced" versus the "naive" subject exposed to similar doses of marihuana. There is no question in my mind that this is something that transcends mere imagination, suggestion, or ordinary learning. It suggests either a sensitization or the induction of a semi-permanent change in the response organ or mechanism.

Many people report being exposed to marihuana a few times without very much effect, but subsequently definite effects are experienced, often with an apparently smaller dose. I don't think this phenomenon can be explained in terms of "learning how to smoke it better." The same thing is reported by youngsters who had never previously learned to smoke anything, even tobacco. Even among teen-agers whose only exposure has been by eating marihuana in cookies, the same phenomenon is reported. Typically, one hears that the first two or three exposures produced nothing very much, perhaps a little dryness of the mouth, dizziness, or time-distortion; but that on subsequent exposures they began to experience the typical "high" effects that we have come to look for, especially the more pleasant aspects, such as euphoria and relaxation.

Furthermore, the experienced subject doesn't need as much to get to the point that he calls his "high" as he did previously. This of course is the opposite of tolerance. I have heard Dr. Kornetsky comment in the past about what this might imply in relation to other mechanisms, linking (at least in theory) the phenomenon of tolerance to the immune response. Sensitization, of course would be logically related. This decreasing dose requirement to get "high" is fairly characteristic of the "pothead."

I'd like to say just a word or two more about the marihuana habitué and others who smoke a lot of marihuana over a long period of time. I approach this question with some trepidation because the times are passing strange. The strangeness was touched upon yesterday by Dr. Osmond. I'd like to return to this issue of the drug, the user, the law, and society.

The marihuana problem has been peculiarly singled out among the many drug problems of our culture. Terrible things are happening to many young people who experiment with the stuff. The smugglers, the peddlers, the pushers, and their peers expose them to it. Their sense of curiosity, adventure, rebellion, or even conformity leads them to try it. Suddenly—by fiat—they are criminals.

Presumably the purpose of the law is to protect these youngsters from such exposure. But along about the time they have been exposed and are experimenting, their lives not yet ruined by the demon drug, along comes the law and completes the process of ruination that the smugglers began. The youngster may find himself convicted of a felony, sent into a dreadful prison situation, with which he's not at all prepared to cope, and stigmatized for life.

Now, some of the people who are perpetuating this unfortunate state of affairs are perfectly willing to pounce upon anybody's statement that there may be dangers in the use of marihuana, even if they are subtle kinds of dangers that can't be picked out of an ordinary experiment like Dr. Domino's. His results seem to suggest a relatively benign set of consequences from the use of marihuana. I like those experiments. But I fear there are dangers that such experiments couldn't be expected to define.

However one speculates publicly about such dangers, the modern day Anslingers (or other marihuanaphobes) are liable to seize upon such speculations and use them to justify the kind of attitude we have just heard from our friends in England. Last week British authorities turned their backs upon the report of a scientific commission to the effect that the drug laws should be made more liberal. Justification for perpetuating the punitive approach was that we already have so much social evil that we shouldn't admit to the acceptability of any more.

Nevertheless, I feel impelled to share with you my growing concerns about psychobiological risks in marihuana use and abuse. There are a great many young people, including some of the brightest and some of the best, who have been using marihuana now more or less regularly for three or four years. Addiction or even habituation is denied. The smoking is said to be simply for pleasure. Untoward effects are usually (not always) denied. But the experienced clinician observes, in many of these individuals, personality changes that may grow subtly over long periods of time: diminished drive, lessened ambition, decreased motivation, apathy, shortened attention span, distractibility, poor judgment, impaired communication skills, loss of effectiveness, introversion, magical thinking, derealization and depersonalization, diminished capacity to carry out complex plans or prepare realistically for the future, a peculiar fragmentation in the flow of thought, habit deterioration, and progressive loss of insight. There is a clinical impression of organicity to this syndrome that I simply cannot shake off or explain away.

As Dr. Teuber can tell us, even people with severe brain damage very frequently will deny there is anything wrong at all. Acid-heads and heavy potsmokers certainly are strong deniers. But the impressions of objective observers should no longer be denied by ourselves.

I have thought of all the alternative explanations. Who are the people who are likely to become heavy marihuana users? Aren't they likely to be suffering from some more basic personality disorder that might account for the foregoing? Aren't some of them schizophrenics? Maybe some of them are using marihuana to treat themselves for symptoms of another psychiatric ailment. And all of these, and other, possibilities are perfectly plausible; furthermore, I think I've seen instances of them all. However, there are simply too many instances of youngsters who should be getting their Ph.D.'s by now, but who are drifting along, smoking marihuana, and gradually developing these symptoms. Some of them, at least, are *not* schizophrenic, *not* psychopathic, *not* avitaminotic, *not* using other drugs, *not* simply "dropping out" by choice. And a few of the brightest ones will even tell you, "I can't even read a book through from cover to cover and grasp its meaning any more. I tell myself that I really don't care what's in it; that these topics are not important. But I really can't do it. Of course, I also really don't care."

Now, it may be that several types of biochemical scarring of the human brain are possible. The term "enzyme induction" was used earlier. It rang a bell with me because I picked up some new ideas about enzyme induction from Dr. Mandell a year ago, and it's been on my mind ever since in connection with the marihuana problem.

Enzyme induction is a biologically important phenomenon. If you induce lots of alcohol dehydrogenase in your liver, adaptation to cocktail parties is improved. It's generally and properly considered a healthy state of affairs that the body can manage this. But suppose a chemical, repeatedly introduced into an organ such as the brain, induces increasing amounts of an enzyme that is atypical, that causes some untoward effects of its own, or that competes too successfully with other enzyme systems for certain materials in the metabolic substrate. If you repeatedly expose the brain to a substance that stimulates the induction of such a new enzyme, is it possible on that basis to effect a changed biochemical state of affairs that would account for a brain that doesn't work quite the same as it did before? If not, are there other biochemical possibilities to explain the syndrome I have described?

I hope that my concern about this whole matter will stimulate some of you, who know a great deal more than I do about biochemistry, to comment.

DR. KORNETSKY: Just one question. Of these drug users, has it been well established that other drugs have not been involved?

DR. WEST: A great many of them have taken other drugs, but not all, by any means. For example, there's a report coming out in the *Annals of Internal Medicine* describing untoward psychiatric reactions among a number of young Americans living in India who have used only marihuana or hashish, never LSD.

DR. KORNETSKY: Even if any part of what you say is correct, the present drug laws are absurd.

DR. WEST: Unquestionably the harshly punitive laws that make felons of youngsters for possession of marihuana are absurd, unfair, unrealistic, cruel and unusual. As I said at the outset, this is also a matter of deep concern, requiring study and, hopefully, reform. Meanwhile, here's what I tell those youngsters who will listen: *Just because alcohol is bad, it doesn't mean that marihuana is good. Just because the present law is stupid, it doesn't mean society shouldn't have some kind of law to control intoxicants. And just because you have been lied to about the dangers of marihuana, it doesn't necessarily mean that the use of marihuana is safe."*

DR. FREEDMAN: I simply listen to Dr. West and say it's perfectly possible there is an interaction between a chemical state, the experience that occurs during a *Cannabis* state, and the observed consequences. But I would be loathe to let seep out at this moment, in the midst of our ignorance, any implication that this is an induction of a chronic organic syndrome. To look for this is facinating, but the range of mechanisms, as you indicated, is immense, and if they're infinite, God help us.

DR. LIPTON: Before going to the last point of our program, the summary of the meeting, I would like to bring to your attention a matter that has concerned us throughout the conference. That is the pending legislation which may permit the Narcotics Bureau of the Department of Justice to control the distribution of psychotomimetics employed for research. This question has alarmed the American Psychological Association and the American Psychiatric

Association, and quite properly alarms us. I think we will all agree that the utility of these compounds for the acquisition of new information about the brain and its functioning have hardly been tapped. Even their utility for therapy is far from clear. I was delighted yesterday to hear Dr. Sim tell us that marihuana may have utility in the management of epilepsy, tetanus and migraine. If this is so, restrictive legislation, generated by social pressures because of the misuse of these agents by youngsters, may seriously impede legitimate medical research. We should individually and collectively through our organizations attempt to recommend a reasonable set of regulations, and these, it seems to me, should be under the control of the National Institutes of Health.

DR. FREEDMAN: I would like to say that to my knowledge, the research people in the Bureau of Dangerous Drugs are concerned with this matter and the problem at this moment, as I see it, is writing a precise bill that makes clear whose functions are what. I say that with respect to Dr. Milton Joffe who sits with us. We don't know the outcome yet.

I don't know what political strategy is advisable. I think everyone should know, though, that a loosely or quickly written bill in this area could have an adverse impact upon us and our research, and that is what we don't want.

DR. JOFFE: This bill has been sharpened up. There was a meeting held about two weeks ago on this subject, and you might ask Dr. Sidney Cohen and Dr. Jonathan Cole who were there as well as numerous other people about the discussion. We agreed to limit our role in conformity with the expressed sentiments of the conference and in accordance with the discussions we had prior to this with Dr. Freedman. We could all see the cause for concern despite our intentions to the contrary.

However, there has never been any intention in our group, in the Department of Justice, or in F.D.A. to "take over," as it's been called, all research and education. Today someone asked me about funds for research because he'd been told by N.I.M.H. that we're going to have all the $25,000,-000 earmarked for this field of research. I would sincerely hope this is so, but I think this is probably the grossest misstatement I have ever heard in my life. We have never had any intention of doing such things as preempting the research and education area. We have no such intentions now.

DR. FREEDMAN: You must understand our concern that Congress not loosely entitle another bureau, whatever it be, let alone a law enforcement bureau, to become the agency of some Congressional struggle whereby they say, "Okay, we're going to punish you guys who publish this dangerous data on pot. We're going to punish you by putting the money in another agency."

Our main aim has been to keep health-related research in the Department of H.E.W.

DR. JOFFE: First of all, I might remind you that this omnibus bill that you are castigating so severely clarifies the confused situation we have right now, and, as you know, it puts compounds such as marihuana, tetrahydrocannabinol, LSD, etc. in a research category. It will, if anything, make this easier to work on. It will enable us to foster research, not to restrict it.

DR. LIPTON: Administered by the Department of Justice or H.E.W.?

DR. JOFFE: Administered only from the standpoint of knowing where the compounds are and who's using them.

DR. LATIES: As of last week that bill contained a clause which gave to the Department of Justice a look at the research protocols for drugs which were on Schedules 1 and 2. Is that still in the bill?

DR. JOFFE: I don't know, but Schedules 1 and 2 are the ones on which we are bound by the Single Convention on Narcotic Drugs of the United Nations, 1961. These are the narcotics.

DR. LATIES: Methamphetamine, morphine, cocaine, and others such as marihuana, are on there. What worries me about the scheduling of drugs like these is that they are put in Schedule 2 because they start getting abused in society. And then, ironically, it becomes much more different for legitimate investigators to study them.

Other drugs can very easily be moved into it, and according to this bill, as soon as something is in Schedule 1 or 2 the red tape increases markedly. It now reads that the Secretary of Health, Education and Welfare shall be asked by the Department of Justice for advice as to whether this research should be done, and then it says that the Secretary shall promptly advise the Attorney General concerning the qualifications of each practitioner, which includes researchers seeking licenses. Before giving such advice the Secretary shall consider the qualifications of the person or persons who will conduct the research, the substances to be used, the place where the research will be performed, and the design of the research protocol.

DR. JOFFE: Which is exactly what the joint advisory committee on psychotomimetics is doing to this day.

DR. LATIES: Yes.

DR. JOFFE: No difference.

DR. FREEDMAN: I don't think we have time to get into this. I think our hope is that this is not an omnibus drug control bill, nor an ominous one, but one that is precise, select, and one in which the community of scientists and physicians will have a chance to help test out the soft spots before it gets to be a public argument, which I hope is not necessary.

DR. JOFFE: If I can say just one more thing. If you people here are worried about this bill, you are not half as worried as I am about it, because if the bill should go through with any of the provisions that you are so worried about (and I feel mistakenly), I will need another job since I would find it impossible to be associated with this sort of repressive activity.

DR. EFRON: The problem is, Dr. Joffe, that we connot vote for you to be a Congressman.

DR. JOFFE: You have a Congressman. You voted for him once. Go tell him what to do, because I have to do the same thing.

DR. EFRON: I would like to ask some questions in connection with the presentation of Dr. Shulgin at the chemistry session. He mentioned different compounds related to tetrahydrocannabinol, and I wonder if somebody could tell us something about the human and animal pharmacology of tetrahydrocannabinols. I think that Dr. Sim is very well qualified to speak about this.

DR. SIM: There are a number of problems related to past history of marihuana and tetrahydrocannabinols which most of us recognize. It is almost impossible to talk about the pharmacology of this group, whether from natural or synthetic sources, unless we use reference samples or reference compounds. The variety of effects reported after oral use and smoking of *Cannabis* of different origin and of different chemical content is to be expected.

Several years ago we obtained a representative sample of a synthetic compound which we called "synthetic red oil"[1] containing:

3-(1,2-Dimethylheptyl)-7, 8,9,10-tetrahydro-6,6, 9-trimethyl-*6H*-dibenzo [*b, d*] pyran-1-ol

---

Monoterpene numbering of Δ^1-THC

[1] The term "synthetic red oil" used herein is rather misleading because it implies that the compound has the same content as the natural red oil but is prepared synthetically. This is not the case, since the natural red oil contains mostly Δ^1-*trans*-tetrahydrocannabinol (Δ^1-THC) (this nomenclature is in accordance with the monoterpene numbering used by Mechoulam and his group). The synthetic compound used by Dr. Sim is, according to this numbering, Δ^3-tetrahydrocannabinol (Δ^3-THC) with a different side chain; C_9H_{29} instead of C_5H_{11} occurring as the side chain in the natural Δ^1-THC. Dr. Sim uses the dibenzopyran numbering. (Ed.)

The compound was the only material used in all research in animals in both acute and chronic studies, and in man in single exposure either by oral or by inhalation in solvents. It is a very viscid material which is only slightly soluble in propylene glycol or 95% ethanol. The effects in man were usually noted within 2–4 hours after oral ingestion of 30–55 μg/kg of body weight.

The acetate of the above compound and its eight stereoisomers were made and tested. The formula of the acetate is as follows:

[Using the R. Mechoulam system this would be referred to as a Δ^3 compound, i.e., a double bond between carbon 3 and 4, using the carbon with the methyl group as carbon 1 and then proceeding with numbering clock-wise.]

At 10–20 μg/kg of body weight mydriasis, thirst, headache, tachycardia, some increase in blood pressure, and colored visual hallucinations were usually noted. At higher doses marked postural hypotension, weakness, giddiness, blurred vision, marked psychomotor retardation, and a decrease in body temperature of as much as 3°F was a fairly common occurrence.

At the present time we have only partially completed the work on the isomers. To date we have not seen any evidence of hallucination at doses up to 10 μg/kg. Isomers 2 and 4, either alone or together, cause rather prolonged postural hypotension at 5–10 μg/kg.[2]

All of this work is being processed for publication and it will include acute, subacute, and chronic studies in cat, dog, and monkey.

DR. EFRON: You mentioned hypothermia and postural hypotension. What compound caused it and how was it administered?

DR. SIM: Oral administration of either the original synthetic compound or of its acetate. Doses required to cause these effects were in the 20–55 μg/kg range. Stereoisomer studies thus far indicate that 5 10 μg/kg of isomers 2 and 4 will cause the same degree of hypotension.

My interest in the natural and synthetic preparations is primarily because

---

[2] Both isomers, 2 and 4, have the α- and β-methyl groups positioned *trans* to each other. The absolute configuration is still unknown. One of the compounds has the

they are interesting from a medical standpoint. There are three areas where they may be of definite use in medicine. Domino, Hardman, Seevers, Heath, Monroe and others have worked with the same original sample, and their work on the cardiovascular and CNS effects is especially noteworthy.

Many years ago, Loewe[3] described the use of similar compounds in prophylaxis for epilepsy. He found these very effective if used in small maintenance doses to prevent grand mal seizures. Unfortunately the addictive question arose, and studies were discontinued. I would like to emphasize and again add that our work has been with Δ^3-THC with a C_9H_{19} side chain and not with Δ^1-THC which has the C_5H_{11} side chain.[4]

The other two areas of medical importance are in the treatment of essential hypertension, and in the possible use of this type of compound in hyperthermia associated with acute sunstroke when other measures fail. The use potential has been severely restricted by the lack of suitable compounds for study as well as by public opinion and the resulting lack of funds to carry out the work unless it has to do with the problem of addiction.

Mr. Chairman, the foregoing appears to be the type of information which is required if we are to be allowed to study these classes of compounds for medical use.

DR. EFRON: I was thinking a long time ago about synthesizing the acetate because of its solubility potential but the information that I had from Mechoulam and his group was that acetate is much less potent than the original tetrahydrocannabinol. I discussed this problem with Dr. Craig from The Rockefeller University. He agreed that from a theoretical point of view it probably would be the case, and this is why I didn't pursue the problem further. But from what we hear from you, it looks more potent than the original compound.[5]

DR. SIM: Your query may have been in respect to the relative potency in causing hallucinations or some other mental aberrations. My impression was that less of this was noted with the acetate. The acetate was slightly more potent as a hypotensive, hypothermic and pulse-affecting agent in man than the original. The answer may be that it is slightly more soluble, and is more stable in storage. The original compound, even when ampuled in

---

α-methyl in the D-configuration; the other has α-methyl in the L-configuration. See: Aaron, H. S. and Fergerson, C. P.: Synthesis of the eight stereoisomers of a tetrahydrocannabinol congener. *J. Org. Chem.*, 33 (2): 684, 1968 (especially Table II). (Ed.).

[3] See Loewe, S. and Goodman, L. S.: Anti-convulsant action of marihuana-active substances. *Fed. Proc.*, 6: 352, 1947, and Loewe, S.: Cannabiswirkstoffe u. Pharmakologie der Cannabinole. *Arch. fur Exper. Path. u. Pharmakologie, 211:* 2, 1950. (Ed.).

[4] See footnote 1 on page 332.

[5] The discussant had in mind Δ^1-THC. (Ed.)

nitrogen and stored in the refrigerator, tended finally to oxidize from a brown to a red color. The acetate was less viscid, slightly more soluble in 95% ethanol and propylene glycol, and could be stored at ordinary refrigerator temperatures without evidence of color change or loss of potency.[6]

DR. EFRON: I would like to stress again the peculiarity of tetrahydrocannabinol (THC). As you know, the difference between THC and Synhexyl, which was synthesized by Adams, is only a difference in the length of the side chain and the position of the double bond, but the activity is completely different. From Dr. Sim's remarks, we see how sensitive the molecule is—the addition of a certain group eliminates the hallucinogenic effects of the compound.

I would like to ask if you could advise us of a good way to administer this compound by inhalation. From what we know, the route of administration is very important and affects the potency of the compounds. Inhalation is probably the best way for administration. Inhalation by smoking is not the best technique for scientific research.

DR. SIM: The two ways we have used for inhalation exposures have been in very small volumes of ethanol either sprayed in solution or dropped on a hot plate for thermal generation.[7]

DR. EFRON: I may add here that extract of *Cannabis* was deleted from the XIIth revision of the *United States Pharmacopeia* in 1942; it had appeared in the XIth revision of 1936.

DR. HOLMSTEDT: I understand that Dr. Sim has done more experiments in man with these compounds than anybody else except, perhaps, the French physician Moreau, who wrote a fascinating book in 1845. Now, I suggest two things: one, that Dr. Sim publish his findings, if he is permitted to do so; and, second, that a translation be published of this very interesting book by Moreau which runs to 400 pages and which treats all aspects of hashish, including a very large series on human experimentation. It is not widely known. The book is difficult to get. As a matter of fact, I had difficulties in getting a microfilm out of the National Library in Paris, but I do have it.

DR. EFRON: I too have a copy of it, and there is much interesting information in it. Recently in our branch Dr. Waskow did some experiments with THC, and I have since found some of them described in this book. I am pleased to report that the publisher of the proceedings of this meeting, Raven Press, has agreed to undertake the publication of Moreau's book.

DR. SIM: The information on most tetrahydrocannabinols has recently

---

[6] The discussant spoke about Δ^1-THC with a C_9H_{19} side chain. (Ed.)
[7] The temperature of the hot plate lies between 400° and 500°F. (Ed.).

been declassified. Since there is a clearance time for publication, I would expect that my report may be released in six months.

DR. OSMOND: I have recently been consulted by a university press about a book consisting of a collection of articles on the use of *Cannabis* in medicine. The articles are clear and well written, the first being that by O'Shaughnessy in 1839. *Cannabis* was used at that time in a variety of conditions, particularly epilepsy, and was considered especially valuable in tetanus, which was described vividly. They saw plenty of tetanus in India in those days and they were excellent clinical observers. Consequently the dramatic response of this terrifying and usually fatal condition to *Cannabis* was a matter of great medical interest. In addition to this, *Cannabis* was used in a number of cardiac conditions. Some of these may have been hypertension. There are several dozen excellent papers in this collection, written by competent clinicians who described real patients with skill and understanding. These papers appeared in reputable journals for a period of many years and they give one a strong impression that *Cannabis* had a variety of useful medical applications. In addition to this, the U.S. Dispensatory has many references to *Cannabis* during the same period. I have urged the editor of this book to make a special section on this. After 1930,[8] for some reason *Cannabis* completely disappeared from the *U.S. Pharmacopoeia.* No explanation is offered for this, and the opinion of several generations of competent medical men was suddenly completely ignored, rather in the way that Stalin rewrote history. It looks as if legal enactments at that time had made taboo what had previously been considered a valuable medicine. This seems a very dangerous precedent which we should examine very carefully. I recall, too, that *Cannabis* was found useful in migraine, which is still a very uncomfortable illness for those afflicted by it. Perhaps we should examine the strange medical history of *Cannabis* carefully, because it seems to be an example of potentially valuable medical substances being lost suddenly and unnecessarily due to the impingement of social silliness and prejudice. I think we will need to develop proper strategies to keep such misfortunes from recurring.

DR. BIEL: I might say we were annoyed with the lack of nitrogen present in tetrahydrocannabinol because most hallucinogens are basic substances. We did make the aza-analogue of the Adams compound and found it completely inert in animal pharmacology.

DR. EFRON: Dr. Sim, did you find in some of your experiments that the mixture of different isomers is more active than any one of them separately?

---

[8] It disappeared from the XIIth revision of *USP* that became official from November 1, 1942. The XIth revision, official from June, 1936 to October 31st, 1942 still contained this entry. (Ed.).

DR. SIM: I would say the mixture of 2 and 4.[9] They were effective in producing marked orthostatic hypotension in man. At doses given thus far we have not seen any hallucinogenic effect. It would appear that this fraction of activity may not be present in these two isomers.

DR. EFRON: Which one of these isomers had the hallucinogenic effects?

DR. SIM: So far, we have not seen these effects with any of them. As I explained, it is probably because we have not gone to a high enough dose with them. We have not gone beyond 10 μg/kg.

DR. DOMINO: You took the original C_9 compound described previously. Could you describe the effects in some detail?

DR. SIM: The material was made up in milk sugar containing one mg in each capsule. Since the oral dose for man had not been previously determined, it was decided to take one capsule each hour, with an upper limit of 5. The experiment started in the evening while we were engaged in conference and film review. By the end of my fourth hour, I was having some difficulty with blurring of vision, my mouth was very dry, and some unsteadiness of gait was apparent. On returning to quarters I asked my associate, Dr. Kimura, to take my blood pressure. It was approximately 85/40 mm Hg. I went to bed and although tired did not sleep. The next morning I decided to walk to the officers' mess for breakfast about a quarter of a mile away. I had difficulty walking, particularly in being able to track in any semblance of a straight line.

On arriving at the mess, which was very busy, I sat down at the table with several of my associates. Despite a rather animated conversation, and a great deal of noise in the room, I became acutely aware of some noise which sounded like someone ruffling paper. Looking around the room failed to confirm this, however. I walked into an adjoining room some 70 feet away which was shut off from the dining area by a partition. Sitting there was an employee thumbing through onion skin inventory sheets. This sudden auditory acuity for specific sounds was most unusual for me.

The effects lasted approximately three days. My blood pressure returned to reasonable figures within 36 hours, but dizziness on first arising persisted longer. The other things which were notable may be worthy of mention. Colors were intensified and landscapes especially delightful. Occasional visual hallucinations of brilliantly colored geometrical designs were experienced. Although aware of all surrounding events, I preferred to be left alone. Even being faced with simple "yes" decisions for certain personnel to leave after completing their work was difficult. There was never any stimulus or inclination for increasing activity. One unusual thing to me was that even the most bland and unappetizing food was very delightful. This change of sensory

---

[9] See footnote 2 on page 333.

awareness of auditory, visual, and gustatory systems was especially interesting.

A VOICE: Did you have any mood changes?

DR. SIM: Experiences were not stressful. There was a distinct lack of need of communication with others; most of the experience was introspective. Time seemed to be interminable. The three days seemed like a much longer period.

DR. HOLMSTEDT: Did you get keener hearing combined with great susceptibility to music and the phenomenon that ordinary noise is enjoyed as though it sounded sweet? Did you enjoy that?

DR. SIM: Yes, music was distinctly enjoyable as long as it was not loud. The ability to pick out instruments in a large group appeared to be facilitated. The incident regarding the discrimination allowing me to hear paper ruffling under very noisy and distracting circumstances was very interesting.

DR. EFRON: I wonder if Dr. Teuber would like to comment from a theoretical point of view.

DR. TEUBER:[10] I wished I could do it introspectively, as others here are able to do. We have heard about various subjective experiences, beginning with Dr. Waser's fascinating description of "recurrent perceptions." These accounts seem to be quite similar to what we have seen in patients with irritative lesions of the brain (perhaps more often in the right than in the left hemisphere) who complain of something that has been, in fact, called *palinopia, palin* meaning again or recurrent, and *opia* meaning vision. Dr. Waser created his own term, echo-pictures, apparently in analogy to such expressions as *echopraxia* or *echolalia*. Obviously, the name does not matter. The reports are so similar, particularly, if they come from patients with episodic or persistent visual disturbances from focal brain irritation, that they seem to refer to essentially the same subjective phenomenon.

In their mildest form, these troubles are perhaps not too different from the vivid visual memories some of use have of microscopic sections after a day of microscopy (the *Sinnengedaechtnis* of the German psychological literature). In its more obviously abnormal form, the experience may be part of an ictal disturbance of perception, in which the ordinary termination of a perceptual process is temporarily lacking. Such a failure of normal termination of perceptual acts can take several forms: A single image may stay with the patients for days, superimposing itself in unvarying shape and color on other things really seen. Alternatively, as in some of our patients with shell-fragment wounds of the brain, one gets the report that on seeing a person rising from a chair, that person would appear simultaneously in different stages of that motion, that is, sitting down, half-risen, and standing up, as if the

---

[10] References for Dr. Teuber's comments appear at the end of his discussion.

motion were dissected into motion-picture frames, and these frames then superimposed (Teuber, 1966; Teuber, Battersby and Beneler, 1960).

We have interpreted such disorders, in our earlier reports, as primary disturbances in the perception of movement, but I believe now that a common feature in such perceptual derangements is an abnormal persistence, or rather, a failure to "clear" the mechanism involved in the individual perceptual process. After all, the visual physiology of perception requires not only the initiation of any given perceptual act but also its termination as we go from one glimpse of a scene to another, and this termination appears to be vulnerable to many of those agents we are considering here, as well as to irritated cerebral lesions, particularly in the temporal lobes and, I should add, probably in the peduncular region of the brain.

To turn to another aspect of the report we have just heard—the problem of hyperesthesia—I should point out that it is rather more difficult to find parallels in abnormal brain states for that particular manifestation of the toxic conditions we have discussed. In fact, until very recently, I would have insisted that the only form of hyperesthesia after focal brain lesions in man would have to be a condition of raised sensory thresholds, in vision, audition, or somesthesis, *i.e.*, an actual reduction of sensitivity, combined with a characteristic hyperpathis, *i.e.*, an over-reaction or enhanced affective response, once threshold values of stimulation are exceeded. This association of raised thresholds and over-reaction to supraliminal stimuli is typical of the so-called thalamic syndrome.

However, there are conditions of genuine hyperesthesia. After perinatal brain injury one finds at times a definite reduction in touch thresholds, a true hypersensitivity, without any over-reaction in these children (see Rudel, Teuber, and Twitchell, 1966), although the site of their cerebral lesions is unfortunately undetermined. Similarly, there are recent reports from the Montreal Neurological Institute suggesting that differential thresholds for tone intensity may be paradoxically enhanced after certain cortical removals.

This enhanced capacity for detecting intensity increments was found in patients in whom left temporal cortex (involving the gyri of Heschl) had been removed (in an attempt at eliminating an epileptogenic focus). Curiously, the heightened sensitivity did not appear when the left-sided removal spared the gyri of Heschl (Swisher, 1967; see also Milner and Teuber, 1968). These are very baffling observations; their interpretation is far from obvious, but they might reflect the loss of some efferent regulation in sensory systems, a regulation in which temporal lobe structures may play a special role.

In this connection, I should remind you of the fact that Klüver and Bucy's discovery of the famous syndrome that bears their names—a syndrome produced by bitemporal lobectomy in monkeys—was prompted (as Klüver once told me) by an interest in mescaline. Klüver had noted in himself and in the reports by others that the perceptual disturbances after mescaline ingestion were quite reminiscent of certain symptoms of temporal lobe irritation in man, including distortions of shape and distance, multiplication of contours and similar derangements. Klüver postulated that removing the temporal lobes in a monkey would remove the anatomical receptor for mescaline, but then found the syndrome resulting from the temporal lobe removal so striking in itself that he concentrated on analyzing what we now call the Klüver-Bucy syndrome; in his published work, in any case, he did not pursue the question of heightened tolerance to mescaline in the temporal-lobectomized animals, although others have picked up that part of the story since (Baldwin, Lewis, and Bach, 1959). In any case, I have always been impressed by the similarity between mescaline-induced states and certain manifestations of temporal lobe epilepsy, particularly those disturbances that arise from a morbid process involving the right side of the brain. One of our graduate students many years ago took mescaline in preparation for his doctoral dissertation (a thesis dealing with the effects of the drug in experimental animals). He complained at first that the drug had no effect, then suddenly reported that the floor was slanting down on his left. A few minutes later, he had a complete left homonymous hemianopia, demonstrable on confrontation tests, and this visual field defect lasted several minutes, as though the right visual pathways had been acting abnormally at first, and then ceased functioning. The hemianopia passed off, much to our relief, without after-effects, but it gave us a healthy respect for what such a drug could do in a presumably normal brain.

REFERENCES

Baldwin, M., Lewis, S. A. and Bach, S. A.: The effects of lysergic acid after cerebral ablation. *Neurology, 9:* 469–474 (1959).

Klüver, H.: *Mescal: The "Divine" Plant and Its Psychological Effects.* London, K. Paul, Trench, Trubner (1928).

Klüver, H.: Mechanisms of hallucinations. In: McNemar, Q. and Merrill, M. A. (eds.), *Studies in Personality.* New York, McGraw-Hill, pp. 175–207 (1942).

Klüver, H. and Bucy, P. C.: Preliminary analysis of functions of the temporal lobes in monkeys. *Arch. Neurol. Psychiat., 42:* 979–1000 (1939).

Milner, Brenda and Teuber, H.-L.: Alteration of perception and memory in man: reflections on methods. In: L. Weiskrantz (ed.), *Analysis of Behavioral Change.* New York, Harper & Row, pp. 268–375 (1968).

Rudel, Rita, Teuber, H.-L. and Twitchell, T. E.: A note on hyperesthesia in children with early brain damage. *Neuropsychologia, 4:* 351–356 (1966).

Swisher, Linda P.: Auditory intensity discrimination in patients with temporal lobe damage. *Cortex, 3:* 179–194 (1967).

Teuber, H.-L.: Alterations of perception after brain injury. In: Eccles, J. C. (ed.) *Brain and Conscious Experience.* New York, Springer (1966).

Teuber, H.-L., Battersby, W. S. and Bender, M. B.: *Visual Field Defects after Penetrating Missile Wounds of the Brain.* Cambridge, Mass., Harvard University Press (1960).

DR. DOMINO: On the basis of your experiences, Dr. Sim, can you say that marihuana compounds are clearly different in every way from mescaline and LSD, and, if so, how?

DR. SIM: There are major differences between the effects of tetrahydrocannabinols and LSD in humans. The extreme degree of sympathetic drive from LSD seems to overwhelm whatever parasympathetic effects and compound may cause. As a result of this, the LSD subject is usually hyperactive and has a great deal of personal anxiety in relation to everything around him. On the other hand, the tetrahydrocannabinol subject tends to be much less anxious, has increased sensory input, but is unlikely to be disturbed by events, and probably will have minimal physical activity because of hypotension. There are similarities in descriptions of visual and auditory hallucinations; the latter appear to be more common in tetrahydrocannabinol intoxication. If the dose of LSD is too high, physiological increases in heart rate, blood pressure, and elevated temperature will occur. In addition, nausea, vomiting, and muscular twitching become prominent. On the other hand, the high dose tetrahydrocannabinol subject has an orthostatic hypotension, slight to no increase in heart rate at rest, and lowered body temperature. I am not prepared to discuss mescaline from a clinical standpoint because we have not studied any compound of reasonable purity.

DR. EFRON: I don't think Dr. Teuber agrees with this. Do you think they are different?

DR. TEUBER: Not having experienced anything but mescaline myself, I cannot say from introspection whether these different agents—mescaline, LSD, and marihuana—are similar or different in their effects. Nor do I have enough experience with others taking it to be sure. I always have the impression that the marihuana experience can be difficult to distinguish from some phases of mescaline intoxication, whereas LSD is somewhat different, as has been pointed out. For one thing, the LSD effect seems to me extremely variable as compared with the mescaline effect, which is more stereotyped.

DR. EFRON: If we are speaking of this compound as one member of a group of compounds, could you define even theoretically some common mechanism of action of this type of drug? I know this is difficult.

DR. TEUBER: I would have to say no, of course I cannot. I would certainly look at this in a manner similar to Dr. Stein's approach to the functions of the median forebrain bundle. He goes after this in an elegant and direct way, fully knowing that he is pushing a special hypothesis as logically and as firmly as he can. I think this is what we might have to do.

I am always impressed, you see, with the way in which these agents seem to overlap in some of their effects with each other, and with those spontaneously rising disturbances we see in people with temporal lobe disorders. This is of course what Klüver had in mind, as I said, when he did his ablation experiments on monkeys. He knew introspectively that some of his own experiences under mescaline were similar to what he had heard and read about various manifestations of irritative temporal lobe lesions in man.

DR. HOLMSTEDT: Can I bring up another question with regard to this echo phenomenon? It is known that in amphetamine psychosis you have this repetitive behavior, and this I experienced with dimethoxy-DMT, or the mixture of the crude drug. I recall it vividly. I kept making my hammock over and over again, and Dr. Shultes at the same time went through his herbarium again and again for about twenty minutes or so. I would like to know from the psychiatrists or the experimental people here whether this is known for any other of these compounds.

DR. OSMOND: Now and again you find patients who have the experience that time has been suspended and the same thing is occurring continuously. They usually dislike this. Our studies suggest that time sense can be disordered in many different ways. Some of them are very difficult to put into words. The enormous extension of time, the contracting of time, the physical appearance of time and its disappearance, all of which are frequently referred to in science fiction novels, occur in illness, but rarely otherwise, fortunately for us. Though, thanks to the use of psychedelics, well people are more familiar with them today than previously.

DR. LEHRER: This repetitive behavior is reminiscent of that seen in people with temporal lobe lesions, except, of course, that the automatic activity in patients with temporal lobe lesions is stereotyped and usually the patient is unaware that he is performing it, whereas in the case that has been described, you were aware of what you were doing, I presume.

DR. TEUBER: As you pointed out, you can have these stereotypes in an epileptic attack. The patient may be in a twilight state in which he rubs his hands over and over, or he twirls his wristwatch around; when you bring this to his attention, he stares at you and goes right on. But there is another phenomenon that is much closer to what you describe. A patient with deep frontal lesions might perform for you any action you might ask him to perform. For instance, you might ask him to tap once with a pencil on the table, and he starts but then goes on tapping; you say "stop," and he goes on tapping—as if he could not terminate the action once it had begun. Then you say "pick up the glass," and he puts the pencil down and picks up the glass, and he picks it up and puts it down, picks it up and puts it down, and so on. You say, "pick up your pencil," and he picks up the pencil. It is a rather frightening picture.

DR. LEHRER: It's not a pure, localized lesion. I think these people also have more generalized brain dysfunction.

DR. TEUBER: Undoubtedly.

DR. LEHRER: Dr. Stein, in your introduction you mentioned one reason for fixing on amphetamine: what is the effect in humans? It struck me this was very similar to the central effect of cocaine. Have you tried cocaine in your system and at what dose?

DR. STEIN: Yes. Cocaine has a moderate behavior-facilitating action on the self-stimulation test itself.

DR. LEHRER: Did it release norepinephrine?

DR. STEIN: I think it might have a small releasing effect. But it's almost the perfect tricyclic antidepressant since it has a potent inhibitory effect on re-uptake of norepinephrine without any receptor blocking action. All of the tricyclics have a chlorpromazine-like receptor blocking action at high doses. Cocaine should theoretically be a good antidepressant, but we heard that from Freud 80 years ago.

DR. EFRON: This will conclude the general discussion. Dr. Freedman will take over the chair for the remainder of the meeting.

DR. FREEDMAN: Now, Dr. Lipton, you can start summarizing the proceedings of this workshop.

SUMMARY OF THE WORKSHOP

Morris A. Lipton, M.D., Ph.D.

*Department of Psychiatry, University of North Carolina
School of Medicine, Chapel Hill, N.C. 27515*

This has been a remarkable conference in many ways. In a two day period, averaging twelve hours a day, we have heard speakers, frequently interrupted by an enthusiastic, informed, and critical audience. I suspect the diabolical hands of Drs. Daniel Efron and Roger Russell in the planning of two days of continued rain. If we had had the typical California sunshine, I doubt that we would have gotten our work done.

This workshop was planned with two purposes in mind. The first was to disseminate information; the second was to communicate across disciplines. If the workshop is to be criticized at all, it might be because we attempted too much in too brief a time. But we shall have an opportunity to digest at leisure.

Psychotomimetic agents have had an enormous impact upon the lay community, especially among our youth, and this has created a set of significant social, moral, and legal problems. This is a matter of concern for all responsible citizens, especially for psychiatrists, psychologists, and pharmacologists, whose opinions will hopefully be sought in the construction of laws and other regulatory devices. Of more immediate professional concern, with these agents we have powerful investigative tools which might offer us insights into many of the puzzling questions relating the structure and metabolism of the brain to the many phenomena of mind. These agents, while they produce somatic peripheral effects, are characterized by their primary action on behavior, and the behavior which they alter is not gross behavior, like consciousness or unconsciousness, but rather the subtle changes involved in alterations of perception, cognition, mood, judgment, and other higher functions. Though agents of this type have been used by men of all cultures for thousands of years, it has only been with their isolation, chemical characterization, and synthesis that their value for knowledge achieved its high potential. The simultaneous discoveries of the nature, distribution, metabolism, and function of the neurohumors have permitted an exciting interaction and the birth of a new discipline, neuropsychopharmacology.

Each new discipline has its problems. Perhaps the most difficult of these are in the areas of communication and methodology. The purposes of this workshop included taking steps towards resolving these problems. Among the participants, we have heard organic and medicinal chemists, pharmacologists, experimental psychologists, neurophysiologists, neurologists, and psychiatrists. Typically, these scientists and clinicians do not speak each other's language nor understand the depth, subtlety, complexity, and even uncertainty of each other's information. In our struggles to understand the relevance of each other's work to our own problems, we too often polarize quickly either by rejecting the other discipline as irrelevant or, alternatively, by expecting a magical answer to our troubles.

This workshop has clearly shown that neither pole is correct, that our various approaches are mutually relevant and that there are no easy answers. It has also shown that we are eager to communicate with each other and able to do so. I estimate that at least one third of our time was spent in discussion of the papers presented. Though this may create an editorial nightmare in the preparation of the proceedings volume, it has led to an exciting and informative workshop.

Dr. Shulgin set the keynote for this position by emphasizing that the action of psychotropic drugs must be examined at the cellular level, animal level and, simultaneously, at the level of man in relation to himself at some other time and in relation to other men. Drs. Harmon and Julesz similarly emphasized that a one-to-one concordance between biological structure and function on the one hand and behavior on the other is not to be expected in the central nervous system any more than it might be in a computer where the nature of the components, their method of linkage, and the programming are all determinants of its performance, and where very different skills are required by those who manufacture it and those who run it. Dr. Kornetsky has emphasized that in such interdisciplinary studies behavior must be characterized and quantified as carefully as the chemistry and pharmacology, and this still poses a major problem for many of us.

It is very difficult to summarize adequately a conference which has touched upon so many disciplines in so short and intense a time, and I am certain that we are looking forward to its publication for more leisurely digestion. Nevertheless, let me attempt to touch on a few highlights. In the opening session in chemistry, Dr. Shulgin offered us an historical survey, a classification and some insights based upon vast experience about the crucial structural characteristics of psychotomimetics and their potentially active metabolites. Dr. Snyder similarly examined the three dimensional structure of the indole and phenylethylamine psychotomimetics and their most crucial characteristics. Dr. Abood, working with a different class of agents, the hallucinogenic glycolate esters of heterocyclics, concentrated on their utility in offering insights into the chemical composition and structure of the synaptic membrane. In the pharmacological section, Dr. Sulser, who professes to know nothing of behavior but nonetheless uses simple behavioral tests in rodents, summarized his work on the mechanism of action of amphetamine, introducing us to new work with halogenated amphetamine derivatives and their effects upon the naturally occurring neurohumors and the adenyl cyclase receptor sites. Dr. Gessner, also using a simple bioassay, that of tremor production in mice, has attempted to correlate this assay with psychotomimetic potency in man. The need for a bioassay of these substances in subhuman species is self-evident, and hopefully his studies and similar ones will offer us one. Dr. Stein has ingeniously combined the electrophysiological techniques of self-stimulation with those of classical pharmacology and shown that in animals in whom the intensity of current stimulation is too low to generate self-stimulation, the administration of amphetamine results in the resumption of self-stimulation. He has used other compounds as well, and this approach offers promise of still further integration and dialogue between the neurophysiologists and the pharmacologists. Dr. Holmstedt, of course, offered us a preview of a very exciting methodological breakthrough in the combined use of the gas chromatograph and mass spectrometer. Since so many of our problems are tied to microanalytical methods, the potential increment of 10,000-fold increases in sensitivity and specificity may be expected to yield much new information. To me, the prospect of seeking interesting metabolites in cerebrospinal fluid rather than in the urinary sewer is most exciting.

In the neurophysiology session, Dr. Aghajanian, who represents the new breed of psychiatrist-scientist, introduced us to his combined electrophysiological and pharmacological approach in which electrophysiological recordings of raphé neurons are taken directly, and the effects of psychotomimetics on the firing of these neurons are explored. Since he is dealing with neurons whose transmitters are chemically defined, his demonstrated effects of LSD in inhibiting their firing are exciting. Even more so are his findings that some neurons respond to LSD and not to mescaline, while others respond to both. I have already referred to the presentations of Drs. Harmon and Julesz. They offered insights into the processing of information in the visual system and into methods for the separation of retinal and central processes in vision. Unfortunately, they have not worked with the psychotomimetic agents which seem admirably suited for their studies, and perhaps this conference will stimulate them to do so. Dr. Winters offered us a provocative paper based on his electrical recordings from the reticular system and the effects of a variety of agents on their synchronization and desynchronization. He described these degrees of hallucinatory activity relating these to the degree of hypersynchrony in the reticular system.

In the fourth session on clinical considerations I attempted to discuss the relevance of the chemically induced psychoses to our theories regarding the etiology of the spontaneous ones. Dr. Snyder discussed the subjective effects of DOET and DOM in man, comparing them to each other and to amphetamine, to which they are chemically related. Dr. Bender reported on her experience with the use of amphetamine (Benzedrine) in the treatment of hyperkinetic, hypersexual, and somnolent children. The results are apparently good, and the absence of psychosis, dependency, and the development of tolerance in children are striking. Dr. Szara reported on the clinical states induced by dimethyl tryptamine and its homologues; and Dr. Griffith, who has administered huge doses of amphetamines to subjects and produced amphetamine psychoses, elaborated on the nature of the amphetamine psychosis and its treatment. Dr. Domino has studied the effects of smoking marijuana on objective sensory visual and auditory thresholds in man and finds no objective changes despite the fact that the subjects felt that such changes occurred. This is a puzzling finding and one which again emphasizes the difficulties in research in this field.

This very brief summary does little justice to the content and quality of the papers and does serious injustice to the contributions of the guests and speakers in the discussion period. Many questions were raised in areas ranging from the molecular to the subjective realm. We have talked and heard not only of new information in our respective and overlapping fields but also of problems ranging from the nature of receptors to clinical problems; we have even heard of some pending legislation which might inhibit the freedom of investigators to work on these fascinating problems. The speakers are to be congratulated for their success in communicating not only to their professional peers but also to those of other disciplines, to whom they addressed themselves lucidly. I think we shall all leave with increased understanding and respect for each other's concepts, methods, problems and limitations.

A final word of thanks should go to Dr. Daniel Efron, who selected the speakers and audience and who will now face the task of trying to organize all of this into a volume. It will be difficult, but fortunately he is a veteran of several such conferences and will undoubtedly drive us to finish our homework.

CLOSING REMARKS

DR. FREEDMAN: Thanks, Dr. Lipton. I agree with all you are saying about Dan Efron. But you didn't really indicate what a task master he also is. I suppose that comes from being a veteran. It's appropriate, I think, that he now be introduced by Dr. Harmon, who has some reflections of his own to offer us:

DR. HARMON: Shortly after lunch I had a revelation, and I set it down on paper for you, Dan:

> *A hallucinogent named Efron*
> *Convened a rainy day session*
> *on LSDelights and unreal affrights*
> *And potsful of psychic regression*
>
> *Our minds were expanded acutely*
> *Our sensory auras aflame*
> *As pharmacological agents*
> *Infiltrated psyche and brain*
>
> *So for Dan's N.I.M.H. hospitality*
> *(T'was psychotomimetically hip)*
> *Great thanks for new lights on mentality*
> *And a most unforgettable TRIP.*

DR. EFRON: I have the privilege of closing this meeting with a few words. I would like to take this opportunity to thank all the participants who so readily responded to our invitation to attend this workshop. *"Neither snow nor rain nor gloom of night,"*[1] and I may add *nor flood nor storm,*[2] prevented you from coming to this meeting.

I must apologize for the compactness of the proceedings, which required that we work twelve hours each day, but it was the only way we could organize the meeting. Perhaps the next time the schedule will be a more leisurely one, especially since I learn that this one earned me the name of

---

[1] Herodotus, *Works,* Book 8, paragraph 98.
[2] During the time of this meeting, California was hit with a severe spell of storms and floods.

"slave driver." But I feel that we all enjoyed this meeting and that we achieved much in reviewing existing information in the field of psychotomimetics, as well as discussing new directions of research in the field.

I would also like to thank you for the kind personal words that were addressed to me. Thank you again.

Appendix

Department of Psychiatry
School of Medicine
University of North Carolina
Chapel Hill, North Carolina

March 6, 1969

Dr. William H. Stewart
Surgeon General
Public Health Service
9000 Rockville Pike
Bethesda, Md. 20014

Dear Dr. Stewart:

The Preclinical Psychopharmacology Research Review Committee understands that the Bureau of Narcotics and Dangerous Drugs of the Department of Justice is drafting legislation to be called the "Controlled Dangerous Substances Act of 1969." We have only incomplete information about its provisions but those sections of the draft that we have examined lead us to question the wisdom of several aspects of the bill.

Most disturbing to us are the proposed licensing procedures. These will apparently call for scientific investigators to submit their research protocols for approval in order to gain permission to work with those high-abuse liability drugs that have approved medical uses. These include such drugs as morphine and amphetamine. We hope the Council will concern itself with the possible consequences of the proposed law and try to minimize its potentially deleterious effects upon research in the field of psychopharmacology.

Sincerely yours,

Morris A. Lipton, M.D., Ph.D.
Chairman, Preclinical Psychopharmacology
Research Review Committee

*Author Index**

Aaron, H. S., 334n
Abood, L. G., 67, 68, 71–76 passim
Abramson, H. A., 239
Adams, R. D., 38, 287, 288, 300
Adamski, R. J., 67
Adey, W. R., 199
Aghajanian, G. K., 44, 161, 166, 167, 252
Amaral Vieira, F. J., 300
Andén, N.-E., 167, 174
Appel, J. B., 165, 168
Apter, J. T., 209
Axelrod, J., 88, 127, 137

Babbini, M., 87
Baldwin, M., 340
Balestrieri, A., 165
Bell, D. S., 102, 287
Bender, L., 265, 268, 269, 270, 272
Bernstein, B. M., 86
Biel, J. H., 76
Bizzi E., 220
Blacker, U. H., 283
Bleuler, M., 235
Borella, L., 88
Boszormenyi, Z., 275
Bowers, M. B., Jr., 237
Bradley, C., 266
Brady, J. V., 138
Brindley, G. S., 184, 318
Brodie, B. B., 113, 123, 268
Brodman, K., 188n
Brune, G. G., 234
Brutkowski, S., 137, 138
Buehler, C. A., 67
Burn, J. H., 83, 123

Carlsson, A., 84, 116, 137, 156
Carlton, P. L., 86
Cerletti, A., 44, 116
Chase, T. N., 167
Chessick, R., 237
Clark, L., 326

Claussen, U., 300
Clemente, C. D., **137**
Cohen, J., 315
Cohen, S., 107
Connell, P. H., 287
Connors, C. K., 267
Consolo, S., 87
Crockett, R., 239

Dahlström, A., 84, 166
Deckert, G. H., 178
de Robertis, E., 92
Dingell, J. V., 84, *85,* **89**
Dooher, G., 272
Dowling, J., 272
Dring, L. G., 89

Efron, D. H., 190, 299
Eliel, E. L., 69
Ellison, T., 89
Eugster, C. H., 155
Everett, G. M., 115

Fabing, H. D., 105
Faillace, L. A., 277
Faretra, G., 269, 270, **273**
Fender, D., 186
Fiden, W. J., 107
Fish, M. S., 275, 286
Fodor, G., 70
Foote, W. E., 167
Freedman, D. X., 166, **167**
Freiter, E. R., 67
Freud, S., 232, 242
Frey, H. H., 89, 92
Friedhoff, A. J., 233, **234**
Fuller, R. W., 90
Fuxe, K., 168

Gabel, N., 67, 68, 71
Gaddum, J. H., 44, 116, 166
Gaoni, Y., 300

* References to source in figures and tables are in italics.

AUTHOR INDEX

Geller, I., 137
Gessner, P. K., 47, 105, 106
Glowinski, J., 83, 84, 123, 131, 136
Godse, D. D., 106
Goldstein, M., 89, 113
Granit, R., 209, 217
Griffith, J. D., 288
Guilford, J. P., 302

Hall, H. K., Jr., 71
Halliwell, G., 86, 87
Hammar, C.-G., 152n
Hanson, L. C. F., 84, 86
Hawkes, D., 295
Heath, R. G., 199, 234
Hernández-Peón, R., 137
Hill, R. T., 86, 141
Hillarp, N.-A., 126
Hively, R. L., 300
Hoch, P., 268
Hoffer, A., 238, 239
Hollister, L. E., 235–36, 239, 287
Hubel, D. H., 183, 188

Isbell, H., 116, 300, 312

Jacob, J., 107
Jacobsen, E., 287
Janssen, P. A. J., 86
Jarvik, M. E., 107
Jequier, E., 111
Johnson, S. C., 186
Jouvet, M., 90
Julesz, B., 184, 186

Kaada, B. R., 137
Kalir, A., 276
Kandel, E., 147
Katz, M. M., 249, 253
Keeler, M. H., 236
Kety, S. S., 235, 288
Killam, K. F., 209
Klüver, H., 340
Koch, R., 232, 233, 234
Koe, B. K., 90, 111
Koella, G., 237
Kopin, I. J., 86, 89
Kornetsky, C., 107
Kraepelin, E., 244, 313
Kramer, J. C., 295
Kurland, A. A., 280, 283

La Rosa, R. T., 107, 108
Laties, V. G., 107

Lessin, A. W., 107
Lewin, L., 22–23
Linton, H. B., 236, 277, 279
Loewe, S., 300, 334

Macdonald, J. M., 287
McGlothlin, W. H., 280
McIsaac, W. M., 29
Mann, P. J. G., 123
Marcus, R. J., 193
Margules, D. L., 137, 138
Mechoulam, R., 27, 311n, 333
Meduna, J., 78
Merril, C. R., 48
Milner, B., 225, 340
Mitoma, C., 49
Moore, K. E., 84
Moreau, S., 238
Mori, K., 194
Morrow, R. S., 300
Musacchio, J., 113
Myers, F., 57

Nielsen, C. K., 89
Nogrady, T., 71, 77

Olds, J., 124, 126

Page, I. H., 105
Palmer, E., 92
Pauling, L., 238
Pickens, R., 138
Pletscher, A., 89, 90
Prockop, D. J., 111
Purpura, D. P., 209

Randrup, A., 86
Rapport, M. M., 105
Rinkel, M., 235
Robison, G. A., 92
Rockland, L. H., 277
Rogeness, G. C., 71
Rome, H. P., 288
Rosecrans, J. A., 167
Rosenberg, D. E., 46
Rudel, R., 339
Rutledge, C. O., 83

Sachar, E. J., 233
Sai-Halasz, A., 273
Sanders-Bush, E., 90, *91*
Sankar, D. V. S., 272
Sargent, T. W., 57
Scheckel, C. L., 86

AUTHOR INDEX

Scheibel, M. E., 209
Schilder, P., 266
Schlag, J., 205
Schweitzer, J. W., 57
Scoville, W. B., 225
Sedvall, G. C., 127
Shakow, D., 236
Sheard, M. H., 167
Shepherd, M., 239
Shulgin, A. T., 35, 49, *50,* 53, 54, *55,* 56, 57, 247, 262
Sigg, E. B., 89
Slotta, K. H., 48
Smart, R. G., 239
Smith, C. B., 83, 123, 146
Smith, K., 234
Smythies, J. R., *50,* 56, 162, 232
Snyder, S. H., 44, 55, 57, 161, 249–57 *passim,* 262
Speeter, M. E., 275
Spengler, J., 87
Stein, L., 83, 86, 87, 123–38 *passim, 139,* 141, 142
Stolk, J. M., 83, 84
Stromberg, V. L., 105
Sulser, F., 84, *85,* 86, 87, 88
Swisher, L. P., 340
Szara, S., 46, 106, 275, 279

Tanimukai, H., 234
Taylor, E. D., 300
Teuber, H.-L., 339
Theobald, W., 155
Thoenen, H., 89
Thudicum, J. W. L., 231
Trendelenburg, U., 83

Turner, W. J., 46, 105, 234
Twarog, B. M., 105

Udenfriend, S., 156
Ursin, H., 138
Usdin, E., 23
Uyeno, E. T., *50,* 57, 65, 256

Valzelli, L., 87
van Rossum, J. M., 83, 123
Vane, J. R., 106, 123

Waser, P. G., 155
Wasson, R. G., 5*n*
Way, E. L., 113
Weil, A. T., 283, 300, 309, 311
Weiner, I. B., 287
Weiss, B., 92, 148
Weissbach, H., 286
Weissman, A., 84, 86, 123, 124, *125,* 127
Wikler, A., 236
Williams, E. G., 300, 309
Wilson, K. M., 78*n*
Winn, D., 272
Winter, J. C., 106
Winter, J. D., 106
Winters, W. D., 193–201 *passim,* 205, 206, 208, 210
Wise, C. D., 127, *128,* 137*n*, 138
Wolbach, A. B., Jr., 169
Woolley, D. W., 44, 166

Young, G. Y., 292

Zalis, E. G., 288

Subject Index*

Acetaldehyde, 29
Acetylcholine, 27, *28*, 77, 146, 176
Acetyldimethoxyphenylethylamine, 234
Adenosine triphosphate (ATP), *72, 73*
Adenosine triphosphatase (ATPase): inhibition of by LSD, 76
Adenyl cyclase, 92, 95, 99
Adrenergic system: blocking properties of chlorpromazine in, 88, 97
  pharmacological action of amphetamine on, 89
Adrenochrome, 232
Adrenocorticotrophic hormone (ACTH), 287
Aldehydes, 123
Alfalfa, 301, 302, *305, 306*, 307
Alkaloids, 24–25, 27–29
Amanita muscaria. See Ibotenic acid; Muscimol
Amnesia, 225, 226
Amphetamine:
  d-, 32, 83, 84, *85, 87*, 88, 89, 92, 123, 127, *135*, 142, 194, 248–54
  l-, 89
Amphetamine derivatives, *51.* See—
  Chloroamphetamine
  Chloromethamphetamine
  Dimethoxyamphetamine
  Dimethoxyethylamphetamine
  Dimethoxymethylamphetamine
  Dimethoxymethylenedioxyamphetamine
  Hydroxyamphetamine
  Methoxyamphetamine
  Methoxymethylenedioxyamphetamine
  Methylenedioxyamphetamine
  Trimethoxyamphetamine
Amphetamine-hydroxylase, 89
Amphetamine-induced psychosis: chlorpromazine or barbiturates in treatment of, 297, 298
  evolution of pre-psychotic to florid phase, 290–91
  resemblance to paranoid schizophrenia, 292
  size of dose a major factor, 293
  study of volunteers, 288–93
  withdrawal syndrome, 292, 297–98
Amphetamines: action of on auditory and visual systems, 205, 209–10
  behavioral effects of, 86, 87, 138–41
  biochemical effects of, 84
  central action of, 83–86
  dopaminergic mechanisms and, 86
  effects on adrenergic systems, 89, 92, 126
  effects on midbrain raphé neurons, 167
  interaction with dopamine-β-hydroxylase inhibitors, 126–30
  metabolic aspects of, 88–89
  modification of central action of by tricyclic antidepressants and chlorpromazine, 86–88, 89, 91, 92
  perfusion experiments, 130–36
  self-stimulation of the brain facilitated by, 124–26, 142
  sympathomimetic action of, 32, 83, 84, 89, 92, 123
  (*See also specific compounds.*)
Anesthetic agents, 201
Anhalonium lewinii (*Lophopora williamsii*): relation to norepinephrine, 30
Anorexigenic activity induced by drugs, 84, 87, 89, 155
Anticholinergics, 77, 78
  hyperactivity peculiar to, 67
Antihistamine: children's reactions to, 267–68
Apiole, 33
Asarone, 34
Atropine, 23, 27, *28*, 78, 176

* References to tables and figures are in italics.

Autonomic drugs: bioassay of, 78n
Ayahuasca, 23, 28

Banisteriopsis, 28, 29
Barbiturates: amnesia or confusion evoked by, 23
   as a specific for amphetamine psychosis, 297
   withdrawal symptoms in users of, 297
   See also Phenobarbital; Sodium amital
Behavioral disturbance index (BDI), 67, 68, 69, 71
Belladonna alkaloids, 28
Benactyzine, 23, 28
Benzoyl esters, 71
Bufotenine (5-hydroxydimethyltryptamine): absence of psychotomimetic effect of, 234
   hallucinogenic effects of, 105, 275
   psychedelic inactivity of, 46
   relation to serotonin, 30

Caffeine, 22
Cahoba, 105
Calamus, 33, 34
Calcium, 71–73
Cannabichromene, 312n
Cannabidiol, 26, 312n
Cannabidiolic acid, 312n
Cannabigerol, 312n
Cannabinoids, 25–27
Cannabinol, 312n. *See also* Tetrahydrocannabinol
Cannabis, Report by the Advisory Committee on Drug Dependence (London), 311n
Cannabis sativa, 25, 312n, 332
   use of in medicine, 336–37
Cat: auditory and visual systems of, 209
   behavior following administration of LSD, mescaline, and psilocybin, 199
   effect of LSD on sleep and wakefulness, 200
   features of visual cortex of, 183
Cataleptoid and epileptoid CNS states, 193
Catecholamines, 86, 88
   amphetamine-induced release of, 92
   drug-induced concentration of in brain, 160
   influence of drugs on function of, 113, *114,* 123
   synthesis of in brain, 83–84
Catechol-O-methyl-transferase, 136

Central nervous system (CNS): action of drugs in, 86, 91, 92, 109
   excitant agents and their effects, 194, *198,* 209–13
   excitation and depression states in, 193, 194, *201, 206*
Chanoclavine, *24,* 25
Chick: behavioral activation of by tricyclic drugs, 98
Children's reaction to drugs: amphetamine, 266–67
   antihistamines, reserpine, meprobamate, energizers, phenothiazines, and anticonvulsants, 267–68
   LSD, 268–70
   methysergide, 270
   psilocybin, 270
Chloranil, 71
p-Chloroamphetamine, 89, 90, *91,* 92
Chloroform, 23
p-Chloromethamphetamine, 89, 91
p-Chlorophenylalanine (PCPA), 90, 108, 109, 111, *116,* 157, 161, 224, 242
   effect of on amphetamine level in brain, 86–88
   effects of DOM accentuated by, 254
   midbrain raphé neurons not inhibited by, 167
   a nonpsychedelic drug, 44
   psychic effects of LSD counteracted by, 116
Cholinesterase inhibitors, 76, 176
Cocaine, 124, 142, 331, 343
Confusion induced by glycolate esters: in human subjects, 67
   performance of mice in a swim maze, 67
   rat behavior characterized by head swaying, 67
Convolvulaceae seeds, 25
Corticosteroids, 287, 288, 293
Crowei, 33

Datura, 27, 39
Deamination, 88
Decarboxylation, 115–16
Delirium: produced by glycolate esters, 67–68
Dementia praecox, 245
Demethoxylation, 33
Depression, 193, 194
Desipramine, 88
Desoxyephedrine, 288
Diethyldithiocarbamate (DEDTC), 86, 127, 129, 142

SUBJECT INDEX

Diethyltryptamine (DET), 105–6, 108
   hallucinogenic action of, 275, 277
   See also 6-Fluorodiethyltryptamine
Digitalis, 152
l-Dihydroxyphenylalanine (l-DOPA), 86, 115, 116
Dihydroxyphenylserine (DOPS). See Threo-3,4-dihydroxyphenylserine
Dillapiole, 33
Dimethoxyamphetamine (DMA), 55–58
   2,3-, 56
   2,4-, 56
   2,5-, 34, 35, 56
   3,4-, 34, 35, 56
   3,5-, 56
   structure-activity of, 56
Dimethoxyethylamphetamine:
   2,5-dimethoxy-4-ethylamphetamine (DOET), 35, 57, 247–48
   comparison with d-amphetamine in effects on normal subjects, 248–54
   effects of on associative labeling of thematic apperception cards, 260–61
   structure of, 248
   subjective effects of varying doses of, 257–60
   as a therapeutic measure in psychiatry, 262
Dimethoxyhydroxyphenethylamine, 37
Dimethoxymethylamphetamine:
   2,5-dimethoxy-4-methylamphetamine (DOM), 35, 36, 56, 57, 247–48
   effects of on associative labeling of thematic apperception cards, 260–61
   effects of low doses of, 254–57
   hallucinogenic effects of, 262
   hippies' use of, 56
   structure of, 248
   See also STP
Dimethoxymethylenedioxyamphetamine:
   2,3-dimethoxy-4,5-methylenedioxyamphetamine (DMMA-2), 33, 54, 55
   2,5-dimethoxy-3,4-methylenedioxyamphetamine (DMMDA), 33, 54
   potency in man, 55
   structure-activity of, 55
Dimethoxyphenethanolamine, 37
Dimethoxyphenylethylamine (DMPEA):
   3,4-, 57
   analog of 3,4-dimethoxyamphetamine, 35
   presence of in schizophrenics, 233
   See also Acetyldimethoxyphenylethylamine

Dimethyltryptamine (DMT):
   4-hydroxy-N,N- (psilocin), 45, 46, 47, 106
   5-hydroxy-N,N- (bufotenine), 46
   6-hydroxy-N,N-, 46
   4-methoxy-N,N-, 106
   5-methoxy-N,N- (5-MeO-DMT), 29, 105–16 passim
   6-methoxy-N,N-, 106
   7-methoxy-N,N-, 106
   duration of action, 247
   hallucinogenic action of, 275
   inhibition of raphé neurons by, 167
   structure of, 29
   See also Bufotenine; Psilocin
Dipropyltryptamine (DPT): chemical structure of, 275, 276
   hallucinogenic effects in dog and human subjects, 276–77
Disulfiram, 113, 127, 128, 287, 288, 293
Ditran, 28, 77, 78
DOET. See under Dimethoxyethylamphetamine
Dog: effect of dipropyltryptamine on, 275
DOM. See under Dimethoxymethylamphetamine
Dopamine: drug-induced concentration changes of in brain areas, 90, 113, 157, 160
Dopamine-β-hydroxylase inhibitors, 86, 115–16, 126–30, 142, 146
Dreams, 222–26
Drug-induced states: similarity and differences between schizophrenia and, 236–37
Drug legislation: dangers in approach to, 327–32, 345–46, 351

Elemicin, 33, 34
Enzymes: action of psychotomimetics on, 76
   in brain, 76, 98
   formation of O-methylated products by, 136
   induction of, 285, 328–29
   result of deficiency in, 232–33
Epéna, 119, 120
Epinephrine:
   dl-, 139
   l-, 138
Ergot alkaloids, 24–25
Ethanol, 23

SUBJECT INDEX

Ether, 23, 194, 199, 204
   action of on auditory and visual systems, 205, 209–10, 211

Fenfluramine, 103
6-Fluorodiethyltryptamine (6-FDET), 276, 277, 286

Gas chromatography, 151–52, 234
Glycolate esters: anticholinergic properties of, 67
   behavioral disturbance character of, 69
   interaction of with calcium, 71–73
   psychotomimetic potency of, 71
Glycosides, 312
Granatol, 70

Hallucination: in animals, 107
   LSD-induced intermittent nature of, 199–200
   produced by glycolate esters, 67–68
   theory of hallucinosis, 204–12
Hallucinogens: ballistic movements in mice induced by, 107–17
   body temperature effects in animals and man, 107, *108*
   tremor effects in small mammals, 107
Harmalan:
   6-methoxy-, 29
Harmaline: resemblance to serotonin, 28
Harman:
   6-methoxy- (aromatic system), 29
   6-methoxytetrahydro-, 29
Harmine (aromatic), 28. *See also* Tetrahydroharmine
Hashish, 238, 300, 325, 326, 329, 335. *See also* Marihuana
Hemp, 300
Heterocyclic imino alcohols, 67, 68, 71
Hexenoic acid:
   trans-3-methyl-2-, 234
   odor of schizophrenic patients ascribed to, 234
Histamine, 272
Human subjects, actions of drugs on:
   acetyldimethoxyphenylethylamine, 234
   amphetamines, 53, 84, 89, 92, 123, 205, 209–10, 287–93
   DPT, 6-FDET, and DET data on hospitalized patients, 277–83
   glycolate acid esters, 67–68
   hydroxybutyrate, nitrous oxide, phencyclidine, pentylenetetrazol, and ether, 205, 209, 211

LSD, 108–16 *passim*, 166, 194, 199–200, 205, 209–10, 275, 277–78, 287
mescaline, 47, 165–69, 194, 199, 205, 209–10, 247, 275, 287
muscimol, 155–56
tryptamines, 46, 105, 106, 157–58, 160, 161, 167, 247, 275
p-Hydroxyamphetamine, 89
γ-Hydroxybutyrate, 199, 201, *207*, *208*, 226
   action of on auditory and visual systems, 205, 209–10, 211
4-Hydroxy-N,N-dimethyltryptamine (psilocin), *47*. *See* Psilocin
5-Hydroxydimethyltryptamine (bufotenine). *See* Bufotenine
Hydroxylation: *p*- and β-hydroxylation pathway of amphetamine, 88–89, 92
   detoxification of amphetamine by, 34–35
p-Hydroxynorephedrine, 89
5-Hydroxytryptamine (5-HT; serotonin), 89, 90, 91, 105–16 *passim*. *See also* Serotonin
5-Hydroxytryptophan, 90, *91*, 111, 112, 167
Hyoscine, 28
Hyoscyamine, 27
Hypnosis: changes in perception effected by, 178–79
   recall of information blotted out by, 221

Ibogaine, 25
Ibotenic acid: influence of on monoamine concentration in brain, 157, 160, 161
   molecular structure of, *156*
   psychotomimetic effects of, 155–56
Imipramine-like drugs, 86–87, 89, 92
Indole alkaloids, 25
Indole metabolites, 234
Indoleacetic acid:
   3-, 281–82, 285
   5-hydroxy- (5-HIAA), 89, 90, 158–59, *160*, 161, 167
Indolealkylamines, 29–30
Ipomoea spp., 25
Iproniazid, 142
Iris of rat: use of isolated preparation for assessment of central-peripheral potency of compounds, 78

Khat, 22

Locomotor activity induced by amphetamine, 86, 87

Lysergic acid diethylamide (LSD):
  l-acetyl-, 161
  2-bromo- (BOL), 44, 57, 116, *117*, 167
  dihydro-, 44, 57
  lumi-, 44, 57
  2-oxy-, 44
  action of on auditory and visual systems, 205, 209–10
  amine concentration changes in brain effected by, 156, 157
  antiserotonin actions of, 44
  cross tolerance between mescaline and, 165, 169
  development of tolerance to, 237
  duration of action, 247, 254
  effects of administration of, 108–16 *passim*, 166, 277–78
  electronic and steric models of, *45*, 57–58
  hallucinogenic action of, 199, 275, 287
  inhibition of ATPase, 76
  LSD-25 action on CNS, 194
  midbrain interactions of 5-HT and, 166–67
  "psychedelic afterglow" in patients, 280–81
  question of chromosome damage in users of, 270
  structure and potency of, 24, 43–44, 57

Man. *See* Human subjects
Marihuana ("pot"): auditory and visual acuity tests on users of, 300–307
  concern over punitive laws on, 329–32
  the "high" effect of, 304, 307, 320, 327
  personality changes in chronic users of, 328
  pharmacological and psychological observations on subjects tested, 303–7
  psychological risks in use of, 310, 325, 327–28
  See also Cannabichrome; Cannabidiol; Cannabidiolic acid; Cannabigerol; Cannabinoids; Cannabinol; *Cannabis sativa;* Hashish; Tetrahydrocannabinol
Mass fragmentography, 151, 152
Mass spectrometry, 151–52, 234
Melatonin, 29
Membranes: drug interaction with, 71–73, 75, 77–78
  model of, 72
Memory, 227–28

Mental illness: possible chemical explanation of, 38, 231
Meprobamate: children's reaction to, 267–68
Mescaline (3,4,5-trimethoxyphenylethylamine), *49*
  α-ethyl, 32, 33
  α-methyl, 32, 33
  action of on auditory and visual systems, 205, 209–10, 211
  brain serotonin concentration influenced by, 161
  as a CNS excitant, 194
  conformation of, 48
  cross tolerance between LSD and, 165, 169
  effects of autonomic function and behavior, 165–69
  hallucinogenic action of, 199, 275, 287
  psychedelic character of, 47, 247
  responses of brain raphé neurons to, 168–69
  sleep states induced by, *202*
  structure and potency of, 33, 34, 43
  tolerance to, 237
Mescaline unit (M.U.): as a measure of relative potency of drugs, 32, 45
Metaraminol, 64
Methedrine, 22
Methoxyamphetamine:
  2-, *61*
  4-, 56
Methoxydimethyltryptamine. *See* Dimethyltryptamine
Methoxymethylenedioxyamphetamine:
  2-methoxy-3,4-methylenedioxyamphetamine (MMDA-3a), 33, 53–54
  2-methoxy-4,5-methylenedioxyamphetamine (MMDA-2), 33, 53
  2,3,4-methoxymethylenedioxyamphetamine (MMDA-3), *55*
  3-methoxy-4,5-methylenedioxyamphetamine (MMDA), 33, 53, 247
  4-methoxy-2,3-methylenedioxyamphetamine, 54
  potency in man, 49, 55
  structure-activity of, *55*
Methoxymethylethyltryptamine. *See* 5-Methoxy-N-methyl-N-ethyltryptamine
5-Methoxy-N-methyl-N-ethyltryptamine, 106
Methyl iodide, 71

Methylenedioxyamphetamine, 33, 55
3,4- (MDA), 247
Methyleugenol, 34
trans-3-Methyl-2-hexenoic acid, 234
α-Methyltyrosine. *See* tyrosine hydroxylase inhibitors
Methysergide, 270, 273
   use of by hippies, 272
Metrazol, 215
Models: Electronic and steric models for predicting psychedelic activity, 44, 57–58
   membrane model, 72
   structural models of psychedelic compounds, 44–46, 50, 70, 72
Monkey: compound in blood of schizophrenics administered to, 234
   impairment of size discrimination in by DOET and DOM, 256
   regional localization of LSD in brain of, 43–44
   response to amphetamines in, 53, 138
   studies on visual cortex of, 183, 184
Monoamine oxidase (MAO) inhibitor: 84, 90, 100–101, 123, 124, 126, *132*, 136, 142, 145, 167
Monoamines: effect of hallucinogens on CNS levels of, 108, 109
Morning glory (*Ipomoea spp.*), 25
Morphine, 152, 331
Mouse: anticholinergic-induced disruption of performance of, 67
   ballistographic activity of after injection of hallucinogens, 107–17
   effects of muscimol, ibotenic acid, and LSD on brain regions of, 156–57, 160
   symptoms evoked by muscimol and ibotenic acid, 155
Muscimol: influence of on amine concentration in brain, 157–58, *159*, 160, 161
   molecular structure of, *156*
   psychotomimetic effects of, 155–56
Mushroom, 29
Myristicin, 33

Nitrous oxide, 194, 199, 204
   action of on auditory and visual systems, 205, 209–10, 211
Noradrenergic transmission, 124, 125, 126, 127, 138, 142
Norephedrine:
   p-hydroxy-, 89, 92

Norepinephrine (NE):
   d-, 128, 129, 138, *139*
   dl-, *139*
   l-, 127, *128*, 129, 138, *139*, 142, 167
   brain levels of, 113, 115, 116
   concentration changes of in brain areas, 157
   as inhibitory transmitter, 124, 130, 137–41
   metabolic effects of amphetamine mediated by, 89, 130–31, 134
   receptors of in brain, 123, 126–27
   release of from the brain by amphetamine, 83–84, 86, 136, 138, 141, 142
Normetanephrine, 84, 136
Norpseudotropine, 70
Nuclear magnetic resonance spectrometry, 234
Numbering systems used for chemical compounds, 25–27, *50, 55,* 332n, 333
Nutmeg, 33

Ololiuqui, 25, 319

Palinopia, 156, 338
Pargyline, 90, *91, 132*
Parsley, 34
Peganum, 28
Pentylenetetrazol, 199, 201, *203*, 204
   action of on auditory and visual systems, 205, 209–10
Peyotl, 30
Phencyclidines, 23, *61, 198*, 199, 201, 204
   action of on auditory and visual systems, 205, 209–10, 211
Phenethylamine, 126, 142
Phenobarbital, 315–16
Phenothiazines, 88, 233, 267–68
Phenoxybenzamine, 107
Phenylethylamines, 32, 47–49
   derivatives, *48*
   molecular model of, 44–45
   See also Dimethoxyphenylethylamine; Trimethoxyphenylethylamine
Phenylisopropylamines, 32
   approximation of the LSD conformation in molecular model of, 44–45
   See also Tetramethoxyphenylisopropylamine
Physostigmine, 78, 176
Piperidine:
   1-methyl-, 68, 69
   1-methyl-4-hydroxy-, 69
   1,2,2,6-tetramethyl-, 71

SUBJECT INDEX

Piperidinol:
  1-methyl-3-, 69
  1-methyl-4-, 69
  1,2,2,6,6-pentamethyl-4-, 70–71
Piperidyl-benzilate:
  N-methyl-4-, 67, *68*, 72
Pipradol, 141
Piptadenia peregrina, 105, 275, 286
Placebo: use of in evaluating hallucinogenic compounds, 276–77
Probenecid, 158, 159
Psilocin (4-hydroxy-N,N-dimethyltryptamine), 29, 45, 106
  4-methoxypsilocin, 57
  molecular model of, *47*
  potency of, 46
Psilocybin, 29, 43, 161, 199, 236, 270
  tolerance to, 237
Psychedelic drugs: compounds embraced in, 247
  molecular orbital calculations for, 57–58
  structural parameters of, *31*, 32–38
  structure-activity relationships of, 43–44
Psychedelic experience: perceptual and thinking disturbances, 276
  phenomenon of the "experienced" vs. the "naive" subject, 326
  resemblance to schizophrenia, 237
  the sense of suspended time, 342
Psychomotor stimulation elicited by amphetamine, 83, 84, *85*
Psychoses: chemical and deficiency models of, 232, 237, 238
  See also Amphetamine-induced psychosis
Psychotogens: endogenous hypothesis of, 37–38, 238
Psychotomimetic compounds: bases of classification of, 21–22
  concern over uses of, 345–46
  defined, 23
  relationship between chemical structures and properties of, 67
  See also Psychedelic drugs; Psychotropic materials
Psychotomimetic families, 24–30
Psychotropic materials: defined by effect on human interrelationships, 21–22
  effectiveness of in children, 268
  Lewin's classification of, 22–23
  new drugs included in, 247–62
  tryptamines with psychotropic activity, 276
Pyrrolidine, 285

Quinuclidine esters, 68, 69

Rabbit: motion perception of in the retina, 188
Raphé neuronal units of the brain:
  5-hydroxytryptophan's slowing of activity of, 167
  inhibitory influence of DMT on, 167
  inhibitory influence of LSD on, 166–67
  noninhibitory effects of amphetamine and chlorpromazine on, 167
  responses of to mescaline, 168–69
Rat: action of esters on brain of, 71
  amphetamine-induced behavior in, 84–90 *passim*, 138
  anticholinergic-induced activity of, 67
  effects of LSD and mescaline on raphé neurons, 165–66, 168, 169
  effects of muscimol, ibotenic acid, and LSD on brain regions, 156–61
  iris preparation of for the bioassay of autonomic drugs, 78 n
  perfusion experiment on, 131–38
  pharmacological effect of *p*-chloroamphetamine, 89
  phenethylamine-induced self-stimulation of, 142
  potency of amphetamine in, 53
  potency of tryptamine in, 105–6
  results of reserpine treatment in brain of, 83–84, *85*
  symptoms evoked by muscimol and ibotenic acid, 155
Receptor sites: action of LSD on, 172–73
  action of tryptamine on, 106–7
  steric effects on, 68, 79
Red oil. *See* Synthetic red oil
Reserpine: action of in depleting the brain of norepinephrine, 83, 142
  behavioral effects of amphetamine in reserpinized animals, 83–84
  children's reactions to, 267–68
  depletion of serotonin in brain caused by, 90
  hallucinogen-induced activity decreased by, 112–13
  receptor sensitivity in animals enhanced by, 83, 86, 92
Resorcinol, 26, 27
Rhombencephalic sleep (RPS), 193, *195*, *196*, *197*, 204
Ritalin, 22
Rivea corymbosa, 25

Safrol, 33
Schizophrenia: chemical compounds unique to, 233–34
  features of in childhood and methods of treatment, 267–70
  lack of a symptomatology in, 213
  models of, 238
  nature of hallucinations in, 235–36
  odor of schizophrenic patients, 234, 244–45, 246
  resemblance to psychedelic experience, 237
  transmethylation hypothesis, 235
Scopolamines, 23, 28
Seizure activity: generalized seizure, 201, 211
  grand mal seizures, 204
Self-stimulation, 87, 124–26, 142
Sensory systems of the brain: modulation control of sensory inputs during drug-induced states, 206–8
Serotonin (5-hydroxytryptamine): action of on rat stomach fundus preparation, 106–7
  antagonism to in muscle preparations, 44, 106
  a component of brain tissue, 105
  drug-induced concentration changes of in brain, 157–58, *159,* 160, 161
  effect of *p*-chloroamphetamine on synthesis of, 90, *91*
  existence of in midbrain raphé nuclei, 166
  interactions with LSD, 166–67
  pargyline-induced increase of in brain, 90, *91*
  resemblance to harmaline, 28
Slow wave sleep (SWS), 193, *195, 196, 197,* 204
Snuffs, 29, 105, 275
Sodium amytal, 221, 268
Stereochemical relationships to drug potency, 68–71
Stereotyped behavior, 84, 86, 87
STP (2,5-dimethoxy-4-methylamphetamine): the hippie population's name for DOM, 56, 247, 254
Sympathomimetic action of amphetamine, 32, 83, 84, 89, 92, 123
Synhexyl, 335
Synthetic red oil, 310, 326, 332

Tabernanthe iboga, 28
Tabernanthine, 25, 28

Taraxein, 232, 234
Teonanacatl mushroom, 29
Terpene, 26
Tetrabenazine, 124
Tetrahydrocannabinol (THC):
  Δ^1-, 26, 27, 311, 312, 326, 332n, 334, 335n
  Δ^3-, 26, 27, 311, 332n, 333, 334
  Δ^8-, 300, 311
  Δ^9-, 300, 302, 307, 311, 316–17, 319–20, 326
  behavioral changes under influence of, 317–18, 325
  differences in effects of LSD and, 341–42
  See also Marihuana
Tetrahydroharmine, 28
Tetramethoxyphenylisopropylamine (TetraMA): 2, 3, 4, 5-, 34
Threo-3,4-dihydroxyphenylserine (DOPS), 116
Tricyclic antidepressants: effect of on central action of amphetamine, 86–87, 92
Trimethoxyamphetamine:
  2,3,4- (TMA-3), 49
  2,4,5- (TMA-2), 34, 49, *52, 53,* 56–57
  3,4,5- (TMA), 32, 34, 43, 49, 50
  potency of in man, monkey, and rat, 49, *50, 53*
  structure-activity relationships of, *50*
Trimethoxyphenylalanine, 40
Trimethoxyphenylethylamine:
  2,3,4-, 48
  3,4,5- (mescaline), *49*
  See also Mescaline
Tropanol, 70
Tryptamine: metabolism of in man, *282*
  molecular model of, 44–45
  receptors of and amphetamine, 123
  resemblance to conformation of LSD, 46–47
Tryptamine derivatives, 45–47. See —
  Diethyltryptamine
  Dimethyltryptamine
  Dipropyltryptamine
  6-Fluorodiethyltryptamine
  4-Hydroxydimethyltryptamine
  5-Hydroxydimethyltryptamine
  5-Hydroxytryptamine
  Methoxydimethyltryptamine
  Methoxymethylethyltryptamine

Tryptophan: effect of *p*-chloroamphetamine on the synthesis of serotonin from, *91*
  See also 5-Hydroxytryptophan
Tryptophan hydroxylase inhibitor, 90, 103, 111
Tyrosine hydroxylase inhibitor:
  α-methyl-*para*-tyrosine, 84, *85*, 86, 91–92, 124, 126, 142, 146
  α-methyl-*meta*-tyrosine, 124

Vision: activation sites of drugs on the peripheral vs. CNS level, 186, 188–89
  "echo pictures" evoked by muscimol, 156, 338
  neurophysiological findings on pathways of cat and monkey visual cortex, 183–84
  random-dot stereograms of images as indicators of mental changes, 184–87
  relation of psychotomimetics to visual perception in human subjects, 183

Wakefulness, 193, *195, 196, 197*